THE
METABOLIC
PLAN

THE METABOLIC PLAN

Stay Younger Longer

Stephen Cherniske, M.S.

BALLANTINE BOOKS • NEW YORK

A Ballantine Book
Published by The Ballantine Publishing Group

Copyright © 2003 by Stephen A. Cherniske

All rights reserved under International and Pan-American Copyright Conventions. Published in the United States by The Ballantine Publishing Group, a division of Random House, Inc., New York, and simultaneously in Canada by Random House of Canada Limited, Toronto.

Ballantine and colophon are registered trademarks of Random House, Inc.

www.ballantinebooks.com

Library of Congress Cataloging-in-Publication Data is available from the publisher upon request.

ISBN 0-345-44101-X

Design by Joseph Rutt

Manufactured in the United States of America

First Edition: March 2003

10 9 8 7 6 5 4 3 2 1

To my best reasons for staying young:
Deborah, Daniel, Misha, Karina, and Ivan

CONTENTS

Acknowledgments

It's difficult to describe how research has changed in the last two decades. With Internet publication, worldwide data reporting, and cyber conferences, the amount of information and the speed at which it is disseminated are truly astounding. This also means that no one scientist can possibly keep up with advances in the life sciences.

I am therefore indebted to hundreds of investigators who have pulled at the threads of this tapestry called aging. I would be remiss not to mention those who have made enormous contributions in the field: Denham Harman, Linus Pauling, Steven Austad, Tom Kirkwood, Caleb Finch, Étienne-Émile Baulieu, Bruce Ames, Lester Packer, Aubrey de Grey, Byung Pal Yu, James Joseph, Barbara Shukitt-Hale, Giovanni Ravaglia, Oasmu Nishikaze, Sam Yen, Henry Lardy, Judith Campisi, James Fries, Jeffrey Bland, the research groups at Unigen Pharmaceuticals in Colorado and Korea, and the Life Extension Foundation.

The fact that this book contains more than four hundred references is an indication of the degree to which we build on the insights and discoveries of others. In reviewing, analyzing, and discussing this mountain of information, I am deeply indebted to research colleagues Michael Schmidt, Michael Zeligs, James Hill, Tom Paquette, Qi Jia, Bruce Burnett, Silvia Jimenez, Don Baird, Bill Hahn, Preston Keeler, Ron Wilson, John Johnson, David Sandoval, and Caroline MacDougall.

I have also gained valuable insights and confirming "real-world" data from clinicians using these principles in their patient care: Doug Pousma, Rhody Edwards, Gary Gordon, Ralph Miranda, Fran Clark, Lawrence Conlan, Jack Woodard, Michael Rosenbaum, Murray Susser, Terry Grossman, Jesse Hanley, Mark Akers, Donald Gay, Rich McBride, Erik Hansen, Ken Power, and Lance Maki.

In the creation of this manuscript, I am particularly indebted to Steve Henne for encouragement and editorial and writing assistance, to Pam Best and Lisa Simone for keeping me on track and taking care of the myriad details, and to David Litt for critical review.

Thanks again to literary agent Robert Stricker, who found the perfect home for this book, and to Ballantine editors Mark Tavani, Tracy Bernstein, Leslie Meredith, and Anika Streitfeld. Also invaluable are living examples of the metabolic model of aging: Eva Cherniske, Gerda Kennedy, Jack La Lanne, Sophia Loren, and others who have tapped into the astonishing power of regeneration.

I am indebted to B. William Lee for putting his money where my mouth is. Mr. Lee's sponsorship of critical research for more than a decade is testimony to his world vision as much as his remarkable generosity.

And because life itself is complex, projects like this require a remarkable cooperative effort. Thanks to my sister Barbara Bischoff, to Stuart Ochiltree, Malcolm Aylett, J. T. Whitworth, Eric Burge, Helen Scanu, Claude Wild, Susan Rampsom, and Geof and Anjila Stimack. Anything worthwhile requires hard work. Thank you all.

Introduction

An amazing thing happens as we grow older. I'm not talking about the appearance of gray hair, expanding waistlines, and a sudden fondness for La-Z-Boy furniture. Far more amazing is the shift in our perceptions and priorities. One day, we are happily oblivious to our own mortality, and then wham, we turn forty and suddenly realize that the fun and games do not go on forever. Then—and this is even more dramatic—we turn fifty, and double wham, we're gripped by the sense that:

1. Our life is more than half over.

2. The half that's over was the fun part.

3. The rest will include progressive disability, degeneration, and decrepitude—in other words, pain and suffering.

These realizations have nothing to do with where you live, how smart you are, or what kind of work you do. They are visceral awakenings that happen on some kind of cosmic schedule. What's more, you cannot explain them to your children or your thirty-year-old colleagues. Again, it's not about intelligence or sensitivity; they simply cannot feel these feelings.

Feelings, of course, do not evaporate. They bring us somewhere. Feelings about mortality commonly lead to one or more of the three Rs:

religion, resignation, or research. As a scientist, I naturally gravitate to research; in fact, I have long applied myself fervently to the study of aging, and I was lucky: I was in the right place at the right time. In fact, for baby boomers, that's been the story of our lives. We've seen more change than any generation in history, and the change has been remarkably favorable.

When we baby boomers were born, life expectancy in the United States was sixty-five years. Today, it's pushing seventy-seven, but that mark hasn't budged in the last decade and a half. What this means is that we've achieved as much benefit as we could squeeze out of advances in sanitation, decreased infant mortality, vaccinations, and antibiotics. In order to get beyond the seventy-seven mark, we're going to need dramatic new developments, but I'm not referring to *genetic engineering*. We've all seen news stories in which some white-coated geneticist proclaims that a life span of two hundred years or more is "just around the corner." Don't hold your breath.

I'm a biochemist, so you might think this is just professional jealousy, but I have some sobering facts for you. Genetic engineering has successfully extended only the lives of fruit flies and worms. Genetically, these are very simple organisms. You are an incredibly complex organism with (at last count) close to one hundred thousand genes. For nearly two decades, optimistic scientists have been making predictions about the eradication of genetic diseases. In some cases, like cystic fibrosis and Down's syndrome, they have even identified the specific gene that causes the problem, and yet these diseases continue to afflict us at the same—or in some cases, increasing—rates. Type-1 diabetes, sickle-cell disease, cystic fibrosis, Down's syndrome, Parkinson's disease, and certain types of cancer are well-known genetic disorders. As of this writing, more than two thousand patients have been treated with gene therapy, and not a single person has been cured.

The problems, although massive, are certainly not insurmountable. It's just going to take *much longer* than anyone imagined. Part of the problem is that genes never work alone. Most cell functions are bewildering and complex chain reactions, so the exact point in the chain of molecular events that causes a disease is not known. It's like a detective arriving at the scene of a crime. There may be evidence everywhere— fingerprints, blood, torn clothing, a weapon—but none of it guarantees that the crime will ever be solved.

Still, the media hypes genetic engineering because the stories sell. I understand the appeal: a genetic fix would enable us to continue to eat the standard American diet (aptly abbreviated SAD), become unfit and overweight, watch 3.5 hours of television every day (the national average), and then, when faced with the terrifying degeneration of aging, simply get our genes tweaked and everything would be all right.

But these are misleading, pie-in-the-sky ideas. Imagine the commander of an army, facing overwhelming odds as the enemy assembles on the opposite ridge. He knows that in the morning he will lead his forces into battle. How should he spend the night?

If you're counting on a genetic or pharmaceutical fix, you are like the commander who does nothing, betting everything on reinforcements' arriving in time. Right now, you face overwhelming odds in your war with time. I urge you to take stock of your situation and, with the help of this book, develop a battle plan. In your camp, there are soldiers with astounding skill, experience, and courage. This army is your immune system. You also have a strategical genius, your mind, and a secret weapon, which I will describe in the following pages. If you are willing, you can win. The fundamental question is this:

What should you do right now?

I'm a late bloomer. It's likely that I'll be in my late seventies when it's time to walk my daughter down the aisle, and I have no intention of doing that in a wheelchair. In fact, I plan to dance at her wedding with the same enthusiasm and energy that I enjoy today. The path for baby boomers like me is thus clearly marked. We must take every prudent step to slow the aging process so that if and when a biotech solution is perfected, we will have a body worth keeping. I cannot think of a more painful situation than seeing the antiaging breakthrough of the century arrive, only to be told that I am too old or too feeble to benefit from the therapy.

Antiaging is a new science, and in any new endeavor, you need a reliable map and a guide who has actually been where you wish to go. My journey on the antiaging trail has taken me to six continents—from the halls of UCLA, where I taught clinical nutrition for a health consultant training program, to the interior of Papua New Guinea, where I examined the diets of hunters and gatherers. I directed the nation's first FDA-licensed clinical laboratory specializing in nutrition testing and a few years later found myself trekking across Nepal studying rare high-altitude botanicals. I've been an adviser to members of the U.S. Olympic team and served on the faculty of the American College of Sports Medicine—and all the while, I was studying aging. Every fact I gathered from the lab or the forest, every second shaved off an athlete's marathon time, provided critical pieces in a stunning puzzle.

It turns out that aging is closely related to human performance, whether that be throwing a discus or a spear, lifting barbells or boulders. In fact, research shows that a major factor in longevity—and more important, your quality of life—is muscle mass.[1] Muscles on your arms appear to be more important than money in your bank. But before you run out to the gym, I should advise you that muscle mass is controlled by something other than time spent lifting weights, and that is your metabolism.

This should be good news to millions of Americans who have made valiant efforts to "get back in shape," only to find that exercise made them feel miserable and sore. After all, who wants to do something three or more times a week that they don't enjoy? And yet the message inherent in advertising slogans like "Just do it" or in the advice of your doctor to "Just get off the couch" is that failing to maintain a high muscle mass is all your fault. Let me make this clear. It's not willpower. It's biochemistry, and you can change that.

You may be thinking, "Wait a minute. Loss of muscle mass isn't everything. There are *dozens* of degenerative changes that occur with aging. We accumulate fat, we lose immune strength, our skin gets dry and thin, we get wrinkles and lines, we experience memory loss and joint pain . . ." Yes, all of that is true—and all of these changes are related to metabolism. *The Metabolic Plan* provides a step-by-step course of action, a metabolic "tune-up" that can dramatically improve the way you look and feel.

The Metabolic Plan is a doorway into a new paradigm. We see all around us glimpses of new possibilities. Jack La Lanne and Bob Delmontique (both in their mideighties) are more fit than most thirty-year-olds. At eighty-seven, Albert Morrow ran the two hundred meter in under forty seconds, and Marjorie Newlin won her twenty-fifth bodybuilding contest . . . at age seventy-eight. Both men's and women's participation in the Senior Olympics is growing by more than 50 percent every year, and on September 24, 2004, a remarkable event will take place: Sophia Loren will celebrate her seventieth birthday.

Futurist and trend watcher Faith Popcorn recently observed that age fifty is now a point of rebirth for millions of Americans. The question is, will you be able to enjoy this new golden age of longevity, or will it merely extend a period of decrepitude and chronic illness? Again, the answer depends on your metabolism.

THE METABOLIC MODEL OF AGING

Draw a horizontal line, on paper or in your mind. At the left end, write *birth*. At the right end, put *death*. Right now, you're somewhere between those two points, but the question is, where? Just about everyone answers that question with a number. They say, "I'm forty-five years old," and assume that this is the most meaningful way to indicate one's age. Wrong! Here's how I know.

I was sitting in a physiology course when the professor put a slide on the screen of two women born in the same month of the same year. Yet everyone was shocked to see that they looked like mother and daughter. At that point, it became perfectly clear to me that one's date of birth is not an accurate way to measure aging. What is?

Well, at the same time that years are passing (the chronology of aging), something else is happening. That something might be called the *biology* of aging. And as the slide of the two women illustrates, the biology of aging is by far the more important factor. Understanding this became my quest.

You see, the professor used this slide to illustrate that people age at different rates, but he had no idea why. In fact, he spent the rest of the class discussing the problems of the older-looking woman. That, after all, is the focus of conventional medicine: "Find a problem and fix it." But I wanted to study the younger-looking woman to discover what she was doing *right*. I remember writing in my notebook:

Goal: Identify the factors that determine one's rate of aging.

Twenty years later, this came into clear focus. Scores of scientific studies pointed to *metabolism,* not genetics, as the primary factor that influences how fast we age. The theory, now known as the metabolic model of aging, identifies two general forces at work in the human body. Anabolic metabolism is the rebuild, repair, and restore activity of your body. Catabolic activity refers to breakdown and degeneration. (When you see the word *catabolic,* think *catastrophic.*) At every stage of life, your health is determined by the ratio of damage to repair.

My young son broke his leg and was in a cast for just three weeks. His rapid healing was accomplished by the remarkably anabolic metabolism we all enjoyed as children. On the other hand, if my eighty-five-year-old mother broke her hip, she would heal very slowly, and perhaps not at all. We know that 40 percent of elderly hip fracture patients require lifelong care. Twenty percent never leave the hospital after the injury. That's because they lack the anabolic drive that is required to heal the bone and connective tissue.

The greater your anabolic drive—your ability to rapidly and efficiently repair and rebuild your tissues—the slower your body ages. And if this were all there was to the metabolic model, it would be interesting in an academic sense. If metabolism were just a matter of "good genes," this would be a very short book. We now know, however, from studies with identical twins, that only about 35 percent of the aging process is genetic. That means 65 percent is in your hands—literally. Antiaging is possible because metabolism can be changed.

Think of the remarkable shift that this creates in the way we experience life. If you just look at chronology, aging can only be de-

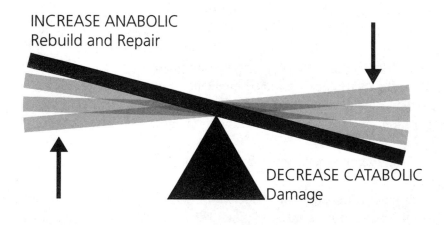

INCREASE ANABOLIC
Rebuild and Repair

DECREASE CATABOLIC
Damage

pressing because nothing can be done about it. Every time the earth circles the sun, we are all a year older. But the biology of aging—the metabolic model—makes chronological age almost irrelevant. It no longer matters how many candles were on your last cake. By supporting anabolic repair and reducing catabolic damage, you can not only slow your rate of aging but even reverse much of the damage that has already taken place. You can, in other words, grow biologically younger.

BODY-MIND KEYS

Restoring youthful anabolic drive is done essentially by resetting the time signals that determine how your brain and body interact. These signals, orginating from a variety of tissues and organs, are sent to the brain, which acts as a data analysis and command center. The brain, in effect, constantly polls the body for information about how the entire organism is performing. This information helps the brain run things at maximum efficiency.

If muscle mass and physical activity are low, for example, the brain assumes that very little energy is required to maintain that system. Consequently, when the brain hears that the stomach has received eight hundred calories (the average dinner), its instructions to the gastrointestinal tract and liver are: "Convert those calories to fat." If, on the other hand, muscle mass is maintained and those muscles are used through regular exercise, the brain's instructions are: "Convert those calories to energy."

The significance of such a dialogue is obvious, in terms of health, fitness, and longevity. *The Metabolic Plan* will explain how this body-mind conversation affects the balance of anabolic and catabolic forces. Importantly, this is not a simplistic view of physiology. The above muscle-stomach-brain dialogue, for example, can be quantified by measuring hormone signals from insulin, cholecystokinin, fatty acid oxidase, carnitine palmitoyltransferase, acyl-CoA dehydrogenase, and lipoprotein lipase. Because you probably don't want that level of detail, I'm going to be translating *biochemicalese* into English to provide an enjoyable lesson in how the human body functions and, more important, to show you how to maximize your health and wellness.

MOTHER NATURE'S GAME

Beyond determining the metabolic fate of dinner, the brain needs to know *how old we are* so that it can most effectively control the vast array of hormones and biochemicals relating to growth, repair, sex, immunity, and energy. This dialogue is *the primary factor that determines how we age and when we die*. The body-mind communications that foster optimal health and maximum life span are known as *longevity signals*. When the brain receives longevity signals from the body, it, in turn, sends anabolic (rebuild, repair, restore) instructions to the cells, tissues, and organs. On the other hand, if the brain receives over-the-hill signals from the body, it responds with catabolic (wear down, tear down, break down) instructions.

You may be asking why. Everyone asks that. You see, life is a game, and it's Mother Nature's game, not ours. Also, this game is much different from the ones most of us are used to. In the games we've invented (sports, education, careers), you first learn the rules, then the fundamentals, and finally strategies for winning. We're so used to doing this that we often think *everything* works this way. Then, one day, you look in the mirror and notice that your hair is thinning, there are deep lines in your face, you don't have the energy or drive you once had, and then it hits you—that there is another game being played here.

Remember that the name of the game is survival. Not your survival, but survival of the species. The flowers that bloom today will die tomorrow, contributing nitrogen and carbon to the soil and thereby supporting thousands of soil-dwelling species. They, in turn, support the growth of plants, which create oxygen, which supports millions of species. All thinking persons at one time or another have marveled at the astoundingly beautiful and unbelievably complex cycle of life.

The problem is that most people fail to understand that they are *part of the cycle*. We think we're different because we own computers, drive cars, walk on the moon, and talk on cell phones. But Mother Nature couldn't care less about technology. She's into survival—the really basic motivation that hasn't changed in millions of years.

This is perhaps the hardest thing for most people to grasp, but we know that the genes that control every cell in our bodies haven't changed a fraction of 1 percent in more than thirty thousand years. Essentially, the brain shifts your body into a catabolic tailspin after age forty because it is simply doing what it was programmed to do many thousands of years ago. Your DNA does not know about hospitals, miracle drugs, and refrigerators packed with food. All it knows is that in the past, when muscle mass and activity decreased and immunity started to fail, it was not a good sign. So the instructions hardwired into your genes initiate the shutdown sequence. Nothing personal. It was fun while it lasted.

Think about that the next time you're sitting on the couch, munching on some high-fat, artery-clogging snack, watching television. You think it's entertainment, but a part of you (the ancient part that hasn't changed in thirty thousand years) is getting a biochemical readout on your heart rate, hormone levels, muscle mass, and respiration and concluding that something is terribly wrong. Thus begins the catabolic spiral that will put you in your grave in your midseventies, terribly premature compared to what you *could* have experienced—if only you had known.

Our technology, in other words, has outstripped our biology. Mankind's technological achievements have led to an arrogant indifference to nature's game. And so we suffer. We suffer with a life expectancy of 76.7 years when our bodies are capable of lasting 120 years or more. We suffer with a host of illnesses that are entirely preventable. We suffer from an excess of fear and a poverty of spirit and enthusiasm. In our blindness, we turn for help in the wrong direction—to technology instead of nature. We behave as though our upset stomach were the result of an antacid deficiency, our fatigue comes from a lack of caffeine, cancer can be cured with poisons, fitness doesn't matter anymore, and unwanted fat will melt away with a diet pill. These are absurd notions, as is the idea that the answer to your stress-filled, maxed-out life is better time management or anxiety medication.

The Metabolic Plan is about learning the rules so you can enjoy the game to its absolute fullest—achieving maximal life span *and* high-level wellness. There are only two rules:

1. You need to restore anabolic metabolism, your astounding capacity for self-repair and regeneration.

2. You have to put the brakes on catabolic activity, the force that is

taking you at full speed down the line we drew earlier that has "death" at the end.

Now, even though there are only two steps to this program, when people hear words like *fitness* and *muscle mass,* many assume that the Metabolic Plan will involve a great deal of work. Here's more good news.

THE PRINCIPLE OF MINIMAL EFFORT FOR MAXIMUM RESULTS (MEMR)

We all know that we could stay *really* fit if we quit our present jobs and became aerobics instructors. But the truth is that we are all *very* busy in our lives. Everybody knows that they should eat a healthy diet, but the nutrition arena is incredibly confusing, and the need for convenience makes less-than-perfect food choices a reality for most of us. We all know that we could be healthier and live longer if we quit our jobs, moved to a pollution-free rural area, and spent hours a day in meditation. But this is simply not possible for the vast majority of baby boomers.

Thus, we look for the most efficient way to exercise, the easiest possible nutrition plan, the most comprehensive and effective antiaging program. In other words, we want to achieve the greatest benefit from the least possible effort. This principle, known as MEMR (minimal effort for maximum results), is built into the Metabolic Plan.

The Metabolic Plan will allow you to maintain a high muscle mass, burn fat, and maintain high-level fitness even while "working out" only about an hour a week. How is that possible? After all, you may be working out far more than that right now and barely maintaining what you perceive as reasonable fitness. That's because you're on the catabolic side of life. As catabolic metabolism increases, you will have to work harder and harder just to stay even, just to keep from getting flabby.

And what of those who are already overweight? I would suggest that their chances of regaining fitness and optimal health are slim—unless they restore youthful anabolic metabolism. Otherwise, the hurdle is too high, the pain is too great, and no matter what program they employ, most will ultimately give up.

The Metabolic Plan is your key to success. Sheila Foster was going to the gym religiously three times a week for a one-hour aerobics class followed by weight training. Still, at the age of forty-two, she felt as if she was losing ground. She rarely felt invigorated by her workout. More and more, she left the gym feeling exhausted, and what brought her to my office was increasing muscle and joint pain. Her friends confided that they were all taking painkillers, but Sheila knew that these drugs all had adverse effects over time.

I congratulated her for her insight and explained that her problem was not an ibuprofen deficiency. Rather, the muscle and joint pain, the fatigue and creeping weight gain were all part of an age-related metabolic shift that was happening in her body. I assured her that restoring a more youthful anabolic metabolism would produce greater benefit with less effort and less time than she was presently expending.

In less than six weeks, Sheila was pain-free, losing weight, and in her words, "feeling better than I've felt in a decade." Importantly, she was getting all of this while decreasing her workout time by 30 percent. How? The Metabolic Plan restored Sheila's body to a more youthful metabolic state. The details are provided in the following chapters. All you have to do is decide what you want to do for the next forty or fifty years. Do you want to work harder and longer for fewer and fewer health benefits? Or do you want to achieve remarkable gains in health and fitness while expending the least possible effort and time? You now have a choice.

MORE THAN A RAY

You may already be experiencing a number of age-related challenges, and even if you're relatively healthy, you may be looking ahead with apprehension. After all, we have been told that degeneration and decrepitude are inevitable and that you're "over the hill" at age fifty. For many baby boomers, trying to cram exercise, healthy eating, and yoga into an already busy schedule just adds to a sense of overwhelm.

The Metabolic Plan will help you relax. Not only will you receive maximal benefit from your efforts, but more important, you will be dealing with the *fundamental cause* of aging rather than running around treating all the individual symptoms. By restoring your body's ability to repair itself, many of the challenges we thought were "inevitable" simply do not arise, and the ones that do arise will be easier to heal. This is more than a ray of hope. It is a whole new way of experiencing life.

THE ROOTS OF THE METABOLIC PLAN

The Metabolic Plan tells a brand-new story because the insights and scientific discoveries that have made this book possible have only recently come into view. What could be called the *antiaging movement* began in the late 1980s with important discoveries about antioxidants, genetic error, nutrition, and stress. My own book *The DHEA Breakthrough* explored critical hormone factors. Then, in 1997, I was asked to head up a research project in Denver on antiaging. This was not the usual kind of inquiry into the treatment of age-related symptoms. The sponsor of this project, a wealthy philanthropist and business leader, wanted go beyond what he called "symptom stomping."

For decades, people have been talking about the *symptoms* of aging. Conventional medicine waits for a symptom to appear and then throws a drug at it. Alternative medicine, for the most part, was not much different, treating age-related symptoms with vitamins, minerals, and herbs. What we were after was a natural approach that could *prevent* the high blood pressure, clogged arteries, memory loss, accumulation of fat, failing immunity, and loss of bone density.

So began the Bioregenics Project, a four-year, multimillion-dollar collaboration that involved more than two dozen scientists from around the world. Our goal was to synthesize all the divergent theories of aging into a cohesive model and then to test—and prove—that model.

The success of this project ignited a new wave of research that has transformed our understanding of the aging process. In the past, most researchers and clinicians looked at age-related disability and said, "Oh, well, that's just the way it is." Many of these same people are now attending conferences and reading journals that explore a new reality, one in which degeneration and decrepitude *simply do not have to be* and, in fact, can be replaced by a long life of vigorous health, creativity, and passion.

THE PROOF

The quest for longevity is as old as mankind, but what's always been lacking is the proof that healthy long lives were possible. Shangri-la claims turned out to be wishful thinking or fabrication. Hundreds of bizarre therapies have come and gone, but the Bioregenics Project included a very important end point: a double-blind, placebo-controlled human clinical trial showing that anabolic repair activity can be improved and independent laboratory confirmation that catabolic damage can be dramatically reduced.

The solid scientific basis for *The Metabolic Plan* is what makes it unique and exciting. Because the book is carefully referenced with some four hundred citations from current medical literature, you can use the references to check for accuracy, for further study, or to discuss with your doctor or biochemist brother-in-law. This book also contains case histories of people who are, in a very real sense, growing younger: they have greater energy, less pain, more muscle, less fat, better sex, and a better outlook on life than they did ten or even twenty years ago.

In addition to careful references and clinical results, this book also presents reliable ways that you can test each facet of the Metabolic Plan *for yourself*. I'm not saying, "Trust me, I'm a scientist," but rather, "Let me prove it to you." At-home tests will enable you to see and measure your progress. Body composition analysis—conducted at any human performance laboratory—will verify by digital readout the changes you'll be seeing and feeling. And finally, a new metabolic profile obtained from a simple urine sample will benchmark your starting point and subsequent success.

If I asked you to think of all the things you wanted to do before you die, you'd probably have no problem coming up with a list. Everything on that list will require three things: energy, health, and time. *The Metabolic Plan* is about regaining youthful energy, maintaining high-level wellness, and then enjoying these blessings for much longer than you've ever imagined. I'm willing to bet that by the time you finish this book, you'll realize that your list is too short. That's because your present mind-set just won't allow for the new possibilities. So my job first and foremost is to change this—to show you a new perspective in which people in their fifties are actually young adults; people in their sixties are approaching "middle age"; the words *elderly, feeble, fragile,* and *decrepit* no longer apply; and we won't consider anyone to be a "senior" until he hits one hundred.

Do you like that picture? It's not just fantasy. I was asked my age on a recent talk show, and I replied, "Well, I was born in 1948, but I'm really only thirty-six years old." Then I explained the difference between chronological age, determined by your date of birth, and *biological* age—the measure of how you look, feel, and perform. You are about to learn how to change your biological age—how to turn back the clock by a decade or more.

Foundations

Although this took place more than thirty-five years ago, I remember it as if it were yesterday. My biology professor was about to give me the key to aging, and I was doodling in my notebook, obsessed with the girl in the blue sweater two rows down.

"Nature," he said bombastically, "doesn't care a *whit* about you and me." The statement jarred me from my musings. "Nature has one goal, and that is survival of the species." Now he had my attention, because that meant *procreation,* which I was contemplating, albeit along different lines.

The argument that he was presenting, which has since been reinforced by decades of research in evolutionary biology, was that aging and death are simply part of the Plan—part of nature's game. Survival of a species depends on its *reproduction.* Through natural selection, traits and behaviors that favor reproduction carry through from generation to generation, while adaptations that don't are selected out. A species that fails to reproduce in adequate numbers to carry on its unique genetic package will become extinct.

Every species has a certain life span and characteristics that maximize its evolutionary success. For humans, this means a fairly slow rate of growth to maturity, with the highest point of energy, vitality, optimism, and sex drive occurring at around age 20.[1] Then we begin to age. It's as if Mother Nature says, "OK, I've flooded every tissue in your body with hormones and maxed out your immune, respiratory, cardiovascular, and endocrine systems. Now procreate!" And of course, the majority of us do. Then, Mother Nature says, "Thanks! I'll give you a few more decades to care for the progeny you've created, and then I'm going to have to get rid of you to make room for a newer, younger model."

Thus, aging and death. Now, I was hearing this at the age of nineteen, not a time when you think a lot about mortality, but the professor had a remarkable way of driving the lesson home. "You," he said, "are filled with energy, while I have to drag myself out of bed every morning. You have strong, muscular bodies, and I have"—here he grabbed his belly with both hands—"fat. You have sex—or at least the contemplation of sex—and I have fading memories." He was fifty-three.

Now, I was on a sports scholarship, so the part about strong, muscular bodies was not lost on me. And I was gripped by the sudden realization that this would not always be the case. If this was nature's game, I decided right then and there to find a way to win: to enjoy what I treasured most—energy, vitality, and enthusiasm—for as long as humanly possible. I was also incapable of imagining life without sex (hey, I was nineteen), and thus began my quest for longevity. I reasoned that success in any game requires that you learn the rules, so I went on to study anatomy, physiology, and biochemistry. I attended graduate school and traveled to six continents to unravel the secrets of aging.

And here I am in my midfifties, *past* the age of my balding, tired, and overweight biology professor; yet I've turned out much differently. My body fat is 9 percent, exactly the same as it was in 1966. My blood pressure is 90/60, *better* than it was back then. My cholesterol is 150, and my immune profile, neurologic scores, and blood tests are about the same as a man in his midthirties.

How did this happen?

I learned the rules to nature's game . . .

And then I figured out how to bend a few.

"That could be just good genes," say the skeptics. But until 1988, I was headed straight for professordom. I was sixteen pounds heavier than I am now, and my body fat was 20 percent and climbing. My cholesterol was 214 and rising; my blood pressure was in the high-normal range. I was tired, and I could read the writing on the wall. Fortunately, an important piece of the aging puzzle was about to be revealed—the piece that would enable me to turn back my biological clock.

Research in endocrinology in the 1980s was showing that metabolism controls aging, life, and death. I was determined to understand this process, not for some abstract academic reason but for a very personal one. A textbook chart illustrating the typical quality-of-life curve for Western man filled me with dismay.

"Normal" Quality of Life

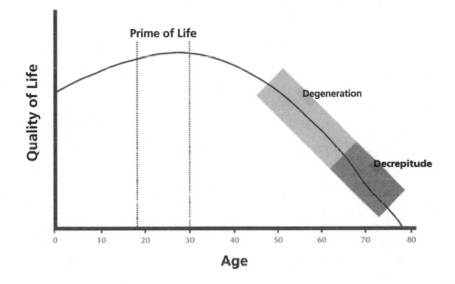

Notice that quality of life rises through childhood as we learn and grow. Then we hit puberty (*yahoo*), and from there, we enjoy a brief fifteen to twenty years known as the prime of life. There's a short plateau when things are OK, but then the downward slope starts, and accelerates as we experience degeneration, decrepitude, and finally slam into the brick wall of death at 76.7, give or take a few years. Take a good look at this graph, because if you do nothing to alter your metabolism, this is pretty much the story of your life. Does it look appealing?

If, however, you understand that something else is happening along with the passage of time, and that that something is actually more important, the graph (and your attitude) can change dramatically. As we've seen, this something is a metabolic shift from the anabolic, high-energy, rebuild, repair, and restore metabolism of youth to the progressively more catabolic (low-energy, break down, wear down) metabolism of old age. At about age thirty, there is a balance of these two forces, so the idea is to maintain anabolic metabolism at about the thirty-year-old level. My research and clinical experience show that this can be done, producing a quality of life that can look more like the accompanying revised chart.

New Possibilities

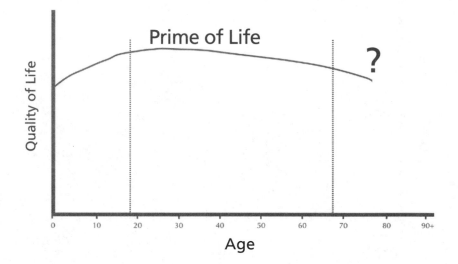

In this graph, we can see that quality of life rises through childhood as we learn and grow. Then we hit puberty, and from there, we enjoy a prime that may last forty years or more. Importantly, rebuild and repair metabolism is maintained, so that there is no sharp downward curve in quality of life. You blaze through life expectancy, discovering to your happy surprise that the wall is really a curtain, and somewhere down the road, maybe at age 120, you die. The most exciting part for me is the absence of degeneration and decrepitude.

If you are willing to attend to your metabolism, you can enjoy this kind of life. The phrase *paradigm shift* sounds trite, but there is no other way to describe this breakthrough. It will forever alter the way that you relate to your body and mind. It will give you a deep sense of hope where before there smoldered only the resignation of being over the hill. Here's the best news you've heard all day: there is no hill. Thousands of people have already discovered this, and you can, too.

Old paradigm: Aging is an inexorable process of degeneration.
New paradigm: Aging is a dynamic process over which we have considerable control.

Old paradigm: The body wears out like our other possessions.
New paradigm: The body has astounding powers of regeneration. We produce billions of new cells every day.

Old paradigm: A life expectancy of 76.7 years.
New paradigm: Life potential of 120 years or more.

FASTEN YOUR SEAT BELT

Research on aging is exploding, and not just because of the *number* of scientists working in this arena; it's the unbelievable acceleration of knowledge that is taking place as a result of technology. I currently utilize analytical equipment that can give me information in forty-five minutes that only a few years ago would have taken a dozen chemists more than a week to produce.

Then there's genomics—the ability to "read" information encoded in DNA—and of course, the Internet. We do indeed live in exciting times, and I believe we are rapidly approaching the point at which the limiting factor is not science but our ability to cope with the breakthroughs, to manage and integrate the massive amount of information into a coherent and practical plan of action.

MOTIVATION AND MEANING

As antiaging research filters down into the public domain, it takes on a certain flavor. This flavor reflects the attitude of those who write articles in the popular press and those who promote various products and programs. At the moment, the sense I get is that the antiaging movement is being fueled mainly by the fear of death. This needs to change if we are to enjoy new paradigm possibilities.

Think about this. Someone who is not fulfilled in his life, who has not found the sense of meaning we all desire, will naturally have an acute fear of death. After all, it represents the buzzer at the end of the game—a game that, as we approach the end, may seem cruel and unfair. But efforts based on fear will produce limited results. Have you ever watched a basketball game in which one team was playing to win while the other team was playing not to lose? It's hard to have fun when you are motivated by fear.

Quality of life, in other words, is as important as longevity, and so I approach antiaging not from a fear of death but from a *love of life,* and this requires that we spend time considering more than facts and hard data. *The Metabolic Plan* will help you examine what may best be summed up in the questions "*Why* do you want to live longer?" and "What will you *do* with the extra years?" Above all, I want to inspire you to have a greater appreciation for who you are and what you are capable of. From there, antiaging takes on a completely new flavor, one based not on fear but on celebration.

We'll start by looking at your relationship to your body. So much of what I read in the popular press implies that the human body is imperfect or limited and that you need some pharmaceutical, genetically engineered, high-tech treatment to enjoy long life. The message is that you are defective and science is going to save you. This is nonsense.

You are a miracle. Science, no matter how well designed and executed, can *never* come close to the astounding capabilities of the human body and mind. To those who put their faith in a pharmaceutical fix, I would like to point out that nature has a perfect track record over millions of years. Not a single biochemical—including *thousands* of enzymes, hormones, amino acids, neurotransmitters, and blood and lymphatic cells—has an adverse side effect. What's the pharmaceutical track record? How many drugs have been recalled because they were shown to have adverse, even fatal, side effects?

My focus, then, is using science to support the body's miraculous *renewal* activity. And this renewal activity can be accomplished deeply and effectively only to the degree that you are aware of what is going on in your body. My motto is, "If people knew better, they'd do better." I believe it is true on the conscious and subconscious levels. That doesn't mean dry and boring Anatomy 101 but rather a new view that begins with the simple but critically important question, "Who . . . are . . . you?"

BUILT TO LAST

What happens in life is determined to a great extent by our attitudes and beliefs. If someone doesn't believe that he could graduate from college, he'll never apply, and sure enough, it won't happen. Likewise, the beliefs we hold about our bodies greatly influence our health and longevity, so it's a good idea to examine some of the assumptions we've made over the years.

Our present mind-set concerning our bodies comes primarily from two places: what we were taught and what we observed. Most baby boomers learned about the human body in the 1950s and 1960s, when the predominant model of aging was that it is a process of wear and tear. So even today, we assume that aging is inevitable because our parts simply wear out, like our cars, houses, and other possessions. This mind-set was strengthened when we observed our grandparents and parents wearing down in their fifties, falling apart in their sixties, and dying in their midseventies.

Millions of people are dying right on schedule because *that is what they expect.* Think of the term *life expectancy*—the age at which most people are *expected* to die. What an absurd concept. Mountains of research show that the human body can last about 120 years, a concept known as maximal life span. Of course, even *maximal life span* is a misnomer. The term implies a biological limit, but it is in reality only a mathematical end point, established for the moment by the fact that we know of only a few people who have lived more than 120 years.

Remember the four-minute mile? When I was a kid, I was told that it was impossible for a human being to run a mile in less than four minutes. Then Roger Bannister showed us that this was not a biological limit at all. In 1954, he shattered—in 3 minutes, 59.4 seconds—a limitation in which people had believed for centuries. Today, of course, the four-minute mile is broken many times every year. Why? Because runners today are not burdened by false assumptions. They allow for new possibilities, new ways of training—and fulfill their dreams.

The wear-and-tear model of aging turned out to be erroneous, but few people know that. So let me be Roger Bannister for a moment. The average adult replaces approximately 300 billion cells *every day*. In the time it takes you to read this sentence (approximately ten seconds), your body will have created more than 30 million cells. This is nearly unfathomable, but just thinking about it will help you to grasp the big truth of human life. You are an extraordinary being with an astounding regenerative capacity. You are *not* like your house or your car—not at all. You are in fact constantly and continually re-creating your body. Once you understand this, you will begin to ask some very important questions, such as, "If I'm capable of this astonishing level of repair, why am I aging and falling apart?"

The answer is simple. You are falling apart because the cells you are making are weaker than the cells they are replacing. This is not inevitable. You just have to learn how to make better cells. Because if the 300 billion cells that you make today are stronger and healthier than the cells they replace, you will, in a very real sense, *grow biologically younger*. Do that consistently, day after day, and every aspect of who you are will improve, including not only your appearance but your biochemical makeup, strength, stamina, immunity, sex drive, memory, mood, and attitude. This is now possible. It's not genes or luck—it's a choice.

MUSCLE MASS AND LONGEVITY

I've explained why Mother Nature pulls the biochemical rug out from under you after age forty. But we all know of people who remained healthy and active into their eighties and beyond. How did they beat the odds? My physiology prof would say that they just had good genes, but that's an unscientific assumption. Even if that were true, the question remains, how exactly does the genetic advantage operate? What functions are maintained in people who live to be ninety in good health?

That question was studied by a team of Italian gerontologists, and the answer was surprising. You would imagine that smoking, exercise, diet, and marital and economic status would all have an effect, but one longevity factor rose above all the others. This factor held true for smokers and nonsmokers, rich and poor, married and widowed, and that was *muscle mass*. In a study of eighty-four men and women aged 90 to 106 years, muscle mass was the most consistent longevity factor.[2] Biochemically, that's reflected in one thing: anabolic metabolism.

When you increase anabolic metabolism, you experience greater energy, you burn fat, and you gain muscle. The muscle creates more energy and makes exercise easy and enjoyable. Anabolic metabolism puts you on an *upward spiral* in which each step builds on the previous step, leading to profound changes in body composition, mental clarity, vitality, mood, and one's sense of power and strength. The operative word here is *strength*.

Pure physical strength is the prime directive hardwired into every gene in our bodies. During 3.5 million years of natural selection, the most critical asset that enabled you to survive (and thereby pass on your genes) was strength. Of course, ingenuity and intelligence play critical roles in survival (thus the development of our large and extraordinarily capable brain), but for the most part, it was sheer strength and power. We forget this to our peril. Because we no longer need to remain physically fit in order to survive, many of us fall into sedentary behavior. But the operating system of human life is still working on the assumption that fitness = survival.

Understanding this solves so many mysteries. Whereas clinicians scratch their heads and wonder why osteoporosis (progressive weakening of the skeleton) cripples or kills more than a million Americans each year, the evolutionary biologist points out that bone strength is maintained by anabolic metabolism. Lose anabolic drive and you lose more than bone density. You lose strength and flexibility in joints, tendons, and ligaments. The loss of muscle mass starts the catabolic break down of all connective tissue.

In fact, the cascade of degeneration affects the entire body and brain, but it is amazing how blind we are to the metabolic answer. Years ago, researchers discovered that elderly people have low levels of cerebrospinal fluid (CSF) compared to young people. This was a valuable finding because CSF is critical to the optimal function of the brain and nervous system. Not only that, CSF also helps lubricate the spongy disks that lie between the vertebrae, thus maintaining the strength, flexibility, and integrity of the spine. But what was the researchers' proposed solution? Their answer to this problem was to create an artificial cerebrospinal fluid.

Think of the market for such a product. Seventy-six million baby boomers lining up for injections. ("Hold still, Mrs. Jones, while I check your oil.") But this approach is nuts. First of all, initial testing of the product was a disaster. All the mice injected with the product died.

Second, of course, no one asked the most important question, which is whether *all* elderly people have low CSF levels. It turns out that only *sedentary* elderly people do. Those who maintain muscle mass (anabolic metabolism) and range-of-motion exercise (twisting and bending the spine) don't have this deficiency.

The bottom line is that anabolic metabolism is a critical key that has been overlooked. One reason is that you can't patent exercise and range-of-motion movement. In the profit-driven research climate, there is no motivation to look at natural therapies. After all, yoga is five thousand years old and hasn't resulted in a single IPO.

But the metabolic solution has been used by a number of remarkable pioneers. Jack La Lanne was born in 1914, but the last time I saw him, he looked like a very fit fifty-year-old, with the spirit and attitude of a thirty-year-old. He'd also done nine hundred push-ups that day, something that most of us couldn't do in a week. Jack has discovered the secret of anabolic metabolism, which is that the brain—which controls every cell of your body—doesn't know how old you are. It doesn't really care, because chronological age is not nearly as important to survival as biological age.

When Jack La Lanne's brain checks in for updated information (so it can operate his body in the most efficient way possible), his muscles report that they just performed nine hundred push-ups. The brain then concludes that the body is superbly fit and quite capable of surviving. It then sends anabolic instructions to every tissue in the body to maintain peak immunity, vitality, bone mass, high metabolic efficiency, mental acuity, and a positive attitude. Included are instructions to convert every morsel of food he eats to energy, so that Jack La Lanne will never—even if he lives to be 120—have to count calories.

As you can see, anabolic metabolism is a cycle. High muscle mass sends longevity signals to the brain. The brain sends anabolic instructions back to the body that maintain muscle mass. All of this communication, of course, is biochemical—a dizzying array of enzymes, hormones, and nerve signals that control life.

THE OTHER SIDE OF THE COIN

Jack La Lanne represents the positive side of nature's obsession with fitness and illustrates the extraordinary rewards associated with this level of motivation. But there's a penalty side as well. Let's listen to the internal dialogue of a fifty-year-old *sedentary* person.

Brain: Good morning, body. I need your month-end reports. Muscles, how are we doing?

Muscles: Zzzzzzzzz.

Brain: Muscles, wake up. How are we doing?

Muscles: Oh, uh, well, not so good. Muscle mass is down 3 percent, and we haven't exercised in weeks. I think part of my problem is that I haven't heard from the endocrine system in a long time. And it's not just me. Bone mass is down, too.

Brain: Gee, not good. Nervous system, how are we doing?

Nervous system: What do you mean, "How are we doing?" Things are changing so fast, I can't keep up, might lose my job, boss is on the warpath. We're barely holding on . . . and I get no support from endocrine anymore.

Brain: Gee, sorry I asked. [Making notes] Nervous system freaking out. Immune system, how are things down there?

Immune system: Not good, boss. We've still got that fungal infection we were dealing with last month; I think the problem in the liver might be serious; we're trying to control a smoldering infection in the teeth and gums; and we're not getting much help at all from the endocrine system.

Brain: Endocrine system, what the hell is going on? Why have you stopped supporting the muscles and the nervous and immune systems?

Endocrine system: Well, boss, I hate to be the one to tell you, but hormone levels are down again this month. My guess is that we're over the hill.

Brain: Of course! Now it all makes sense. Muscles mass is down, the nervous system can't cope, immunity is failing, and hormone levels are falling. We are over the hill. All right, listen up! My instructions are to put this body into shutdown mode. Catabolic city. OK, let's see, turn down metabolic efficiency; no need for much energy. We can start making fat; it's so much easier than muscle anyway. Immune system, you've done a splendid job all these years, but it's time to give up. Whatever comes along—pneumonia, hepatitis, whatever—just let it come. And nervous system, stop worrying so much; the show's about over . . .

If that dialogue sounds a bit chilling, it ought to be. After all, it's taking place in more than 70 million Americans, and you might be one. Again, it is the over-the-hill message that starts the programmed shutdown sequence. The brain, concluding that the organism is beyond reproductive age and therefore of little evolutionary value, initiates the cascade of catabolic breakdown activity. The question for you right now is, where would you intervene in the above scenario?

If you answered endocrine system, you're right on target. If you said take piles of nutritional supplements—echinacea to shore up immunity, kava and valerian to manage stress, calcium to build bones, ginkgo for memory, and creatine for muscle—you've fallen into the trap of what I call *symptom stomping*. Last year, more than $9 billion was spent on these remedies, and studies show that in terms of longevity, they're not working. People who take nutritional supplements, even in high doses, die at about the same age as people who take no supplements at all.[3]

It's not that these products are worthless. It's just that without dealing with the underlying *cause* of aging, symptom stomping will not produce the rewards you're hoping for. Your endocrine system is the key to reaching the underlying cause.

THE WHEEL OF LIFE

The endocrine system maintains and controls the exquisitely complex function of the human body. Six major glands—the hypothalamus, pituitary, thyroid, adrenals, pancreas, and sex organs (testes or ovaries)—secrete hormones that act as chemical messengers to regulate every aspect of metabolism. This includes growth and development; rebuild-repair-restore functions; temperature regulation; energy metabolism; heart, lung, and kidney functions; and a host of feedback mechanisms that keep us in a state of homeostasis, or balance.

It's important to note that the endocrine system is a closed loop, meaning that changes in one glandular function will affect the others to some degree. The adrenals play a key role because of the range of hormones they produce. Each of the two adrenal glands, located on the upper part of the kidneys, produces hormones with a vast array of functions. The outer part of the gland produces hormones that control the fluid and mineral balance of the body. The inner part of the adrenals produces a group of hormones known as *glucocorticoids,* so named because they help control glucose metabolism (energy). Glucocorticoids also include the stress hormones epinephrine (adrenaline), norepinephrine, and cortisol.

Finally, the adrenals produce DHEA (dehydroepiandrosterone). Although DHEA is produced in amounts *hundreds of times greater* than any of the other hormones, it received very little attention until the 1990s. The physiology text that I studied in college (published in 1973) never mentioned DHEA. Other texts on my bookshelf published in the late 1980s include nothing about DHEA. How did this happen?

There's a saying in research that "you only see what you're looking for." Because no one could pin down a narrow function for DHEA (unlike aldosterone, which balances sodium and potassium, or epinephrine, which initiates the flight-or-fight stress response), it was considered a "junk hormone." Even after it was determined that DHEA levels plummet after age thirty, the most common response was, "Oh, well, that's what happens when you age." I was among a small group of researchers in the 1980s who said, "Wait a minute. Perhaps the sharp decline in DHEA levels, unparalleled in human physiology, is not an effect of aging at all. Perhaps it is a *cause* of the aging process."

What a concept. Several years and more than three thousand scientific studies later, here is the leading view of DHEA:

1. DHEA contributes to more than 150 different metabolic functions. As such, it is the most comprehensive anabolic influence in human biochemistry.

2. When we're under a great deal of stress—that is, when the adrenals are pumping out stress hormones—DHEA levels fall. This is one reason stress is so damaging to the body. It may be that the adrenals simply cannot produce large amounts of both stress hormones and DHEA.

3. Falling levels of DHEA and other anabolic hormones are responsible for much of the catabolic downward spiral (a.k.a. the shutdown sequence) that we've been talking about. Low DHEA is associated with impaired immunity, rising cholesterol, increased risk for cancer and cardiovascular disease (America's first and second leading causes of death), low energy, declining sex drive, accumulation of excess fat, depression, and memory loss.

4. Restoring DHEA levels appears to provide a tune-up for the adrenals and may have a ripple effect of benefits throughout the endocrine system, but it is not a magic bullet. Other critical factors, essential for restoring anabolic repair or reducing catabolic damage, are presented in Chapters 2 and 3.

The Metabolic Plan is a comprehensive and proven system designed to reset your biological clock. In so doing, the effects of aging can be postponed, diminished, or in some cases, entirely eliminated. In other words, you can avoid the catabolic cascade that leads to degeneration, decrepitude, and death at the current life expectancy of 76.7 years. There are actually two ways to accomplish this: the hard way (the 900-push-ups strategy) and the easier way. Which would you prefer?

THE EASY WAY (WELL . . . THE *EASIER* WAY)

If you're like me, no matter how motivated you might be, it would be impossible to do nine hundred push-ups a day. The good news is that you don't have to. I realized decades ago that my life path (research, teaching, and writing) would take a great deal of time and attention. I currently review fifty scientific and medical journals each month and sort through another three hundred to five hundred studies published on the Internet. I run a growing biomedical business and have a growing family (four kids under the age of ten). Last year, I flew more than sixty thousand miles. So my first prerequisite for a successful antiaging program was that it had to be *time-efficient.*

Remember that the degeneration associated with aging is caused by a decline in anabolic repair and the accumulation of catabolic damage. So antiaging, quite simply, is the reverse of that. You support or promote anabolic repair, and you take steps to reduce the damage to which you are exposed on a daily basis. This is not terribly time-consuming, but there's a fair amount of new information you will need to learn.

DEFINITION OF TERMS

It is important to understand that I am using the term *metabolism* to refer to the process of anabolic repair and catabolic damage within the body. Widespread confusion has been created by a raft of weight-loss products with names like Metabolift, Metaboblast, and Metaborama. Invariably, these pills contain stimulant drugs such as caffeine, ephedrine, or both. They induce appetite suppression by an amphetamine-ike effect and are dangerous. Stimulant weight-loss products do not enhance metabolism any more than pressing harder on the accelerator will improve your engine's performance. In fact, these products are highly catabolic and can actually accelerate aging. What's more, the labeling of these products is often deceptive, with the caffeine and ephedrine hidden by the use of "all-natural" herbs such as guarana, kola nut, bissy nut, maté, ma huang, and Chinese ephedra. But whatever names you want to use, the active ingredients in these products are still caffeine and ephedrine.

We also have to be precise about what we mean by antiaging. If a person eats a well-balanced diet, exercises regularly, doesn't smoke, and drinks but a glass of wine a day, is he practicing antiaging? No. He is practicing prudent lifestyle or optimal self-care, but it is not antiaging. That's because none of these measures (or taking megadoses of vitamins and minerals) has any bearing on longevity. Don't get me wrong. People who practice optimal self-care are likely to reduce their risk for cardiovascular disease and cancer, and that is *extremely valuable*. I'm all in favor of doing that—the reduction of pain and suffering is a good thing—but it is not antiaging.

Antiaging is not simply decreasing your risk for the diseases associated with aging. It is the alteration of the *fundamental cause* of aging, which is progressive degeneration. I'm not splitting hairs by making this distinction. This is an important part of the confusion that exists in the health care arena today. There are a hundred steps you can take to optimize your current metabolic state, but the only strategy that will enable you to slow the aging process is one that shifts metabolism back to *a more youthful anabolic state*, restoring the body's ability to heal and repair itself. I'll detail the numerous advantages of this strategy in the following chapters, but here are the top three:

1. Muscle mass is restored and maintained. Solid research has shown that this is one of the most important factors determining quality of life and longevity. Why? Because it translates into greater functional ability, the ability to take care of oneself.[4]

2. Immunity is maintained. Restoring anabolic drive has profound effects on the immune system. Evidence suggests that natural

killer (NK) cell numbers and activity against viruses and cancer will be maintained.[5] The balance of cytokines (biochemicals that control immunity) can be restored.[6]

3. Rebuild-repair-restore biochemicals, most notably IGF-1, are restored to youthful levels. This translates to more rapid healing, stronger bones,[7] decreased risk of injury, and according to the latest studies, sharper memory, better mood, and accelerated learning.[8]

Review the two charts on pages 17 and 18. There are two very unattractive aspects to normal aging: the steep decline in quality of life and that brick wall at 76.7 years. I'll say it again: the idea is not simply to postpone death. We all know people as young as forty who are walking and breathing but aren't truly enjoying life. No, what I'm after could be called an *ecstatic* life—one filled with the exuberance, vitality, and passion we normally associate only with youth. To merely stay aboveground, all you need is technology and wonder drugs. To live an ecstatic life, you have to maintain high-energy anabolic metabolism. And now you can.

Restoring Your Anabolic Power

As a graduate school instructor, I had a tremendous responsibility. After all, many of my students were going on to medical school, and if I didn't instill in them a sense of the miraculous nature of the human body, chances are they would graduate knowing the facts but missing the inspiration.

Clearly, one of the most astonishing aspects of human physiology is the body's ability to repair, rebuild, and restore itself. This anabolic activity goes on twenty-four hours a day and is the most intense during deep sleep. As I've mentioned, your body replaces approximately 300 billion cells every day. Perhaps a more familiar visual image will help you to grasp this. A thousand dollar bills would form a stack about two feet high. A stack of 1 million dollar bills would be three times as tall as the Washington Monument. A billion dollar bills would extend way beyond the stratosphere, and a stack of 300 billion dollar bills would reach halfway to the moon.

The wear-and-tear model of aging gave people the impression they were falling apart just like their possessions. But your body is *not* like your house or your car. Imagine living in a house that grew a new roof before the old one started leaking, that painted itself every two years, repaired its plumbing, and washed its own windows.

You live in a miraculous body, and as with home improvement, you can do a great job or a lousy job, depending on three factors.

ANABOLIC FACTOR 1: RAW MATERIALS

Only about forty-two nutrients are required to keep you alive, but hundreds are required to optimize cellular repair. Practically every month, another nutrient (or an entire group of nutrients) is highlighted in the biomedical literature for its role in supporting anabolic repair or reducing catabolic damage. Invariably, these nutrients—including polyphenols, flavonoids, isoflavones, carotenoids, vitamins, and trace minerals—are found in whole grains, fresh fruits, and vegetables. And yet surveys show that Americans are consuming fewer of these foods than ever before.[1] It's hard for people to understand how Americans could be malnourished—we suffer no beriberi, scurvy, or pellagra, after all—but once again, it comes down to the difference between adequate and optimum. If you want to maximize your body's youthful anabolic metabolism, you'll need more than the standard American diet.

What's Missing?

You've no doubt heard the bad news about America's depleted soil. Plants cannot take up nutrients that aren't in the soil, and thus, even a "well-balanced" diet may be deficient in essential minerals such as selenium and zinc.[2] Then there's food processing, which strips away critical nutrients. Chromium, for example, is essential for muscle synthesis and the body's production of energy; yet the U.S. Department of Agriculture reports that up to 90 percent of Americans have insufficient intake of this essential anabolic trace mineral.[3]

Storage and cooking deplete still more nutrients, and recently, an overlooked aspect of nutrient depletion came to light. Researchers at the University of Washington and the Fred Hutchinson Cancer Research Center in Seattle report that important plant nutrients known for their anticancer activity have been effectively removed from American foods by processing and selective breeding.[4] Why? Many of these health-promoting compounds are bitter or astringent, and in an effort to enhance flavor, growers and manufacturers dramatically reduced the foods' nutrient value.

The National Academy of Sciences has issued an alert that it takes twice as many vegetables to get the daily requirement of vitamin A as previously thought.
> —Life Extension, *March 2001*

The Vicious Cycle

Depleted soil produces deficient plants. Combined with poor food choices, cooking, and selective breeding, many of the nutrients critical for anabolic repair are simply unavailable to most Americans. This accelerates the aging process as unrepaired damage contributes to further catabolic breakdown. To make matters worse, surveys show that older Americans (those with the greatest need for anabolic repair) are the ones suffering the most from malnutrition.[5]

You can overcome this obstacle by incorporating what I call *longevity foods* into your diet. Chapter 8 explains how this can be done quickly and easily, by making better food choices and taking advantage of superfoods that provide literally hundreds of anabolic nutrients to meet your body's repair and rebuild needs. Chief among these nutrients, and one that deserves attention here, is protein.

The Critical Role of Protein

Without a doubt, protein is the raw material most needed for repair and rebuild functions. Now, most people think immediately of meat, poultry, fish, milk, and eggs, but few people are deficient in *dietary* proteins. The problem with aging is at the *cell level*, where tens of thousands of proteins must be synthesized around the clock. This ability to create, transport, and metabolize proteins decreases with age. Imagine again that you're building a house. In youth, it's as if every nail, beam, shingle, windowpane, and light fixture is at your fingertips the minute you need it. As we age, however, the truck from the lumberyard takes longer to deliver the materials we need, and then shipments start arriving incomplete, with "back order" or "out of stock" written all over the invoice.

Most builders can make do. They'll work on another part of the house while they wait for the needed part. They might even fashion or jerry-rig a part from available materials. But at a certain point, your house is going to start looking rather strange. In life, that's called middle age. Suddenly, lines and wrinkles start appearing on your face. Hair turns gray. The clear definition of muscle is lost, and in its place, we see flab. We find that a late night with too much alcohol (something we used to do with impunity) knocks us out of commission for an entire day. We might become allergic to things that never bothered us before. Exercise tolerance declines, meaning that the same amount of exercise that used to invigorate us now produces a sense of exhaustion. Even worse, we start to experience fatigue even when we've done nothing strenuous. All of these changes are due in great part to the impaired ability to create and deliver the myriad proteins that our bodies require for optimal function.

Proteins come from two sources. Each cell manufactures a dizzying number of proteins, and the liver plays a central role as the protein "lumberyard" to the body. As we age, both of these functions are compromised, and to understand the solution, you really need to have a clear idea of the problem. Hang in there. This is not complex. The next few pages will give you important insights into how your body works and how to make it work better and last longer.

Inside the Cell

Continuing with the construction analogy, imagine the architect's office. This is the cell nucleus. The blueprint on the table is DNA. All day, contractors (RNA) are coming in and out of the office, studying the blueprint, and then giving instructions to the builders (ribosomes), who create all of the proteins that the cell needs to function, grow, protect itself, and replicate. Now imagine this happening at high speed with almost unfathomable complexity—like Grand Central Station times a thousand—*and* it's happening in 100 trillion cells throughout your body. Amazing.

Over time, however, the office gets cluttered, and somebody spills coffee on the blueprint. The contractor gets the wrong information, and the builder does a completely botched job: he puts the garage door on the roof. ("Hey, I was just following instructions.") Aging is like that. The DNA blueprint is damaged, and erroneous instructions are sent throughout the cell. Proteins don't work, and as this general sloppiness accumulates, entire tissues and organ systems start to fail. We'll cover this in more detail in Chapter 3, but for now, consider that Mother Nature knew this would happen.

You can't have 300 billion cells replicating a billion DNA strands (do the math and you get a 3 with twenty zeros) every day without error. So this construction company placed a bunch of guards all around the blueprint to protect it. The most important guard, interestingly, is another protein known as glutathione.

The bad news: Glutathione levels decline with age.

The good news: You probably know this by now. The answer is the mantra of this book: restore anabolic metabolism. There is solid evidence that increasing anabolic metabolism increases glutathione levels,[6] which is good because that's one of the *only* ways to increase levels of this extraordinarily important substance. Contrary to popular belief (and the claims of glutathione pill manufacturers), you can't raise glutathione levels by eating it. Glutathione is manufactured *within the cell.* It's not obtained from food and transported to the cells like glucose or potassium. Of course, you can eat the raw materials from which glutathione is made (see Chapter 8), but the critical factor once again is metabolism. If you are highly catabolic (over the hill), your body will simply say, "Why should I bother producing glutathione? We're in shutdown mode; plummeting glutathione is just a part of the degeneration."

Additional Protein Factors

Two of the most important repair proteins produced by the body are glucosamine and chondroitin, responsible for the structural integrity and flexibility of joints, tendons, and ligaments. These connective tissues act as shock absorbers in the weight-bearing joints of the body—including the knees, hips, and fingers—and morning stiffness is often an early signal that our body is not able to keep up with the repair. What is often happening is that the body is losing the ability to manufacture adequate levels of glucosamine and chondroitin.

Fortunately, you can deal with this on two levels. First, research suggests that improving anabolic metabolism will stimulate production of repair proteins,[7] and you can also take glucosamine and chondroitin as nutritional supplements. Studies have shown that these compounds are incorporated into the joint tissues, where they help to stimulate repair functions.[8] Unlike aspirin and other analgesics, which help with the pain of cartilage destruction but actually inhibit cartilage repair, glucosamine and chondroitin help alleviate joint stiffness and pain by repairing the connective tissues at the cellular level.[9]

Outside the Cell

If you will allow one final construction analogy, imagine a building supply warehouse that is never out of stock on any item, for the simple reason that the owner is a magician. If he runs out of rain gutters, he simply takes some scraps of lumber or a handful of nails and—*poof!*—

turns them into the precise rain gutter that you require. When it comes to protein, the liver does stuff like that every day. If it runs out of a specific protein, it can take apart another protein and reassemble the amino acids to produce whatever the body needs.

In fact, the liver performs an enormous range of tasks. It was a common joke among my students that you could write "the liver" for any question on a physiology exam and be correct most of the time. Among more than sixty different metabolic functions, the liver is in charge of collecting and distributing nearly every nutrient from every bite of food you will ever eat. Imagine this astoundingly busy supply depot, providing a constant stream of building materials to 100 trillion customers. At the same time, it is being asked to double as the police station, recycling plant, and garbage disposal. And all the while, it's being assaulted by alcohol, caffeine, drugs, food additives, environmental toxins, and potentially exposed to six or more types of hepatitis, any one of which could cripple or destroy it completely.

The liver constantly monitors the bloodstream for compounds that might pose a danger to a body's overall health. When possible, it simply removes the offending substance and eliminates it through the digestive tract. If removal is not possible, the liver will try to break down the dangerous compound or alter its chemical structure to render it harmless. If even that is impossible, the liver will surround the toxin with a layer of fat and send it to remote areas of your body for indefinite storage.

TOP TEN LIVER FUNCTIONS

The liver performs more than sixty metabolic functions. Here are the "top ten" that relate directly to longevity:

1. Detoxification

2. Cholesterol production and control, including conversion of cholesterol to bile acids

3. Blood sugar control

4. Circulation and blood pressure

5. Hormone and enzyme production

6. Critical role in immunity

7. Digestion and metabolism of carbohydrates, fats, and proteins

8. Clearinghouse for virtually all nutrients that you consume

9. Protein synthesis for all tissue repair

10. Production of critical anabolic repair biochemicals or growth factors (GFs), including IGF-1, IGF-2, TGF, and EGF

Clearly, if you're interested in living a long and healthy life, you've got to start thinking of ways to maintain optimal liver function. Surprisingly, this critical factor is largely ignored in the antiaging arena. Dozens of books, scores of articles, and hundreds of product brochures all promote ways to restore youth, but in fact, *nothing*—no hormone, herb, injection, amino acid, vitamin, pill, or potion—will work if your liver is not in top shape. Once again, the deck is stacked against you if you're over forty and living in a polluted metropolitan area. Even in the best environment, the average American will lose 40 percent of liver function by age seventy. That's simply part of the catabolic downward spiral. If you're a smoker, your liver is suffering dearly for the habit, and if you have chronic hepatitis, your chances for success in any longevity program are markedly reduced. Thus, the next chapter includes a four-step "protect-your-liver" program.

ANABOLIC FACTOR 2: ENERGY

"Well, I just don't have the energy I used to." Doctors hear this complaint more than any other, and until recently, they had no response other than to say (and perhaps you've heard these words yourself), "You're just getting older." Or how about this one: "You're going to have to learn to live with it."

You see, after ruling out anemia or a disease-related cause of fatigue, physicians had no solution. And because they themselves were most likely experiencing the same thing, they thought it was pretty much hopeless. All of that has changed, as scientists have started to unravel the mystery of age-related fatigue. For more than two decades, Bruce Ames and his colleagues at the University of California, Berkeley, have been looking at the connection between declining energy and reduced anabolic metabolism. In a paper just published in the *Proceedings of the National Academy of Science*, Ames and his group report on a fundamental cause of aging.

Background

The Ames group began by comparing the activity levels of young rats versus old rats. To no one's surprise, they found that young rats were far more active. And here's where the new paradigm of aging comes in. While others made these observations and said, "Oh, well, that's just the way it is," the Ames group looked for the *reason* for this decline. In the metabolic model of aging, in other words, there are no assumptions. If aging is associated with increasing fatigue, we can learn the *cause*—and find a cure.

Breakthrough

Cells make energy through oxidation, a biochemical combustion of the fuel you eat and the oxygen you breathe. The energy "factories" within the cell where this takes place are known as mitochondria (my-toe-KON-dree-ah). The Ames group theorized that over time, the by-products of oxidation might damage the mitochondria, resulting in lower energy production. Think of a factory where the product being produced also causes the machinery to rust. At a certain point, the factory will grind to a halt, and that's exactly what happens to mitochondria. As cellular energy declines, so does organ function. As organ function declines, so does your health. It used to be inevitable, but thanks to Ames and his crew, this critical facet of aging can now be reversed.

In a series of experiments, a team of scientists from five research organizations[10] gave acetyl-L-carnitine and alpha lipoic acid—nutrients found in small amounts in red meat and milk—to older rats. Within seven weeks, they saw dramatic improvements in mitochondria function and energy production.[11] This not only led to increased activity levels, but as Dr. Ames stated, "With the two supplements together, these old rats got up and did the Macarena. The brain looks better, they are full of energy—everything we looked at looks more like a young animal."[12]

Ames's last point is perhaps the most compelling. Because restored energy is important, but to achieve dramatic improvements in memory as well was an unexpected and exciting "side effect." In other words, increasing cellular energy production appears to improve *everything,* and follow-up research is under way to look at immunity, strength, endurance, and cardiovascular health.

Not Just Happy Rats

Acetyl-L-carnitine boosts the activity of a mitochondrial enzyme that is critical for energy production. Alpha lipoic acid is a powerful antioxidant that protects the cell from the by-products of oxidation. You'll learn more about oxidation in Chapter 3 and even how to create more mitochondria energy "factories" in Chapter 7, but for now, the important point is that this mechanism of action is perfectly applicable to the human condition. Moreover, these nutrients are safe and available at your local health food store. Antiaging specialists recommend a daily intake of 200 milligrams to 500 milligrams of acetyl-L-carnitine and 100 milligrams to 500 milligrams of lipoic acid.

ANABOLIC FACTOR 3: HORMONE SIGNALS

If you give an elderly woman handfuls of calcium, will her bones get stronger? Probably not. Even if she has a lot of energy, we know that a third factor is required for successful anabolic metabolism, and that is a hormone signal that tells her body *what to do* with the raw materials. In youth, these signals—coming from growth hormone, DHEA, estrogen, testosterone, and progesterone—produce a loud and clear message throughout the body that says, *"Rebuild, restore, repair."* In middle age, the message is reduced to a whisper. And in old age, the message becomes "Why bother?" For effective antiaging, the anabolic signal must be amplified. The good news is that there is now a safe and effective way to do this.

Background

When I turned forty, I looked in the mirror and didn't like what I saw. Even though I was exercising, had been eating a good diet, and was taking nutritional supplements, I was aging just like my father. Because he had died nine years before, the face in the mirror was quite a wake-up call, and I decided to shift into antiaging research in earnest.

Talk about being in the right place at the right time. A week later, I received a flyer about a conference on DHEA, the first of its kind as far as I know. Now, keep in mind that this was a scientific symposium, not an antiaging conference—*antiaging* was not even a popular term—and I was intrigued by the range of data that was to be presented, having to do with decreased risk of cardiovascular disease, cancer, and obesity as well as the enhancement of immunity, insulin sensitivity, and memory. Granted, the vast majority of the data was from animal experiments, but I was particularly struck by one abstract from a human study that concluded: "In normal men DHEA administration reduces body fat, increases muscle mass, and reduces serum low density lipoprotein cholesterol levels."[13]

At that very moment, I was losing muscle and gaining fat, and my cholesterol level was 214 and rising. Provided this stuff was safe, I was *very* interested. At the conference, I saw pieces of the metabolic model of aging everywhere. Of course, no one was *using* that term. But the data on cardiovascular disease, cancer, diabetes, body composition, immunity, and stamina was all related to the balance of anabolic repair and catabolic damage. Speaking with the presenter of the only human trial, I asked the big question, "Is DHEA safe?" to which he answered, "It's too early to tell. Our experiment lasted only twenty-eight days, and although there were no adverse side effects, long-term risks are unknown."

The Researcher as Guinea Pig

So I did what scientists have been doing for thousands of years: I started taking it myself. First, I had my DHEA blood levels measured and found that I was "normal" for a forty-year-old. Swell. I knew all too well what "normal" means (see the " 'Normal' Quality of Life" chart in Chapter 1 if you've forgotten). No, I wanted to be normal for a twenty-five-year-old, so I had to learn how much DHEA the average twenty-five-year-old produced. That turned out to be about 50 milligrams per day, and that became my experimental dose.

Over the next eight years, I kept track of blood chemistry, body composition, and hormone levels, comparing notes with a small fraternity of biochemists around the world who were doing the same thing. Gradually, an important facet of the metabolic model of aging began to take shape. Each of us was noticing a decrease in body fat without drastic dietary change. At the same time, even a modicum of strength training—such as moderate weight lifting or Nautilus machines—produced visible results. I looked in the mirror on my forty-eighth birthday and then sifted through a drawer of old photos to find one from eight years earlier. The difference was striking. I'd lost about fifteen pounds, but the most noticeable difference was in my face. At age forty, my complexion was starting to get "blotchy," and I had lost the strong lines of my jaw and cheekbones. Eight years later, I looked more like I did in college. Even more striking was the reduction in my cholesterol and blood pressure.

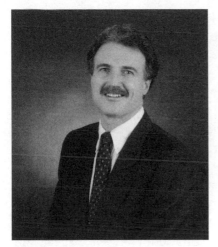 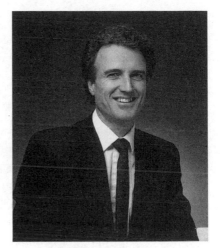

1988: Cholesterol: 214
blood pressure: 140/80

1996: Cholesterol: 165
blood pressure: 90/60

I kept looking for adverse side effects. Indeed, many of my colleagues promised as much. "DHEA will give you prostate cancer," said one endocrinologist, but my prostate-specific antigen (PSA) level (indicating risk for prostate cancer) went down 35 percent. "DHEA will mess up your liver," advised an internist, but my liver functions improved. "That stuff won't do you a bit of good," scoffed my thirty-three-year-old tennis partner right before I beat him for the third time that week.

At the same time, DHEA research was accelerating rapidly, and the body of knowledge was all supporting the metabolic model of aging. Many experts were saying that DHEA—and not human growth hormone (hGH)—was the most comprehensive anabolic influence. The debate was intriguing but came down to a fairly simple observation: restoring DHEA levels caused improvements throughout the endocrine system, including increased growth hormone, whereas raising growth hormone had no such beneficial effect on DHEA.[14] What's more, both hormones stimulated the production of growth and repair factors by the liver, such as IGF-1. DHEA was readily absorbed from an oral dose. Growth hormone had to be injected. A month's supply of DHEA cost about $25. Growth hormone was runing around $800 per month, and adverse side effects, including abnormal growth of joints and impaired glucose metabolism, were disturbingly common. For me, the matter was pretty much closed. DHEA was the anabolic key.

Mixed Signals

The metabolic brain-body dialogue is incredibly complex, and to alter the aging process, the "youth" signal has to be consistent. It makes no sense to eat well and work hard at maintaining muscle mass if these longevity signals are canceled out by the powerful over-the-hill signal represented by low levels of DHEA.

Remember that DHEA is produced by the body in enormous quantities until about age thirty. Thereafter, the body's production of the hormone declines rapidly, until, at age seventy, most people are producing only 15 percent to 20 percent of what I refer to as *prime peak*. There is no biochemical in the human body that declines as rapidly, nor one whose decline can have such catastrophic consequences. Restoring DHEA is like amplifying the body's most powerful longevity signal, and it can be done safely at any age. This alone will not make you younger, but it is, for most people, a critical step to restoring youthful anabolic metabolism. If you do nothing, the brain is programmed to initiate the shutdown sequence at about age forty.

Knowledge Without Action Is Folly

The question is, what are you doing about this? Conventional medicine simply waits for the consequences of this metabolic shift to become severe. If your blood pressure is rising, chances are that your doctor won't do anything until it gets to the threshold level of 140/90. At that point, he or she will diagnose hypertension and write you a prescription for a drug to lower blood pressure. The same is true for blood sugar. Deteriorating glucose metabolism is common after the age of forty, but conventional medicine does nothing during what may be decades of degeneration. It waits until your blood glucose level is pushing 140. Then a sticker with the word *diabetic* is placed on your chart, and you are given another prescription.

Rising cholesterol is considered to be a "normal" consequence of aging, and when it gets to about 220 milligrams per deciliter, a drug is prescribed. Even obesity is treated with symptom stomping. Do physicians routinely perform comprehensive body composition analyses to measure body fat, hydration level, muscle mass, and metabolic rate? Such a test would reveal a tendency toward obesity at an age when patients would actually have a good chance of doing something about it.

But this is rarely done. Instead, the doctor looks at the patient once he or she is obese and writes a prescription. This in the face of clear evidence that weight-loss drugs have *the worst* track record of all pharmaceuticals, in terms of success rate and adverse side effects.

You have to admit this is crazy: to ignore a fundamental cause of aging—which is the loss of anabolic metabolism—and spring into action only when a treatable symptom appears. But you'd have to be pretty naive to ignore the fact that treating the symptoms of aging is big business: it's approaching *$1 trillion a year,* roughly one-seventh of our entire gross national product.

The DHEA Backlash

In 1995, I learned that the FDA was going to approve DHEA for over-the-counter sale. I had mixed feelings about this. On the one hand, it would make an extremely valuable antiaging product available at an affordable price, but I also knew that it would be hyped to the sky and used unwisely in huge doses. "Someone's going to have to tell people how to use this stuff safely," I thought, which led me to write *The DHEA Breakthrough,* released in September of 1996.

The DHEA Breakthrough presented a program for longevity and optimal health—basically what was known at that time about the metabolic model of aging. It advised caution regarding DHEA supplementation and provided dose guidelines and information on side effects. It offered a carefully referenced and balanced point of view and frequently reminded readers to work with their doctors to take advantage of this remarkable hormone. I fully expected that the book would stimulate debate and further study. But by the spring of 1997, anyone with something negative to say about DHEA was on the evening news.

In one televised debate, a DHEA critic started by claiming that DHEA causes liver cancer. When I asked for evidence to support such a claim, I was told there were studies. I asked what *species* the studies were conducted on. My opponent finally admitted that the data was from trout, an organism that doesn't even manufacture DHEA.[15] When I suggested that this was a red herring, he presented a study conducted with mice. Allowing that at least this study was conducted with a mammal, I asked what dose was used. My opponent claimed not to remember, so I produced the study, revealing that the poor animals were given more than two thousand times the dose they would normally produce—the human equivalent of 10,000 milligrams per day.[16] I reminded viewers that the recommended human dose was 10 to 50 milligrams per day.

I then presented studies done with humans in which DHEA was shown to *improve* liver function. One group of researchers at the University of California in San Diego even concluded that DHEA's ability to enhance liver detoxification "may contribute to the anti carcinogenic (cancer-fighting) and chemoprotective (cancer-preventing) properties of this intriguing class of endogenous steroids."[17]

In the summer of 1997, I was invited to a scientific conference to present the latest research on DHEA. I arrived with a briefcase brimming with extraordinary studies from around the world, including:

- A yearlong study with postmenopausal women[18] illustrating that DHEA:
  Increased bone density
  Improved glucose tolerance
  Enhanced feelings of well-being
  Decreased body fat
  Increased muscle mass
  Raised growth hormone levels
  Improved vaginal tone and moisture
  Produced no deleterious side effects

- A six-month study with men[19] showing that DHEA:
  Significantly increased blood levels of IGF-1, the body's main rebuild-repair-restore biochemical
  Produced dramatic improvements in immunity
  Produced no deleterious side effects

- Studies with depressed patients showing that DHEA improved not only mood but memory and learning ability as well.[20]

- A study evaluating men in nursing homes, which found that their level of independent functioning was *directly related* to their DHEA levels. Men with lower DHEA levels were more dependent and had greater difficulty carrying out daily activities.

I also brought an editorial from a leading journal in the field, the *Journal of Clinical Endocrinology and Metabolism,* which stated the case for DHEA supplementation as clearly as it could be made: "Logic pleads in favor of oral administration of DHEA at a dose that provides so called 'young' DHEA levels in the blood. . . ."[21]

Normally, such a presentation would have a significant impact in the health care arena. My presentation, including all of the above references, would be published in the conference proceedings and read by thousands of physicians. But this never happened. At the last minute, I was informed that the DHEA module had been deleted from the program. Here was one of the most controversial subjects in antiaging medicine, but no reason was given for its complete omission from the program. In similar medical conferences nationwide, there was nothing but stony silence about this critically important topic.

Becoming a DHEA Detective (Follow the Money)

I was dumbfounded. Everyone I knew in the field wondered what was going on. Then a friend suggested that we might think of who stood to benefit from the disappearance of DHEA from the clinical radar screen.

We learned that patentable DHEA analogs (altered forms of DHEA) were in development at a dozen pharmaceutical companies. These included DHEA-based drugs to accelerate wound healing and to treat AIDS, cancer, and autoimmune disorders such as lupus. One company even had a patent pending on an electronically "improved" DHEA. Having low-cost DHEA available in health food stores along with reliable instructions on its effective use would take a lot of the wind out of the sails (and sales) of these drug companies.

But you can't stuff a genie back in the lamp. All over the world, research was being published showing that DHEA could help restore peak immunity, improve mood and memory, reduce risk for the leading causes of death, burn fat, build muscle, and ignite sex drive. The only way to stop the DHEA movement would be to make people afraid to use it.

Thus, in 1997, "experts" appeared all over the country crying "The sky is falling." Government and private institutions filled the airwaves with an anti-DHEA chorus, and in a matter of months, health food stores were taking down their WE HAVE DHEA banners; many actually put up signs proclaiming WE DON'T SELL DHEA.

Just for fun, I went into one of these health food stores and asked why it would make such an announcement. "Because DHEA is dangerous" was the reply. "And precisely why is that?" I queried. The manager sifted through a pile of papers and took out a university health letter. Handing it to me, he announced, "DHEA causes cancer." "Sure it does," I said, "when fed in massive amounts . . . to trout."

Fast-Forward

All of this took place in 1997, so you might be wondering what actually came to pass. Were the naysayers right? Did people using DHEA get liver cancer? Did their bodies stop making DHEA? No. Since 1997, more than eight hundred new studies on DHEA have been published, and not a single one validates these dire predictions. In fact, new evidence has created an avalanche of support for this anabolic hormone:

- Alcoholics in recovery are vulnerable to relapse resulting from depression. Researchers found that the incidence of relapse correlates strongly with low DHEA levels.[22] This was followed by confirming, double-blind, placebo-controlled studies showing that DHEA is an effective antidepressant.[23]

- This, in turn, was followed by research showing that DHEA supplementation restored beta-endorphin levels in postmenopausal women. Endorphins are feel-good biochemicals produced by the brain and may be responsible for the improvements in well-being reported by these women.[24]

- A six-month study found that DHEA produced remarkable improvements in libido and sexual function in men with erectile dysfunction.[25]

- A landmark review of eight separate studies published in the *British Journal of Cancer* found *no association* between DHEA and the incidence of prostate cancer.[26]

- A breakthrough study on nearly a thousand subjects published in the prestigious *Journal of Epidemiology* clearly demonstrated that

DHEA not only reduces risk for atherosclerosis (arterial block-age—the leading cause of death in Western nations) but may help to treat the disease in its early stages.[27]

- A landmark Harvard study showed that DHEA supplementation restored normal bone growth and hormone balance in women with anorexia.[28]

- Convincing evidence was published showing that abnormal DHEA metabolism contributes to chronic fatigue syndrome[29] and rheumatoid arthritis.[30]

- It was discovered that DHEA is actually *manufactured in the brain* and plays a critical role in maintaining peak memory and learning ability as we age.[31]

- Research showed that DHEA may be protective against Alzheimer's and other forms of brain degeneration.[32] Brain tissue contains up to six times more DHEA than any other tissue in the body, but Alzheimer's patients had only half as much DHEA in their blood compared to age-matched controls.

- It was found that raising DHEA levels appears to stimulate glutathione production in laboratory animals, thereby enhancing critical detoxification and immune functions.[33]

- The influence of DHEA on cellular energy was confirmed when researchers discovered a relationship between DHEA and L-carnitine. They concluded that "L-carnitine and DHEA independently promote mitochondrial energy metabolism.[34]

- The list of positive effects derived from DHEA supplementation was expanded. Restoring DHEA levels in postmenopausal women produced improvements in *other* critical hormones (17-OH progesterone and allopregnanolone), which, in turn, produced additional benefits related to hormone balance, mood, memory, and anabolic metabolism.[35]

- Yet another antiaging benefit of DHEA was discovered when researchers found an inverse relationship between DHEA levels and inflammation, meaning that as DHEA levels increased, a primary marker of inflammation known as IL-6 decreased. The authors of the study concluded that the increase in inflammatory disorders associated with aging might very well stem from declining levels of DHEA.[36]

There's not space in this book to catalog all the benefits associated with optimal levels of DHEA. Documented effects include the entire range of immune, energy, body composition, mood, memory, and longevity benefits. Researchers at the National Institute of Mental Health even used DHEA to treat what they termed *midlife dysthymia*, otherwise known as the "blahs." They conclude: "A robust effect of de-hydroepiandrosterone on mood was observed. . . . The symptoms that improved most significantly were anhedonia [lack of pleasure], loss of energy, lack of motivation, emotional 'numbness,' sadness, inability to cope, and worry."[37]

And yet, as the mountain of data grew even larger, critics continued to complain that the studies weren't long enough, big enough, or ad-ministered by experts with sufficient standing in the international sci-entific community. Thus it was that Étienne-Émile Baulieu, one of the world's foremost hormone biochemists, decided to create what was called The DHEAge Study.

This yearlong trial included nearly three hundred men and women ranging in age from sixty to seventy-nine. Baulieu assembled a team of twenty-two researchers that reads like a Who's Who in European en-docrinology, geriatrics, immunology, and human performance. The study was double-blind and placebo-controlled (the gold standard of scientific methodology) to eliminate any conceivable bias in observa-tions or effects. The results, published in the prestigious *Proceedings of the National Academy of Science*, were dramatic. First and foremost, there were no adverse effects and no potentially dangerous elevation of DHEA, testosterone, or estrogen. The benefits? Increased bone density in women, improved libido, and marked improvements in skin tone, hydration, thickness, and color.[38]

The Real Problem

Dr. Sam Yen, a leading DHEA researcher at the University of California at San Diego, concluded that "DHEA in appropriate replacement doses appears to have remedial effects with respect to its ability to induce an anabolic growth factor, increase muscle strength and lean body mass, activate immune function, and enhance quality of life in aging men and women."[39]

But although Yen, Baulieu, and many others have proved that DHEA is a safe and effective metabolic enhancer, one has to admit that well-controlled scientific studies are one thing, and unbridled use by the American public (motto: If a little is good, a lot is better) is something altogether different.

DHEA is a powerful hormone. As I've mentioned, it influences more than 150 metabolic functions throughout the human body. It's not like vitamin C, which is easily excreted in the urine. If you take too much DHEA, you can experience adverse effects.

That's because the body converts some DHEA to testosterone and estrogen, two powerful sex steroids. Thus, one must be careful—something that is rather difficult to get across in a health food store when the product is right next to the organic corn chips. I spelled out the appropriate cautions quite clearly in *The DHEA Breakthrough* but still received reports of overdose symptoms, such as acne, even in people who were taking a reasonable (25- to 50-milligram) dose. Well, I have good news.

The 7-Keto Breakthrough

About the time that American pharmaceutical companies were pulling out their hair at the FDA's decision to release DHEA as a nutritional supplement, Dr. Henry Lardy and his research group at the University of Wisconsin were finalizing work on what was to be the most important DHEA analog of all, 3-acetyl-7-keto DHEA, or 7-Keto[40] for short.

Dr. Lardy determined that 7-Keto was a natural metabolite of DHEA. Importantly, it was "downstream" from the sex steroids and therefore could not be converted to testosterone or estrogen. But when he went shopping for an interested pharmaceutical company, he got no offers.

That's because Big Pharma still didn't understand DHEA, did not realize that conversion to testosterone and estrogen was only a minor effect. Far more important was the anabolic signal that it sent throughout the body—the message that the body was getting younger. All I needed was a way to prove that Dr. Lardy's compound did the same thing. In 1998, researchers in Japan identified a group of anabolic biomarkers that appear in the urine when the body shifts into rebuild-repair-restore activity. I saw this not only as an interesting metabolic profile but as a way to gauge a person's rate of aging and a way to evaluate the antiaging benefits of 7-Keto.

Remember, aging is fundamentally a metabolic shift from youthful anabolic metabolism to a progressively more catabolic state characterized by low energy and degeneration. I knew that DHEA could help restore anabolic metabolism, but could the same results be obtained with 7-Keto? If so, given 7-Keto's enormous safety profile, the naysayers would finally be silenced.

In 1999, a joint research project was launched to evaluate the effects of DHEA, 7-Keto, and their combination on the anabolic metabolism of seventy-six volunteers. You can find the details of this important antiaging research in Appendix B, but here is the bottom line. In a double-blind, placebo-controlled study, the combination of a small daily amount of DHEA (12.5 milligrams) and 27.5 milligrams of 7-Keto produced dramatic improvements in anabolic metabolism. A separate lab, measuring a different anabolic biomarker known as IGF-1, was used to confirm the results. Here also, the treatment group experienced remarkable improvements compared to the placebo group.

Today, we know a great deal about hormone therapy. Yet some doctors are saying, "Wait." The question is, how long? For people over forty, waiting even a few years may be costly in terms of the loss of anabolic drive. I believe that the combination of DHEA and 7-Keto is a safe and effective way to maintain or regain anabolic metabolism as we age. Abundant evidence exists to show that this can enhance quality of life by optimizing the body's own repair and rebuild activity.

A major challenge in preventing an epidemic of [muscle loss]–induced frailty in the future is developing public health interventions that deliver an anabolic stimulus to the muscle of elderly adults on a mass scale.
—R. Roubenoff, "Sarcopenia: A Major Modifiable Cause of Frailty in the Elderly." Journal of Nutrition, Health, and Aging

CONSUMER EDUCATION

Some People Should Not Take DHEA

These include:

- People under age thirty-five (unless following the advice of their physician). In general, young people are already producing adequate DHEA. Since the hormone can be converted to testosterone and estrogen, taking DHEA can produce symptoms associated with excess sex hormones, such as acne and (in women) facial hair growth from elevated testosterone. Obviously, women with a tendency to grow facial hair (often indicating a high testosterone level) would not want to exacerbate this condition.

- Pregnant or nursing women.

- Men with prostate cancer. A common medical treatment for prostate cancer is testosterone blockade, in which all sources of testosterone are suppressed. Taking DHEA in this case would be counterproductive.

Easy Does It

We live in an instant-results society. The benefits of DHEA and 7-Keto, however, tend to be experienced *gradually* as tissue levels are optimized. Unfortunately, the hype surrounding DHEA has set up an expectation that you can take it and instantly feel twenty years younger. When this doesn't occur, people often assume they need to take more. Remember that the human body, even at age twenty-five, produces only 40 to 60 milligrams of DHEA per day. A sensible replacement dose should therefore stay within that level, and research suggests that 10 to 25 milligrams of DHEA and 25 to 50 milligrams of 7-Keto will be sufficient for most people [41]

No Place for Guesswork

Before starting on DHEA or 7-Keto, obtain an anabolic/catabolic index (ACI) from a urine sample or have a blood or saliva test to find out how much DHEA your body is currently producing (see Appendix A). If levels are below prime peak (the amount produced at about age twenty-five), supplement at the above dose and retest in sixty to ninety days to evaluate the results.

DHEA SULFATE (DHEAS) BLOOD TEST

Unit of measure		PRIME PEAK	GOOD	DEFICIENT	WORRISOME
mcg/dL	men	450–600	300–450	125–300	less than 125
	women	280–380	150–280	45–150	less than 45

Note: The unit of measure mcg/dL is the same as mcg/100 mL and µg/dL.

If your results are reported in ng/mL (nanograms per milliliter), simply divide your result by 10 and use the above chart to see where you fit in.

DHEA SALIVA TEST

Unit of measure		PRIME PEAK	GOOD	DEFICIENT	WORRISOME
pg/mL	men	200–300	100–200	70–100	less than 70
	women	125–170	70–125	35–70	less than 35

Source: S. Cherniske, The DHEA Breakthrough, *(New York: Ballantine, 1996), 255.*

If retest shows that you are at or near prime peak, that is your appropriate dose. If your levels have not significantly improved, talk with your physician to determine if you should increase your daily intake or work some more on stress management and exercise. Research shows that reducing stress and increasing exercise can boost anabolic metabolism by 50 percent to 100 percent.

BEYOND DHEA: OTHER CRITICAL ANABOLIC FACTORS

The Role of Growth Hormone

Human growth hormone, or hGH, is produced by the pituitary gland. Like DHEA, it has many anabolic influences, but unlike DHEA, most of these, as the name implies, are related to growth and development. Also unlike DHEA, growth hormone cannot be administered in an oral dose. It must be prescribed by a physician and injected. And because these injections far exceed the level of growth hormone produced by the body, such therapy causes the pituitary to cease producing the hormone. Should one have to discontinue growth hormone injections (for medical or financial reasons), it may take many months for the pituitary to get back up to speed. No such "rebound" is seen when people stop taking DHEA.

Still, higher levels of growth hormone are associated with significant antiaging benefits; and fortunately there are natural ways to restore this important anabolic signal.

Natural Ways to Optimize Your Body's Production of Growth Hormone

- *Minimize your consumption of refined sugars.* We'll discuss the catabolic influence of refined sugars (white sugar, brown sugar, corn syrup, fructose, high-fructose corn syrup) in the next chapter, but the bottom line is that eating sweets raises insulin levels, and elevated insulin is associated with decreased GH and DHEA.[42]

- *Be moderate with alcohol.* Here's another reason to drink in moderation. Too much alcohol accelerates aging by disrupting the growth hormone anabolic signal.[43]

- *Build up to strenuous exercise.* If you can get beyond moderate exercise by lifting weights or increasing the duration or intensity level of your workout, you can stimulate very significant increases in hGH release.[44]

- *Sleep deeply.* Growth hormone is released from the pituitary during deep sleep (also known as stage 4, or slow-wave sleep), and studies show that the declining sleep quality associated with advancing age contributes to growth hormone deficiency.[45] Conversely, measures to improve sleep quality can produce significant increases in growth hormone. Snoring, for example, reduces your ability to get into deep sleep. The use of a nostril dilator to treat snoring has been shown to increase growth hormone release and produce more restful sleep.[46]

- *Optimize DHEA levels.* I've already described how improving adrenal function via the administration of DHEA produces benefits throughout the endocrine system. This includes pituitary release of growth hormone.

CONCLUSION

You now know that anabolic repair is the key to both quality of life and longevity (quantity of life). You are capable of replacing 300 billion cells every day, but this astonishing renewal starts to slow and sputter after age thirty-five. This chapter described three critical steps that you can take to restore anabolic drive to more youthful levels:

1. *Provide optimal levels of raw materials.* Depleted soil, extensive processing, cooking, and poor food choices result in widespread malnutrition. Today, even a "well-balanced diet" cannot provide levels of nutrients critical for optimum anabolic metabolism. We can now provide hundreds of repair nutrients from nutritional supplements and longevity foods (Chapter 8).

2. *Boost energy.* The association of aging with fatigue is so common, we assume that it's inevitable. By restoring mitochondrial efficiency, you can increase cellular energy production, which, in turn, fuels regular exercise, which generates more energy and puts you into an upward spiral—at any age. As you will learn in Chapter 7, increased energy and vitality is usually the first benefit that people experience on the Metabolic Plan.

3. *Restore the anabolic repair "signal."* Decreasing production of anabolic hormones such as DHEA, growth hormone, and IGF-1 results in a weakened anabolic signal. We now know that restoring anabolic hormones can amplify this biochemical signal to every cell of the body and brain. Now it's time to look at the opposite side of the coin, to learn how to reduce catabolic damage.

THREE

Putting the Brakes on Catabolic Metabolism

When my physiology professor was trying to explain the complexities of human metabolism, he summed up the lecture very effectively. "Look," he said, "it's rather simple. The day that your total catabolic activity exceeds your anabolic activity is the day you begin to die."

In the last chapter, we focused on ways to support anabolic repair. Clearly, it's just as important to push down on the other side of the seesaw—to reduce catabolic damage. That's because damage is cumulative, which means that the older you get, the faster you age.

Reducing the damage to which we're exposed on a daily basis is not an easy task, considering that environmental pollution, ultraviolet radiation, highly processed food, dehydration, stress, obesity, and a sedentary lifestyle are all catabolic accelerators. An action plan is available, however, once you understand that 90 percent of catabolic damage stems from four basic factors.

CATABOLIC FACTOR 1: OXIDATION

Scientists have been studying oxidation reactions for centuries, observing how oxygen combines with—and alters—an enormous variety of substances from metals to fats, oils, and proteins. Oxygen combines with iron to make rust (ferric oxide). It combines with fats and produces the characteristic rancid butter smell of butyric acid. When you go to correct a mistake on your crossword puzzle and the eraser only smudges the word (I hate that), it's because the eraser has been oxidized.

By now you've got the point that oxidation doesn't generally *improve* things. When your windshield wipers don't really wipe, but streak and squeak, it's because the proteins in the rubber have been oxidized. When you bought the car, the blades were new and supple. After a few years—especially if you live in a sunny climate—they become brittle. And guess what? So do you. The tan you got last summer was created by billions of dead skin cells that were darkened by an oxidation process known as *browning*. That's why bread is darker and harder on the outside crust and softer and lighter on the inside. When it was baking (as you were in the sun), the outside was exposed to more oxygen.

The paint on your house fades and flakes off—oxidation. Oxidation cracks the asphalt in the street. Your contact lenses get cloudy; your Tupperware gets stiff. Newspaper clippings turn yellow. Garage sales and flea markets are chock-full of stuff that's falling apart because of oxidation. And so are you.

Aside from tanned skin, oxygen is damaging your blood vessels, the neurons in your brain, your heart muscle, and your liver. It's blowing holes in cell membranes. Oxidation is the coffee stain on the DNA blueprint that I talked about in the last chapter. Bottom line: it's the catabolic downside of life—life that was made possible, of course, by . . . oxygen. What an astounding paradox.

So here it is in a nutshell (and by the way, nuts get rancid, too): energy is created when oxygen combines with fuel. In your car's engine, oxygen combines with gasoline, and the spark plug ignites this mixture to propel your car. We learned in Chapter 2 that the oxidation of fuel in your body takes place in the mitochondria within your cells. And in both cases—your car and your body—the process is incomplete. There's some exhaust. The incomplete by-product of human energy production—what might be called cellular "exhaust"—is what chemists call a free radical.

Free What?

Free radicals are atoms or molecules that contain an unpaired electron. They're called radicals because this imbalance causes them to be extremely unstable. To become stable, a radical must steal an electron from a neighboring atom, and this causes a chain reaction that results in cell death and tissue damage.

You've most likely heard the term *free radical* before. If you're a health-conscious person, you may have heard this term dozens of times. Now, be honest. Do you really get it? Since this is one of the major causes of aging and death, since free radicals are known to cause or contribute to most diseases, including cardiovascular disease and cancer—don't you think it would be a good thing to understand? I promise I can make this simple.

Imagine there's a dance where everyone has a partner. The room is "stable," and everyone is happy. Suddenly, the door opens, and here's this fellow without a date. Not only is he alone (unpaired), but he's incredibly good-looking. So this guy goes over and steals some other guy's date. That guy is now unpaired (and angry), so he tries to cut in on another couple. And before you know it, the entire dance floor is filled with guys fighting over the available girls. In your body, free radicals wreak similar havoc.

But Mother Nature has a way of protecting her creations. In this case, she goes up to the unpaired fellow and says, "Do I have a date for you!" and introduces him to a beautiful partner named Ann T. Oxidant . . . OK, I'll stop. All you have to know is that antioxidants neutralize free radicals by donating an electron.

So what's the big deal, you ask? If oxidation produces free radicals but antioxidants stabilize them, why is everybody so concerned? Why are there now more than a dozen scientific journals devoted entirely to free-radical chemistry? Why has every medical school in the world added courses (and sometimes entire departments) to study free-radical pathology? It has to do with something we'll come back to over and over in this book: the peculiar predicament of modern man.

You see, for millions of years, the balance of oxidants and antioxidants was kept pretty even. Free-radical production was controlled by antioxidants produced by the body and obtained from the plentiful fruits and vegetables in a hunting-and-gathering diet. Again, the hunting-and-gathering diet was largely comprised of plants in their raw natural state. But then what happened? About ten thousand years ago, everything started changing. Agriculture enabled people to stop foraging and stay in one place. Unfortunately, they tended to grow only a limited number of crops, and so the highly varied diet of raw plants was replaced by a few staples such as wheat, rice, corn, and beans. These foods contain only a fraction of the antioxidants of fruits and vegetables, and most of that was destroyed by milling, bleaching, and cooking.

So the agricultural revolution was, in one important sense, a disaster, in that it dramatically reduced mankind's intake of high-antioxidant foods. But it gets worse. Because then came the industrial revolution, and suddenly, machines and factories were creating massive amounts of free-radical pollution and spewing it into the air. This has continued—and in most respects, has become progressively worse—for centuries.

But that's not all. About a hundred years ago, all this pollution started to destroy the protective ozone layer of the atmosphere, so you and I are exposed to a great deal more ultraviolet radiation than our ancestors. And UV radiation dramatically accelerates the production of free radicals.

Are you beginning to grasp the enormity of this problem? Our genes haven't changed in more than thirty thousand years. That means we are genetically designed to live in a pristine, pollution-free environment with a high level of UV protection, consuming a highly varied, antioxidant-rich diet of unprocessed and uncooked fruits and vegetables. Since we no longer live this way, we face almost *impossible* odds when it comes to protecting our bodies from the damage of free radicals.

Perhaps you're familiar with the device that is used to measure automobile emissions. It's an instrument that traps and measures the various levels of pollutants coming from the tailpipe of a car. Well, a few years ago, I took a more sophisticated version of this instrument and stood on a street corner as a city bus went by. After measuring the pollution level, I was able to calculate that in the ten seconds it took for that bus to pass in front of me, I was exposed to a higher level of free radicals than most of my ancestors experienced in their entire lifetime.

Now imagine what cigarette smoking does. It has been calculated that every puff on a cigarette sends tens of billions of free radicals deep into the most sensitive tissue of the body. Even standing *near* a smoker can result in massive free-radical exposure—which accounts for the National Cancer Institute estimate that more than fifty thousand Americans are killed by secondhand cigarette smoke every year.

All in all, Bruce Ames, one of the world's leading free-radical experts, estimates that in the body of an average *non*smoker, every cell suffers more than 10,000 free-radical hits every day. That's about 100 trillion cells times 10,000—a bombardment of 10 quintillion free radicals. Every day. The question is, what kind of damage does that do?

Scientists today are finding that free-radical damage contributes to nearly all disease states. It is a causative factor in most types of cancer and is probably the single most important factor in age-related degeneration of the brain. Free radicals are in great part responsible for the wrinkles and lines on your face, but go *beneath* the surface to find the real damage caused by exposure to the sun's ultraviolet rays. Free radicals produced by UV radiation damage the DNA—the genetic blueprint of the cells—and cause these cells to start dividing abnormally. In time, if not repaired, this results in skin cancer. According to the American Cancer Society, more than 1.4 million Americans were diagnosed with basal cell and squamous cell carcinoma in 2001. The American Academy of Dermatology reports that malignant melanoma, a more lethal type of skin cancer, claims the life of one American every hour.[1]

Free radicals also damage the lining of your arteries, causing microscopic lesions. These tiny rips and tears attract repair cells and result in scarring that starts to accumulate plaque at the injury site. This is the beginning of cardiovascular disease, the number one killer in the Western world. If the blocked artery leads to your brain, you have a stroke. If it leads to your heart, you have a heart attack. Either event can easily kill you or leave you paralyzed. Last year, 950,000 people died of cardiovascular disease; more than 45 percent of all heart attacks occur in people under sixty-five. So much for antiaging.

Imagine that every day three jumbo jets crashed in the United States, each one packed with 450 passengers, and there was never a single survivor. That's the incredible toll that cardiovascular disease takes in this country, day after day.

Follow the Money

Did you know that bypass surgery (in which a blocked coronary artery is replaced by a clean artery obtained from the thigh) is one of the biggest growth industries in the United States? Would it surprise you to learn that this procedure, together with other surgical treatments for heart disease, brings in more money to metropolitan hospitals than any other type of care? Bypass surgery is often referred to as "preventive care," even though studies show that the procedure does not extend overall life expectancy. (That's because the newly grafted artery usually starts clogging right away.)

Then there are the drugs used to lower blood pressure and cholesterol—another growth industry. These drugs are also called "preventive care," even though there are studies showing that individuals treated with them have *increased* overall mortality[2]—and even though an entire class of blood pressure medication has been shown to *increase risk for heart attack*.

There's an astronomical amount of money being made on treatments that provide only symptomatic benefit, while prevention is largely ignored. And given the fact that cholesterol itself does not appear to cause heart disease but rather the *oxidation* of cholesterol, what do you think would be the best preventive strategy? *Antioxidants,* of course.

Where Antioxidants Come From

Again, I want you to think hunting and gathering. I studied a tribe of present-day hunters and gatherers and cataloged seventy-five species of plants in their daily diet. What's more, these plants comprised 70 percent of total calories, the equivalent of twenty servings per day. That is a high-antioxidant diet.

At the same time, they didn't smoke (didn't know what a cigarette was), were not exposed to urban pollution, drank from clear mountain streams and deep springs, and enjoyed the benefits of a close community. You and I, however, face free-radical exposure hundreds of times more lethal than what these tribespeople face. We "civilized" folk eat few antioxidant-rich foods, we're stressed to the max, and we think we can compensate for all of this with a multivitamin or a fortified breakfast cereal containing a smattering of vitamins C and E. That's like tossing a cup of water on a forest fire.

The average American consumes fewer than ten species of plants, most of which are antioxidant-poor. For decades, the U.S. Department of Agriculture and national health agencies have been begging Americans to eat at least five servings of fruits and vegetables every day, but surveys tell us that less than 8 percent of Americans actually do this. What's more, when you look at the data, you find that the number one fruit is bananas and the most commonly consumed vegetable is potatoes, usually fried. White foods are poor sources of antioxidants, even when eaten raw.

Quite simply, there is no substitute for a highly varied natural foods diet. Look at the numbers: the quarter of the population that eats the fewest fruits and vegetables has more than *triple* the heart disease rate compared to the quarter with the highest intake.

The $64,000 Question

If we're exposed to thousands of times more free radicals than our ancestors, would even a hunting-and-gathering diet provide adequate levels of antioxidants? Of course not. Nature could not predict that in the short span of a few centuries, free-radical exposure would increase to astronomic levels. The solution proposed by a growing number of scientists is to take additional antioxidant supplements. Note that "supplement" implies that these are *supplemental* to a natural foods diet.

In 1993, two remarkable studies were published in the *New England Journal of Medicine* showing that supplemental antioxidants can decrease heart disease risk by 26 percent to 46 percent.[3] Additional research suggested that antioxidant supplements could also reduce risk for certain types of cancer.[4] In the last chapter, I described how Bruce Ames used acetyl-L-carnitine to improve cellular energy production, but this dramatic success could only be achieved by the addition of alpha lipoic acid, a powerful antioxidant. Others have demonstrated similar benefits of these two nutrients on the heart.[5]

Alpha lipoic acid (also known as lipoic or thioctic acid) is a remarkable nutrient. While not exactly a vitamin (because the body can manufacture it), lipoic acid possesses remarkable antioxidant activity. Not only does it play a critical role in cellular protection and repair, but it also helps to improve energy metabolism, increases stamina, and helps to recycle other antioxidants by restoring their ability to perform their jobs.[6]

There isn't room in this book to catalog all the conditions that are relieved or resolved with antioxidant therapy, but several of those with specific relevance to the aging process deserve mention. Following this review, I'll provide an antioxidant supplement guide to get you started.

DNA Damage

Imagine that your boss at work asks you to "make some copies" and then takes you outside and shows you a stack of paper as tall as a twelve-story building. Shocked, you ask how many copies he wants, and he says 300 billion. That's the task that your body performs every day. The information in your DNA, if printed out, would be a stack of paper more than 150 feet high, and every day, you have to make 300 billion copies of this incredible molecule as part of your rebuild-and-repair metabolism.

The issue here is genetic error. We all know what happens when we make a copy of a copy. Because every generation reproduces the smudges, hairs, and specks of dirt that fell on the copier glass, ultimately, the page we produce is not even readable. Likewise, cumulative genetic error is a fundamental cause of aging. Your DNA contains all of the information that every cell in your body needs, but as you age, the damage to this master blueprint results in increasing error and impaired cell function.

You've probably guessed that the major cause of DNA damage is free radicals, and research shows that the older the cells, the greater the damage.[7] That means you don't want to wait until you're sixty-five to do something about this catabolic disaster.

Fortunately, antioxidant supplementation has been shown to reduce DNA damage,[8] and the strategy must include multiple types of antioxidants (see the "Supplemental Antioxidants" table later in this chapter).

Nutritional compounds have been identified that enhance mitochondrial function and reverse several age-related processes.
—M. D. Seidman et al., "Biologic Activity of
Mitochondrial Metabolites on Aging and Age-Related
Hearing Loss," American Journal of Otology

Joint Inflammation and Pain

Arthritis is a condition that causes pain and stiffness and sometimes redness or swelling in one or more joints. Two common forms are osteoarthritis (OA) and rheumatoid arthritis (RA). Both diseases are three times more common in women than in men.

OA is caused by the breakdown of the cartilage cushion in joints and can cause the bones in the joints to become rough. OA occurs most often in weight-bearing joints, such as the spine, knees, and hips. It also often affects the fingers. Most people over the age of sixty have some OA, although they may not have symptoms.

Rheumatoid arthritis affects the lining of the joints. It is thought to be an autoimmune disease, which means that the body's immune cells attack the body's own tissue. The disease causes inflammation, stiffness, and deformity—particularly in the joints of the hands, arms, and feet—and usually starts in early adulthood or middle age.

Recent research has identified a significant free-radical factor in most types of joint pain. What's more, it has been shown that taking antioxidant supplements not only reduces pain but may actually help to reverse the underlying degenerative condition.[9]

Mind, Memory, and Learning

A study of free-radical biochemistry will show that the greatest danger is found at the points of highest oxygen use. So you would naturally think of the skeletal muscles, which burn tremendous amounts of oxygen to enable us to work, play, run, jump, and do all the things we do. You think of the heart muscle, contracting with remarkable force every minute of every day throughout life. But you might not think of the brain because it involves no obvious movement or force. Yet the brain, which comprises only 2 percent of the body's weight, uses more than 20 percent of the oxygen you breathe. In fact, the job of managing every cell in your body requires massive amounts of energy. Have you ever found sweat glistening on your forehead even when you weren't doing any physical work? That's the heat given off by the brain.

And sure enough, when researchers began to look at the aging brain, they found that antioxidants played a critical role in maintaining optimal function. Research presented at the July 1997 meeting of the American Society for Neurochemistry revealed that schizophrenic patients had far lower levels of antioxidants in their brain tissue than healthy controls. It is unknown whether the antioxidant deficiency is a causative factor in the disorder or whether it results from the schizophrenic condition.

Importantly, memory, learning ability, and even mood are affected by antioxidant nutriture. We'll talk more about this important topic in later chapters, but here is the bottom line, Metabolic Plan good news. Much of the degeneration that has been considered "normal" for centuries is now considered treatable. Breakthrough research conducted by scientists from Tufts University has shattered old assumptions regarding the age-related decline in brain health.

Previously, scientists had been able to postpone brain degeneration in lab animals to a small degree using a variety of experimental drugs. The Tufts University team, however, *restored normal brain function* in old animals that already had deficits in balance, coordination, learning, and memory. And the agent used to accomplish this extraordinary feat was not a pharmaceutical or high-tech treatment—it was blueberries. The authors conclude: "These findings suggest that, in addition to their known beneficial effects on cancer and heart disease, phytochemicals present in antioxidant-rich foods may be beneficial in reversing the course of brain and behavioral aging."[10]

Beyond Berries

How many times have adult children complained that a grandparent or parent was forgetting things, acting strangely, or getting depressed, only to have the doctor say, "Well, what do you expect? That's old age." I figure it's happened millions of times, and every time that phrase was uttered, people were harmed. The grandparents or parents were harmed because their condition went untreated. The adult children and the doctor were harmed because a completely unscientific assumption was accepted as fact. Fortunately, this is changing.

The change started when research was published showing that vitamin E supplements could slow the progression of Alzheimer's disease. The study, reported in 1997 at the annual meeting of the American Academy of Neurology, confirmed a great deal of previous test tube (in vitro) research. "The results of the study will change the way we treat

Alzheimer's disease," predicted one of the study coauthors, Dr. Leon Thal, professor and chairman of the department of neurosciences at the University of California, San Diego.

Dr. Thal was correct—at least, in part. Since he made that statement, hundreds of new studies have been conducted to examine the way that antioxidants protect the brain. Further studies with Alzheimer's patients have shown increased free-radical damage and lower blood levels of *many* antioxidants compared to healthy individuals of the same age.[11]

The question is, however, when was the last time your doctor had your blood level of vitamin E tested? Heck, when was the last time your doctor even asked you about your intake of antioxidant-rich foods?

Also commonly overlooked are folic acid and vitamin B_{12}. Both are absolutely essential for the health of the brain and nervous system, and even a slight deficiency can dramatically affect mood, memory, and mental clarity. It is now known that folic acid (also known as folate) does quadruple duty in the body, having vitamin, antioxidant, detoxification, and enzyme activity. As the name implies, it is derived primarily from foliage—the dark green, leafy vegetables that most people don't eat.

Equally important is vitamin B_{12}, which becomes more difficult to absorb the older we get. As a result, studies show that as many as 20 percent of elderly individuals are deficient in one or both of these critical nutrients.[12] What's more, we now know that many more people are affected by low or suboptimal levels of folate and B_{12}, and serious symptoms can result long before a clinical deficiency. Most of these symptoms are silent and invisible to both doctor and patient, such as increased DNA damage, impaired DNA repair, damage to the brain and nervous system, and increased risk for cardiovascular disease, dementia (including Alzheimer's disease), and cancer.[13] Unfortunately, few physicians screen for folate and B_{12} deficiency. In the absence of pernicious anemia (a severe deficiency), they assume the patient is adequately nourished. Since even blood tests for these critical nutrients are not reliable, the only rational course of action is to eat a highly varied, natural foods diet and to take B_{12} and folic acid supplements. For millions of Americans, this step alone will reduce catabolic damage significantly.

Note: Please understand that it is not my intention to bash doctors. Over the years, I have worked side by side with more than fifty physicians. I know how dedicated and hardworking they are and how much they care for the welfare of their patients. I also know, however, that nutrition was largely ignored in medical school and that unless they take valuable time away from their practices and families to seek out this information, they just won't get it. No drug company representative will visit their office to talk about antioxidants, and there is no blueberry, broccoli, spinach, or carrot special-interest group lobbying in Washington. But something must be done to narrow the gap between research and clinical practice. In Appendix A, you'll find a list of organizations that are active in this regard, and it is my sincere hope that this book can serve to educate and inspire patients and physicians alike.

Vision and Hearing Loss

About seven years ago, a colleague of mine went in for an eye exam, and the optician described a new test in which a photograph is made of the macula (the portion of the retina responsible for fine vision). After the photo was developed, the optician remarked with surprise, "This is amazing. You're nearly seventy, and there's no macular degeneration whatsoever." "Of course not," said my friend, a biochemist specializing in free-radical research, "I've been taking antioxidants for thirty years." "Why would that help?" asked the optician. My friend explained that macular degeneration is caused primarily by free-radical damage to the retina from exposure to ultraviolet (UV) sunlight.

About three years ago, I went in for an eye exam and had macula photographs taken. The results were the same, but the response was different. Said my doctor, "I was going to tell you to supplement with antioxidants, but I see that you must already be doing that." It's good to see that research is making its way to the practitioner level, at least in the field of ophthalmology. And it couldn't come too soon. Macular degeneration and cataracts (clouding of the lens of the eye) are the leading causes of age-related vision loss. Both are primarily caused by free radicals and thus can to a great extent be prevented.[14] There is even evidence that the conditions can be reversed with antioxidant therapy.[15]

Then there's hearing loss, another "normal" consequence of aging. Current research shows that supplementation with N-acetyl-cysteine (NAC), alpha lipoic acid, and acetyl-L-carnitine can help prevent hearing loss by protecting ultrasensitive mechanisms in the inner ear.[16]

Periodontal (Gum) Disease

Gum disease (also called periodontal disease or gingivitis) is an infection of the tissues surrounding and supporting the teeth. It's caused by plaque, a sticky film of bacteria on the teeth. As part of their life cycle, these bacteria create toxins that damage the gums and erode the teeth. And yes, your dentist was right. Daily brushing and flossing are essential for gum disease prevention, but so is nutrition.

Most people know that a deficiency of vitamin C causes scurvy, which is characterized by swollen and bleeding gums. And preventing scurvy requires only a modest amount of vitamin C–rich fruits and vegetables or a modest amount (50 or 60 milligrams) of vitamin C in pill form. According to conventional medicine, that's the end of the story. In reality, however, oral health is not a black-and-white issue in which you have either scurvy or perfect gums. There is a tremendous "gray area" in which individual needs, habits, diet, and lifestyle factors may create antioxidant needs that far exceed the reference daily intake (RDI) for vitamin C.

What Does This Have to Do with Aging?

Today, periodontal disease affects three out of four adults over the age of thirty-five. It is a major cause of tooth loss as we grow older and constitutes a major stress on the immune system. A smoldering infection in the gums essentially "uses up" major immune cell resources that would be much better applied to fighting more serious infections and watching out for nascent cancer cells. What's more, the presence of open wounds (no matter how small) in the oral cavity greatly increases your risk for a host of infections, from the common cold to herpes and hepatitis.

In fact, secondary infections that develop from gum disease are now known to contribute to a number of serious conditions, including heart disease, stroke, and lung disorders. In 1998, a breakthrough research project opened the eyes of longevity and health experts throughout the world. The study, conducted by the U.S. Department of Veterans Affairs, was remarkable not only for its findings but for its design and scope. Starting in the mid-1960s, researchers followed more than eight hundred healthy men to assess the relationship of periodontal health status to all-cause mortality. You can imagine that many factors would help to determine who would die within the twenty-five-year study period. So the researchers controlled for smoking and alcohol use, education, weight, cholesterol, white blood cell count, blood pressure, and family history of heart disease. And when all those factors were eliminated, the most striking factor contributing to death from all causes was gum disease. Those who started with significant gum disease had nearly *twice* the death rate of men with healthy gums. In fact, the report concludes that "the increase in risk attributable to periodontal status was found to be similar in magnitude to that attributable to cigarette smoking."[17]

Help from Antioxidants

I want to restate that the first line of defense against gum disease is daily flossing and brushing, along with regular professional care. But clinical and experimental evidence is mounting that antioxidant supplementation can be of significant value. Vitamins with reliable research support include vitamin C, coenzyme Q-10, and a group of phytonutrients found in cranberries.[18]

Cancer

People who consume ample amounts of fruits and vegetables tend to have a lower cancer rate than people who eat few fruits and vegetables. But the benefits afforded by a high-plant diet don't affect cancer risk nearly as much as they do for heart disease. This is because heart disease mainly occurs outside the cells—in the blood vessels—while most cancers start *within* the cell. New research shows that a dramatic reduction in cancer risk will only be achieved by restoring intracellular antioxidant levels, which effectively prevent DNA damage.[19]

The problem is that you cannot benefit by eating intracellular antioxidants. They have to be made by the body at the site where free radicals are produced. Fortunately, there are steps you can take to stimulate intracellular antioxidant production, and this represents the cutting edge of cancer prevention. Data on intracellular antioxidants is now being presented at biomedical conferences, and it's having a tremendous impact in the scientific community. In the last three years, in fact, there has been a widespread shift in our understanding of the nature of cancer, its cause, prevention, and treatment. Physicians are realizing that it is ridiculous to wait until a palpable tumor is present before mentioning the word *cancer* to a patient.

Some might say that cancer prevention has been on the topic list of medical conferences for a decade, but the discussions have been limited to new mammogram techniques, more sophisticated pap smear analysis, and information on prostate-specific antigen (PSA). That's not prevention; it's early detection. The last time I looked in the dictionary, prevention meant stopping something from occurring. That's the promise of intracellular antioxidants.

You see, cancer starts when a cell's DNA is damaged (the spilled coffee on the blueprint). If the damage affects the normal quality-control functions of the cell, it can go through uncontrolled growth to become a cancer cell. If this mutation is not discovered and destroyed by the immune system, it can become a tumor. Taking action at that late stage is like a fire department's ignoring a smoldering brushfire, then having to mobilize all of its resources to fight the ensuing five-alarm blaze.

The key is therefore to deal with the brushfire—the event that altered the cellular DNA and set the carcinogenic wheel in motion. Many things can cause this damage, such as ionizing radiation (people who get sunburned have a greater risk for skin cancer), pollution (people who smoke have a greater risk for lung cancer), chemical exposure (agricultural workers exposed to pesticides have increased risk for cancer), a high-fat diet, and a high-fat body (obesity increases risk for many types of cancer).

What do all of these risk factors have in common? They initiate or accelerate free-radical activity. To be sure, there are non–free-radical causes of cancer, such as genetics and certain viruses (hepatitis C, Epstein-Barr virus, human papilloma virus, and HIV), but the most preventable are free-radical–mediated. That's more than 80 percent of all cancers. Preventable, not just early-detectable. Here's a practical and research-proven action plan:

Action Plan to Reduce Free-Radical Damage

Things to Stop
• *Cigarette Smoking* As I have already mentioned, every puff on a cigarette sends tens of billions of free radicals deep into your lungs. If you smoke, it's time to quit. Time to do *whatever* it takes—nicotine patch, nicotine gum, hypnosis, acupuncture, counseling. If you're not willing to quit, you have to ask yourself why you're reading this book.

Things to Limit
• *Barbecuing and Charring Foods* High-heat cooking, especially foods high in fat, produces a number of cancer-causing compounds (collectively known as polycyclic aromatic hydrocarbons, or PAHs). Catabolic damage to your body increases the longer the food is cooked and the higher the temperature.

• *Carbohydrates Prepared with High Heat* In April 2002, a Swedish study was presented at a biomedical conference that created a stir among toxicologists around the world. Scientists testing a long list of starchy foods cooked with high heat found extremely high levels of acrylamide, a cancer-causing chemical.[20] They proposed that the toxin is formed whenever starches are exposed to high heat.

Weeks later, a British team confirmed the findings, looking at fried, baked, and processed foods, such as French fries, potato chips, corn chips, biscuits, and "puffed" breakfast cereals. The results so alarmed health experts—they found acrylamide levels 1,280 times higher than international safety limits—that as this book was going to press, the World Health Organization was calling for a special meeting in Geneva to discuss what should be done.[21]

Certainly, it seems prudent to reduce intake of highly refined carbohydrates, no matter what the World Health Organization decides. Most of these fall into the category of "junk food" because they are high in fat (often the most damaging kind of fat), high in sodium, and provide no significant vitamins, minerals, or fiber.

• *Chemical Exposure* I grew up in a housing development that was built on a filled-in swamp. Every summer, volunteers (including my father) would ride a tractor around and "fog" the entire area with DDT. The riders never wore protective gear, but even worse, we kids would delight in following the tractor around, running through the pesticide cloud. Today, my risk of cancer is increased because of foolish behavior more than half a century ago.

Of course, we now know better. It is important to reduce your exposure to pesticides, herbicides, household chemicals, and cleaning supplies. I encourage the use of environmentally safe alternatives whenever possible and have been active in getting my local garden supply store to stock alternatives to the chemical frenzy that occurs every spring as homeowners start the battle for greener, weed-free lawns and insect-free patios.

Things to Do

• *Increase Your Intake of Fruits and Vegetables* Vegetables and fruits contain a cornucopia of lifesaving compounds collectively known as phytonutrients. These include antioxidants, vitamins, minerals, and thousands of flavonoids and flavones with potent anticancer, energizing, and heart- and brain-protective benefits.

> *The protective effect of fruits and vegetables against cancer is well established. It is believed that this effect is mediated by antioxidants and decreased oxidative damage to DNA.*
> —Y. T. Szeto and I. F. Benzie, "Effects of Dietary Antioxidants on Human DNA ex Vivo," Free Radical Research Communications

As I've mentioned, maximum benefit will be gained from eating these foods in their raw, natural state. Making fresh juice is also beneficial, as are powdered deep-green vegetable products (so-called green drinks) if they are carefully processed at low temperatures.

Cooking will reduce the nutritional value of fruits and vegetables, but keep in mind that the damage done depends on the amount and type of cooking. Lightly steaming vegetables does very little harm, while deep-fat frying or overcooking by any method will severely deplete critically important nutrients. Interestingly, most frozen vegetables (including peas, green beans, and spinach) come out with nearly the same vitamin and mineral content as fresh. Just remember to cook them lightly if at all.

From these results, it is evident that healthy centenarians show a particular profile in which high levels of vitamin A and vitamin E seem to be important in guaranteeing their extreme longevity.

—P. Mecocci et al., *"Plasma Antioxidants and Longevity: A Study on Healthy Centenarians,"* Free Radical Biology and Medicine

• **Use Sugar-Free Berry Concentrates** Berries (especially blueberries, bilberries, black cherries, and cranberries) are loaded with powerful antioxidants and hundreds of other phytonutrients. Research at the University of Illinois shows that blueberry inhibits an enzyme necessary for the initial stages of cancer development, and cancer researchers at Rutgers University have found that berries and cherries act to induce enzymes that protect against cancer and reduce rapid tumor growth.[22]

Research at the University of Western Ontario demonstrates that cranberry may also have anticancer potential.[23] Mice fed cranberry extract had remarkably reduced incidence of breast cancer, and the tumors they did create were delayed and smaller compared to controls. Moreover, the cranberry group showed a lower rate of metastasis, lending support to the theory that the spread of cancer is dependent to some degree on free-radical activity.

In addition, you'll remember the remarkable research by Tufts University scientists who restored balance, coordination, and memory in old rats just by giving them blueberries.[24] I recommend berry concentrates because few people will consume one and a half to two cups of berries every day. These are nutraceutical products (as opposed to grocery items) with no added sweetener and quality controls that maintain the highest levels of antioxidants and other beneficial compounds.

• **Optimize Glutathione** Glutathione is the primary intracellular antioxidant responsible for preventing DNA damage. What's more, it enhances the protective effect of other antioxidants, including lipoic acid and vitamins C and E. Glutathione also plays a critical role in the body's detoxification of a wide range of carcinogenic compounds, including some of the worst—aflatoxin, benzopyrenes, and nitrosamines. In the last twenty years, hundreds of studies have been published dealing with glutathione's triple-duty anticancer activity.

As we age, however, levels of glutathione decrease as part of the catabolic spiral. But you don't have to take it lying down. Although you can't benefit from eating glutathione, you can supplement the raw materials your body uses to make and utilize this critical protein. These include the amino acids glutamine and L-cysteine, a related compound known as N-acetyl-cysteine (NAC), the mineral selenium, lipoic acid, and undenatured (minimally processed) whey.

Importantly, there are also nonnutritional ways to optimize glutathione synthesis. As you would expect from our discussion of the metabolic model of aging, restoring anabolic power can help a great deal. Studies show that exercise and increasing muscle mass can raise glutathione levels.[25]

• **Optimize Superoxide Dismutase (SOD) and Catalase** Like glutathione, SOD and catalase are powerfully effective enzymes produced by the body to neutralize the free-radical by-products of cellular metabolism and environmental exposure. And like glutathione, they cannot be directly supplemented, although optimizing levels of SOD precursors can help. To optimize SOD and catalase production, the body requires adequate zinc, copper, and manganese. (*Note:* Adequate doesn't mean enormous. Guidelines for supplemental intake of these critical minerals are provided in the "Supplemental Antioxidants" table.)

Current research is confirming that SOD and catalase levels are primary biomarkers of aging. As such, they can even predict to a significant degree one's risk for cancer.[26] This being the case, wouldn't it be great to be able to increase your body's production of these powerful antiaging enzymes? Maintaining adequate levels of precursor minerals is important, but new research suggests that something else may help as much. It's absolutely safe and costs nothing.

It's the experience of joy. Researchers have found that happiness stimulates production of a biochemical known as lymphotoxin (LT). LT induces the production of a specific SOD enzyme known as manganese superoxide dismutase (MnSOD), which is an incredibly powerful antioxidant specifically targeted at protecting DNA.

• **Drink Green Tea** Green tea contains powerful antioxidants known as polyphenols, shown to be more potent than vitamins C or E. These compounds provide a wide range of protection, which may include significant enhancement of the immune system.[27]

• **Spice It Up** Before refrigeration, mankind used spices to preserve food. Today, modern science is finding that many spices contain powerful antioxidants. Since different spices contain different antioxidant compounds, the best strategy is to use cayenne, garlic, turmeric, cumin, rosemary, oregano, and paprika liberally in your diet.[28]

• **Monitor Your Iron Level** Iron is an amazing substance and the perfect example of a double-edged sword. It's responsible for the evolutionary development of hemoglobin, which carries oxygen to the cells of all animals, birds, reptiles, and fish. And because it's so important, the body has multiple ways of storing and recycling iron. In fact, the body holds on to the mineral so jealously that nearly none is lost in urine, stools, or perspiration. The only way to lose iron is through blood loss. Thus, the problem for menstruating women is most often iron deficiency, while many men tend to accumulate an excess.

What's the problem? Iron is a pro-oxidant element, meaning that it catalyzes and accelerates oxidation reactions, which produce free radicals. So the trick is to have enough in your body but not too much, and that ideal range appears to be rather narrow. Scientists first started focusing on the iron issue when studies revealed that men with excessive iron stores had greatly increased risk for heart disease. Since then, there has been a flurry of iron-related research, but nothing in regard to public health directives. This is appalling, because we have all the information we need to determine optimal iron nutriture and the consequences of excess or deficiency are catastrophic in magnitude. In another breakthrough study looking at mitochondria and the aging process, researchers from the departments of molecular and cell biology and nutritional sciences at the University of California, Berkeley, found that iron deficiency and iron excess both produced cellular malfunctions that accelerate aging.[29]

Too Little Iron

For generations, doctors have been measuring iron adequacy by looking at a complete blood count (CBC). This is like measuring for water adequacy when the reservoir is bone-dry. That's because a CBC only reveals the end-point disease state of iron deficiency known as anemia. A person will typically be iron-deficient for three years before becoming anemic. The preanemic state has come to be known as iron *insufficiency*.

The tragedy is that iron insufficiency is fairly easy to correct, while anemia is not. Thus, out of pure negligence, we have created a situation in which nearly a third of all American women spend most of their lives suboptimally nourished in iron. Research shows that this can significantly reduce a woman's energy, stamina, vitality, mood, memory, and learning ability. Remember that I am not talking about anemia. We know that anemia can produce all of those deficits. But what is not widely understood is that mere iron insufficiency can have similar effects.

How to Measure Iron Status Accurately

So far, we know that a CBC is not a sensitive measure of iron adequacy. But neither is a serum iron test. In fact, serum iron merely tells you how much free iron was in the blood at the time of the test. What you're looking for is the level of iron in the tissues of the body, and this is indicated by a test called *serum ferritin*.

For thirty-five years, doctors have been able to measure serum ferritin. For over a decade, research has been available to show that it is the best and most reliable indicator of iron status.[30] But when was the last time you had a serum ferritin? Chances are you never have, and that's critical information that everyone (especially a woman) needs to have. If your ferritin is less than 20 micrograms per liter, you're iron-deficient. Greater than 20 but less than 40 indicates iron insufficiency. Optimal is somewhere between 40 and 150 micrograms per liter.

Testing for Anemia

You may be surprised to learn that even anemia (the disease state of iron deficiency) is often overlooked, especially in the elderly, because it is considered a "normal" consequence of aging. By now, you know to vigorously question assumptions like this and pay careful attention to your CBC. If you are even *borderline* anemic, it is important to follow up with a nutritionally oriented physician to find the underlying cause and correct the disorder. Because anemia, in effect, produces oxygen deficiency throughout the body and brain, it is associated with increased mortality. A recent study in the *New England Journal of Medicine* found that heart attack victims who were anemic were more than twice as likely to die within thirty days than patients who were not anemic.[31]

DETECTING ANEMIA

Your complete blood count (CBC) includes a red blood cell count and levels of hemoglobin and hematocrit. The following are the reference ranges for men and women:

Test	Normal Range for Men	Normal Range for Women
Red blood cell count (RBC)	4.10 to 5.60	3.80 to 5.10
Hemoglobin (HGB)	12.5 to 17.0	11.5 to 15.0
Hematocrit (HCT)	36 to 50%	34 to 44%

Too Much Iron

When body stores of iron are excessive, the production of free radicals accelerates dramatically. To illustrate this, cut an apple in half. Rub lemon juice on the cut surface of one side and stick an iron nail in the other half. Come back the next day and compare the pieces. The half that was rubbed with lemon juice will look pretty much the same as it did when cut. That's because the lemon juice contains vitamin C, which protects the "flesh" of the apple from oxidation. The cut surface of the other half, however, will be visibly browned by oxidation. Then remove the nail and cut through the nail hole. There, the apple will be dark brown or nearly black from the extraordinary free-radical destruction.

Such accelerated destruction (while not this fast or dramatic) can take place in human tissues. We know, for example, that the oxidation of cholesterol in the blood is one of the primary causes of cardiovascular disease, the leading cause of death in Western nations. Studies show that in the presence of excess iron, this process can be increased by as much as 70 percent[32] and the amount of free radicals produced is truly astronomical.

Equally important is the damage that occurs in the brain, and here again, iron is a key factor. In fact, new research shows that degeneration of cognitive and motor skills is directly proportionate to the level of iron accumulation in the brain.[33] This is extremely important information, because it reveals two positive steps we can take (at any age) to minimize brain degeneration in later years:

1. Keep a watch on your ferritin level by having it checked at your yearly physical. If you see that your ferritin level has climbed above 180 micrograms per liter (rarely a problem for pre-menopausal women), consider giving blood every ninety days to bring it down. In addition, reduce your intake of high-iron foods such as red meat. Make sure that your multivitamin does not contain iron. Avoid occupational exposure (carpenters: keep those nails out of your mouth).

2. Maintain high levels of antioxidants in your brain and bloodstream. The next subsection explains how.

• *Take a Variety of Supplemental Antioxidants* The accompanying table summarizes current research on antioxidants and provides a general dose range. Because everyone is different (in size, weight, metabolism, habits, lifestyle), I encourage you to confer with a prevention-oriented physician for individual guidance. Many of these antioxidants can be obtained in a comprehensive antioxidant formula, but remember that you cannot benefit from oral intake of glutathione, SOD, or catalase. These intracellular antioxidants are manufactured within the cell.

SUPPLEMENTAL ANTIOXIDANTS		
Antioxidant	*Natural Source*	*Prudent Supplement Range*
Vitamin C	Citrus fruits	200–1,000 mg
Vitamin E (d-alpha tocopherol)	Raw nuts, seeds, and unprocessed oils	30–1,000 IU
Vitamin A	Fish oil	2,500–5,000 IU

Carotenoid complex (e.g., beta carotene, lycopene, lutein, zeaxanthin)	Orange, yellow, and red fruits and vegetables	20–50 mg
Flavonoids	Wide variety of fruits and vegetables	50–100 mg
Anthocyanins	Berries, cherries, grapes	100–500 mg
Proanthocyanidins	Pine bark, grape seed extracts	20–100 mg
Coenzyme Q10	Whole grains, nuts, seeds	20–200 mg
NAC*	No natural source	100–200 mg
L-cysteine*	Eggs, garlic, onions	—
Polyphenols	Green tea, red wine, rooibos tea	—
Selenium*	Selenium yeast, wheat germ, nuts	50–100 mcg
Ginkgo biloba	Ginkgo biloba extract	50–250 mg
Alpha lipoic acid*	Liver, yeast	50–200 mg
Zinc†	Shellfish, fish, red meat, pumpkin seeds	10–30 mg
Copper†	Shellfish, beans, nuts, seeds	1–3 mg
Manganese†	Nuts, whole grains, green leafy vegetables	5–15 mg

* Supports glutathione production.
† Supports SOD production.

Point 1: More is not necessarily better. Optimal health is a balance between oxidation and antioxidants. For example, your immune system uses free radicals to kill bacteria, and megadose consumption of antioxidants has the potential to disrupt this important function. What's more, too much of one may create an imbalance. Taking more than 60 milligrams of zinc per day, for example, can impair copper absorption and metabolism. Still another reason not to overdose is potential toxicity, in which excessive levels can actually be poisonous. Selenium is used slowly by the body, and daily intake of more than 500 micrograms will tend to accumulate in the kidneys and other tissues, potentially leading to selenium toxicity.

Point 2: Different antioxidants protect the body in different ways. Some prevent free radicals from forming. Some work in lipid areas of the body. Some work in the water compartment. Some, like lipoic acid, work well in both areas. Some antioxidants prevent free-radical penetration into the cell or cell nucleus, and yet others accelerate cell repair after the damage has been done. Beware of anyone who tells you that one particular compound (such as pine bark or green tea) is *the* best antioxidant; the prudent and most effective approach is to take a variety of antioxidants in each of these categories. Even within the same category (berries, for example), different berries have widely different protective benefits.[34]

This does not mean taking handfuls of supplements. Today, comprehensive antioxidant products are available that provide many, if not most, of the listed nutrients.

Point 3: DHEA possesses significant antioxidant activity but is not included in this chart because it is not appropriate for those under thirty-five years of age. Recent evidence also suggests that DHEA may be a powerful antioxidant stimulator. Researchers at Stockholm University in Sweden have found that feeding DHEA to animals stimulates the synthesis of coenzyme Q10 in the blood, brain, and internal organs.[35] This may account for many of the extraordinary benefits achieved by DHEA supplementation.

CATABOLIC FACTOR 2: GLYCATION

Closely related to free-radical activity is a process known as glycation or glycosylation. Those are actually fancy words for a process that food chemists and bakers have known for a century, only they call it *browning*. Browning, or glycation, takes place when sugars (primarily glucose and fructose) combine with proteins. Take a look at the steaks in the meat aisle next time you go shopping. The steaks on the bottom will be uniformly pink, while those on top (exposed to the air) will have turned slightly brown. Some of the protein has been glycated. Take one home and cook it and it will turn brown rapidly, and the longer you cook it, the browner it will get. The same thing happens to us as we age, only the "cooking" is a matter of time, not temperature.

Actually, some of us brown a whole lot faster than others, a fact that was discovered about thirty years ago in studies with diabetics. Since a diabetic will tend to have higher levels of glucose in the bloodstream, researchers noticed that some of that glucose was binding to hemoglobin, a blood protein that carries oxygen to the cells. The first indication that this was not a good thing was that glycosylated hemoglobin didn't work, leaving the individual in a perpetual state of relative oxygen debt. That's one reason diabetics have low exercise tolerance.

Further research confirmed that glycosylation was accelerated elsewhere in the diabetic's body, and the higher the person's blood glucose, the greater the damage and the faster it was taking place. We now know that uncontrolled diabetes is like high-speed aging. People with diabetes are at greater risk for atherosclerosis, cataracts, heart disease, stroke, lung disease, joint disorders, and brain degeneration, all related to the intense catabolic process of browning.

And of course, it's not just a problem for diabetics. In 1987, Anthony Cerami, a biochemist at Rockefeller University, suggested that glycosylated proteins accumulate in all of our tissues and contribute to the aging process.[36] He called these altered proteins AGE, short for advanced glycation end products. The essential AGE problem is that the affected protein no longer functions as it should. The seriousness of this problem is apparent when you look at the astounding range of protein activity in the human body.

Proteins do more than make muscle. A major portion of every metabolic process in the human body depends on the perfect timing of more than fifty thousand proteins. Enzymes are proteins that catalyze chemical reactions in every cell and tissue of the body. Glycated enzymes don't work. Proteins turn genes off and on, ferry nutrients and other essential biochemicals throughout the body, help balance blood chemistry, play an integral role in the immune system, and direct the entire process of cell repair and replication. When these proteins are glycated, they become less soluble and tend to clump. In fact, glycated proteins appear to be a major component of the plaque that causes Alzheimer's disease.[37] Even the collagen fibers in a man's penis are susceptible to glycation, and this may be a hidden cause of erectile dysfunction.[38] We get a hint of a solution from the data I discussed earlier concerning the ability of antioxidants to put the brakes on degeneration.

How Antioxidants Help De-AGE Your Body

In 1992, scientists discovered that lipoic acid could arrest the glycation process in a test tube.[39] Five years later, endocrinologists at the University of Heidelberg, Germany, took the experiment an important step further with a research model of blood vessel deterioration.[40] When they introduced AGE material to blood vessel tissue, glutathione and vitamin C were both severely depleted. As a result, free-radical activity increased, leading to a cascade of damaging effects typical of atherosclerosis. In effect, they had identified glycation as an important factor in cardiovascular disease.

But they didn't stop there. They then added lipoic acid and found that glutathione and vitamin C were *completely restored*. More important, this restoration put the brakes on the destructive effects of glycation. Researchers from the Mayo Clinic found that lipoic acid conferred similar protection on nerve tissue.[41] Research has confirmed that flavonoids (found in fruits, vegetables, and whole grains) significantly reduce the glycation of hemoglobin, and researchers at Tokyo University School of Medicine found that N-acetyl-cysteine (NAC) also slows glycation.[42] I'm willing to bet that in the next few years, we'll find that *most* antioxidants help, but although glycation is accelerated by free radicals and can be slowed, the battle cannot be won with antioxidants alone.

The Bitter Truth

Aside from free radicals, the other factor that accelerates glycation is the presence of glucose and other simple sugars. As you'll see, there's an intriguing similarity between glycation and oxidation. Here are two essential substances (glucose and oxygen)—in simple terms, the chemical basis for all life—and both act as poisons when not properly managed by the body. We talked about the balance of free radicals and antioxidants, and how that balance has been hopelessly destroyed by our exposure to massive levels of free radicals in the postindustrial world. Well, guess what. The same thing has happened to the food we eat.

For millions of years, glucose was delivered in complex "packages" known as starch. These starches or complex carbohydrates were found in a variety of roots, tubers, fruits, and vegetables, and nature developed taste buds, a sensitive mechanism for the detection of starch. Because starch was so important as a fuel supply, the taste buds to detect its sweet taste covered two-thirds of the tongue. And therein lies the problem.

For hunter-gatherers, the predominance of sweet taste sensors was a lifesaver. Not only did it tip them off to the presence of starch (which they desperately needed), but it also gave them information about food safety. Poisonous plants are never sweet.

But then, about seven hundred years ago, people figured out how to refine two particular starches (cane and beets) down to a very simple substance known as sucrose, or table sugar. No longer were complex starches releasing glucose slowly into the bloodstream. Sucrose is digested by enzymes in saliva and raises glucose levels in a matter of seconds. Not only that, but the amount of glucose available is nearly unlimited. As Europeans quickly discovered, one could eat sugar by the pound, and they did, knowing nothing about the disastrous consequences to their health.

You have to understand that the effect of this discovery was literally earthshaking. Sugar produced an energy rush and a taste impact that fueled centuries of wars and colonial expansion. Sugar was the prime reason for the African slave trade, as vast areas of the Caribbean were destroyed to create sugar plantations.

Biochemically, sugar is also a disaster, primarily because it raises glucose levels so fast and so high. This not only accelerates aging via skyrocketing glycation but contributes to obesity, heart disease, osteoporosis, and a raft of other disorders associated with altered blood sugar metabolism. Remember that elevated blood glucose is quite dangerous, and so the body responds by secreting insulin, the hormone responsible for taking glucose out of the bloodstream and into the cells. This mechanism, however, was designed for slowly digesting starches. The massive increase in glucose resulting from sugar consumption overwhelms the body's ability to maintain this critical balance, producing a roller coaster of energy followed by profound fatigue. When blood glucose and insulin levels are high, brain biochemistry may be altered, producing mood swings and confusion. When blood glucose levels drop, symptoms of fatigue, anxiety, depression, irritability, disorientation, and headache are all intensified.[43]

The issue here is metabolic stress. Biochemically, the body is simply not equipped for the intake of pure glucose, and although it will adapt and function, the liver, adrenals, and pancreas will be strained in the process. All of this accelerates aging.

Dr. Sheldon Reiser, former head of the carbohydrate lab at the U.S. Department of Agriculture's Human Nutrition Institute, points out that two early signs of diabetes develop when people consume excess sugar: high insulin and high glucose levels. Dr. Reiser has recommended drastic reduction of refined sugar intake, suggesting that "a national campaign be launched to inform the populace of the hazards of excessive sugar consumption."[44] That was in 1978, when the per capita intake of sugar was about twelve teaspoonfuls per day. Nothing was done. Twenty years later, a coalition of health agencies and public health experts petitioned the USDA to review escalating sugar consumption, citing medical evidence that it poses a national public health threat. Nothing was done.

Today, the average American consumes about twenty-four teaspoonfuls of refined sugar (table sugar, corn syrup, and so forth) per day, amounting to well over one hundred pounds of sugar per person each year.[45] Anyone serious about antiaging cannot consume twenty-four teaspoonfuls of sugar every day and hope to succeed.

Antiglycation Action Steps

Reduce Consumption of All Refined Sugars

Refined sugars include sucrose, glucose, dextrose, fructose, and corn syrup. I was going to include a detailed chart listing the sugar content of commonly consumed foods. Then I thought it might be easier to tell you to read labels. But food labels are confusing, and manufacturers often provide misleading information. For example, the "sugar" listing includes *all* sugars, some of which are complex starches inherent in the food. Far more valuable would be disclosure of *added sugar,* but the processed-food industry has refused to provide this information.

Finally, I realized that the simplest and easiest action step would be to *reduce your consumption of foods that require labels*. Think like a hunter-gatherer. Avoid packaged and processed foods. As much as possible, eat food in its natural state.

FRUCTOSE FOLLIES

For years, the health food industry has been telling us that fructose is a safe and beneficial sugar. But while it is classified as a "natural" sweetener, I would argue that the enormous amount of fructose contained in many foods and beverages would be nearly impossible to get from nature. The 18 grams per serving provided by a leading "energy drink" is the fructose equivalent of approximately ten apples. Remember also that there are no foods in nature that contain just fructose and that fructose only contributes to energy production after metabolism by the liver.

Essentially, fructose accelerates aging in well-defined ways:

• It promotes glycation at nearly seven times the rate of glucose.[46]

• Fructose contributes to an increase in total cholesterol and LDL (the "bad cholesterol"), especially in diabetics.[47]

• Research has shown that administration of fructose at 5 grams per day (certainly obtainable from a fructose-sweetened food or beverage) can disrupt mineral metabolism and lead to depletion of iron, magnesium, calcium, and zinc.[48]

Avoid Glycated Proteins (AGE-Laden Foods)

These foods accelerate aging.[49] Thus:

• Limit browned or charred foods. This includes grilled or barbecued meat, poultry, and fish as well as well-done broiled meats. Evidence is mounting that consumption of well-cooked (not even charred) meat is associated with increased risk for breast cancer.[50]

• Don't overcook eggs. This doesn't mean you should eat eggs raw or runny (that increases risk for salmonella), but avoid cooking them to death. Skip the eternally reheated scrambled eggs at breakfast buffets.

- Most foods contain some protein that can be glycated. Thus, even burned toast contains significant levels of AGE material.

- Cook foods at the lowest possible temperature. Deep frying is the worst, not only because of the excessive heat but because of the incorporation of high amounts of fat. Thus, poaching, microwaving, steaming, stir-frying, and careful broiling (to avoid charring) are the way to go.

Get Regular Exercise

Exercise influences blood sugar almost as much as diet. As you'll see in Chapter 7, you don't have to work out strenuously. The key here is *consistency*. You were designed to move, and everything including glucose metabolism works better when you exercise regularly.

Drink Green Tea (Again)

Breakthrough research just published demonstrates that, in addition to its potent antioxidant activity, green tea may directly inhibit glycation.[51]

CATABOLIC FACTOR 3: WEAR AND TEAR

So now you're getting the picture that life is a balance (or a battle) between anabolic repair and catabolic damage. You understand that for optimal results, you need to deal with *both* sides of the equation. Nevertheless, you cannot expect to look and feel like a thirty-year-old when you're eighty. My eighty-five-year-old mother is presently aging at the rate of a sixty-year-old. She's not complaining. In other words, some things are going to wear out no matter how well you've followed the Metabolic Plan. One of those is collagen.

A Collagen Education

Collagen is a protein that holds you together. It's an important component of bone, tendon, ligament, and joint tissue. It forms the foundation for your skin and arteries and keeps your internal organs in place. After water, collagen is the major constituent of your body, and for good reason. Because of the way it's constructed, collagen has a "springy" quality that lends both strength and flexibility to your body. In time, however, we tend to lose that flexibility. Collagen becomes stiff, and so do the tissues that contain this valuable protein.

And it's not simply that you can no longer bend forward and touch your toes. The reduced flexibility is far more damaging to your arteries, which need to expand when the heart pumps and relax between beats. As blood vessels lose this flexibility, blood pressure rises, and they become damaged. Reduced flexibility means increased risk of injury and slower healing.

Of course, this was once assumed simply to be part of the aging process. ("Oh, well, collagen gettin' stiff.") Because the turnover rate for collagen is so slow, scientists thought for a long time that it was inert. We now know that collagen cells are replaced, only very slowly, which makes rebuilding difficult but not impossible. Athletes who tear a ligament, for example, have to have it surgically repaired because it would take years for the body to create enough collagen to mend a wound of that kind. Thus, protecting collagen becomes a top antiaging priority.

We've discussed oxidation. Free radicals attack your collagen every day. For some people (such as those with arthritis), this damage can be severe and painful. The solution is to maintain adequate antioxidant protection.

We've discussed glycation. Since collagen is a protein, it's a primary target for this catabolic process. But this can be avoided if you maintain adequate antioxidant protection, avoid refined sugars, and get regular exercise. Particularly helpful is range-of-motion exercise, in which the joints are moved through their full rotation, because it keeps collagen lubricated with synovial fluid. We now know that this thick fluid contains antioxidants and a variety of restoring and rebuilding biochemicals like chondroitin sulfate and that exercise dramatically enhances the protective and restoring capacity of synovial fluid. New research, in fact, shows that exercise alters the composition of synovial fluid to increase levels of antioxidants and anabolic repair biochemicals (including IGF-1) to support healthy joints.[52]

More Good News

Collagen is manufactured by cells known as fibroblasts. Decreased collagen production was once assumed to be an immutable part of the aging process. ("Oh, well, fibroblasts not showin' up for work"), but recent research shows that fibroblast production of collagen can be increased. Is it by taking a new prescription drug? Using a high-tech electronic stimulation device? No, it's something people have been using for five thousand years: aloe vera.

You probably know that aloe vera applied to a wound accelerates healing. Researchers were intrigued not only by the speed of healing but by the fact that the healed tissue was stronger than before it was injured. This led to the discovery that aloe stimulated collagen synthesis by fibroblasts in the skin. Great, but what about other parts of the body? Here's where we get to the really good news. Researchers then *fed* aloe to the test animals and got the same results. Faster healing, stronger tissue, increased collagen production.[53]

Aloe, of course, has been used topically for five thousand years, but nobody ever drank it. That's because the rind contains bitter compounds known as anthraquinones, which have a strong laxative effect. In the last twenty years, however, processing techniques have been perfected that completely remove these harsh compounds, producing a gel or juice that is palatable and extraordinarily healthful. Such products have been used with great success for people with gastrointestinal illness, but current research shows that drinking aloe can produce anabolic and anticatabolic benefits throughout the body by supporting:

Immunity
Healthy cell proliferation
Collagen production
Detoxification
Antioxidant activity
Intestinal health

We need to understand collagen metabolism in order to understand how we grow, adapt to the environment, maintain our adult shapes and then wrinkle and crumble as we age.
—M. J. Rennie, "Teasing Out the Truth about Collagen,"
Journal of Physiology—London

Reducing the Catabolic Phase of Exercise

As you follow the Metabolic Plan, you'll experience greater energy, improved stamina, and renewed feelings of vitality. This will no doubt lead to the desire to exercise more strenuously, and activities like weight training, resistance machines such as Nautilus, and vigorous walking will result in greater gains—even more energy and well-defined reductions in your biological age.[54]

At that level of exertion, the muscles go through a catabolic phase following exercise. When you are in your twenties, this normal metabolic stage lasts only thirty to sixty minutes. As oxygen and glucose are restored to the tired muscles, they regain their anabolic strength. As we age, however, this catabolic stage tends to last longer. It may take many hours for the muscles to recover from strenuous exercise. Thus, a fifty-five-year-old is likely to feel less invigorated by exercise and more tired than she did thirty years before. Ironically, exercise is more important for her than for the twenty-five-year-old, and this loss of exercise tolerance is an important part of the downward catabolic spiral. What's more, muscle soreness may dampen her enthusiasm for vigorous exercise even further.

BCAAs to the Rescue

Branched-chain amino acids (BCAAs) have been shown to enhance recovery after exercise.[55] The catabolic stage can also produce a feeling of "the blahs," which is partly but not entirely related to fatigue. BCAA supplementation has been shown to counteract this effect, leaving people feeling "pumped and powerful" after their workouts.[56]

And for those who get *really* inspired and go into triathlon-level competition, BCAAs have been shown to completely abolish the catabolic-induced immune suppression that typically follows ultra-endurance exercise.[57]

How Do They Do This?

BCAAs (leucine, isoleucine, and valine) are metabolized differently from all other amino acids in that they can be incorporated directly into the muscle without going through the clearinghouse function of the liver. To a tired muscle, that's like getting an immediate boost rather than having to wait for normal metabolic functions to restore protein and fuel for the anabolic building process. The effective dose depends on your weight. If you weigh from one hundred to two hundred pounds, try three or four 500 milligram capsules (available in health food stores) immediately after a workout.

Additional Anticatabolic Support

In your efforts to minimize the catabolic response to exercise, you'll get additional help from antioxidants (especially, vitamins C and E),[58] the amino acid L-carnitine, and the glutathione precursors N-acetyl-cysteine and alpha lipoic acid.[59] Dosage recommendations are listed in the "Supplemental Antioxidants" table.

The Thyroid Factor

Both hypo- and hyperthyroid conditions affect exercise tolerance by impairing energy metabolism,[60] and the incidence of thyroid disease increases as we age. Thus, if you experience a persistent inability to exercise, have your physician conduct a complete thyroid panel to check this important endocrine function.

CATABOLIC FACTOR 4: DECLINING LIVER FUNCTION

In the last chapter, I discussed the importance of the liver in maintaining peak anabolic repair. Since aging is associated with declining liver function, a catabolic spiral results. Hormones like DHEA, thyroid hormone, and growth hormone send the anabolic signal, but the liver is responsible for actually carrying out those instructions. If the liver is impaired, anabolic activity declines. Studies show that if mice are given a toxic load that stresses the liver, even the direct injection of growth hormone will not restore essential anabolic functions.[61]

You're right, it isn't fair. Just when our repair needs start to increase, the building supply goes out of business. Fortunately, there are a number of steps that you can take to restore and maintain liver function.

How to Care for Your Liver

Consume Alcohol in Moderation

Limiting alcohol consumption is important to liver health, and if you have liver disease or even impaired liver function, don't consume alcohol at all. What's moderation? That's determined primarily by your size, because large livers can detoxify more alcohol. The *general* guideline for a person from one hundred to two hundred pounds is that fewer than two drinks per day constitutes moderation.[62] One drink is equal to:

- 12 ounces of beer

- One 6-ounce glass of wine

- 1.5 ounces (one jigger) of distilled spirits

Anything more than moderate intake is defined as *excessive consumption*. If this describes you, I strongly suggest that you consult with your physician to evaluate the risks and develop a treatment strategy.

Avoid Hepatitis Like the Plague

With more than 11 million Americans infected (and 500,000 new cases each year), that's exactly what hepatitis is—a plague. Regarding this epidemic, C. Everett Koop, former U.S. surgeon general, has stated, "We stand at the precipice of a grave threat to our public health. . . . It affects people from all walks of life, in every state, in every country. And unless we do something about it soon, it will kill more people than AIDS." (quoted in *The Times* (UK) April 19, 2000)

There are basically two types of hepatitis, or inflammation of the liver. *Toxic hepatitis* is a noninfectious condition caused by exposure to alcohol or other chemicals that damage the liver. *Infectious hepatitis* is caused by a group of viruses that attack the liver, each designated by a letter from A through G. We'll discuss the most prevalent forms, hepatitis A, B, and C. Recovery is possible, and most patients improve, but nearly 80 percent of hepatitis C cases will develop into a chronic and often lifelong condition.

• *Hepatitis A (HAV)* Hepatitis A is the one most often contracted by international travelers, usually from feces-contaminated food or water. Fortunately, it rarely becomes chronic, and most people recover completely in one to three months. About one-third of Americans test positive for hepatitis A antibodies, indicating previous infection. Because the virus is contagious for two to four weeks *before* symptoms appear, those returning from overseas can infect family members if careful hygiene is not followed. Anyone with hepatitis A should not prepare food for others.

Precautions: Those traveling to areas where hepatitis A is endemic should be vaccinated. When traveling in these areas, fruits and vegetables should be peeled and washed carefully with purified water. Obviously, meat, poultry, and fish should be well cooked and drinking water purified or bottled.

• ***Hepatitis B (HBV)*** Historically, hepatitis B was transmitted through contaminated blood. Thus, people who received transfusions before 1990 ran a significant risk. Today, blood is carefully tested for hepatitis, but you can still be exposed through body fluids in unprotected sex or even cuts, scrapes, and other breaks in the skin. Hospital workers exposed to blood products are at risk, as are the staff and residents of mental institutions and prisons. Roughly 10 percent of hepatitis B patients carry the virus throughout their lives, and about 25 percent of these carriers progress to chronic disease.

Precautions: Several vaccines have been developed, and public health experts are recommending immunization for all children who may have routine contact with immigrants from countries with high incidence of hepatitis B. In adults, safe sex practices can reduce risk considerably.

• ***Hepatitis C (HCV)*** Like hepatitis B, hepatitis C is transmitted through the blood. Thus, shared hypodermic needles, unprotected sex, and pre-1990 blood transfusions are the most common modes of transmission. What is most alarming is the rise in new cases to more than 100,000 per year in the United States alone. Worldwide, it is estimated that more than 200 million are infected.

You may be wondering why I'm spending so much time talking about hepatitis. After all, you're not an intravenous drug user, and you don't have sex with strangers. But HCV is far more easily transmitted than HIV (the virus that causes AIDS). You can be exposed to HCV through injuries in the skin or *indirect* contact with blood or blood products. Shared razors or toothbrushes, poorly sterilized medical instruments, blood spills, unbandaged cuts, and tattooing are all possible routes of infection. For this reason, and because it so often leads to chronic disease and cirrhosis, HCV is one of the greatest public health threats of the century. Talking about antiaging without careful attention to this global epidemic is like a swimming instructor's ignoring nearby sharks.

Precautions: There is no effective vaccine for HCV, the primary reason being that it is remarkably different from the other hepatitis viruses. Hepatitis C is an RNA virus that can outmaneuver the human immune system (and vaccine strategies) through rapid mutation. This also makes the infection hard to treat. The current strategy (a combination of interferon and ribavirin) is successful in less than 20 percent of cases—thus, the critical importance of prevention.

Clean Up Your Act

Remember that the things that damage and tax the liver are primarily the noxious substances that we eat, drink, and breathe. Thus, the best liver-protection strategy is to reduce your exposure to car exhaust and other pollutants, drink only purified water (bottled or filtered, not tap water), and avoid the use of pesticides, herbicides, and other agricultural chemicals. Choose occupations that have no exposure to chemical fumes. Hair and nail stylists are especially vulnerable due to daily exposure to solvents, styling chemicals, and dyes. If you live in a highly polluted area—for example, near an oil refinery—you need to know that breathing the air can be injurious to your liver.[63]

Eat a widely varied natural foods diet, with approximately 70 percent of total calories coming from fresh fruits, vegetables, and whole grains. As much as possible, choose organically grown foods. Foods that have specific liver-support benefits include artichoke, Brussels sprouts, cabbage, broccoli, and carrots.

Be moderate with coffee (one cup a day max) and remember that all drugs—recreational, over-the-counter, and prescription—are detoxified by the liver. Long-term use of acetaminophen (Tylenol, Excedrin, Lortab) is especially hard on the liver, and overuse may result in acute liver disease.

Note: There are probably more than a hundred herbs, tablets, powders, and capsules that have been touted as "liver cleansers." Over the years, I've contacted nearly every manufacturer with a simple question: "What evidence do you have that your product does in fact cleanse, protect, or improve the liver?" Although this data should be easy to obtain (more than a dozen liver-function tests can be inexpensively performed), I have received reliable evidence for a total of four: Milk Thistle (and an extract from milk thistle known as silymarin), Wolfberry, Fo-Ti, and Schizandra. In addition, there is promising data on the value of anthocyanins derived from blueberries, cranberries, bilberries, black cherries, and red or purple grapes.

Why am I so skeptical? Because a number of "natural" products have been shown to actually *damage* the liver. Numerous herbs—including comfrey, mistletoe, germander, and chaparral—can actually *interfere* with normal liver function and, used in excess, may contribute to serious liver disease.[64]

What about the popular "liver-flush" program, wherein large amounts of lemon juice and olive oil are consumed for a number of days, followed by a coffee enema? I would ask the same question—namely, "What evidence exists that such drastic measures improve liver function?" One liver-flush enthusiast presented me with a vial of "sludge" that he claimed was liver toxins. Undaunted by the fact that this material had been recovered from a toilet, I had it (carefully) analyzed. Turns out the major constituent was olive oil.

Glutathione (Again)

I was tipped off to the bona fide liver-support benefits of glutathione when reviewing a hospital protocol for acetaminophen overdose. Step one was administration of N-acetyl-cysteine, a variant of the amino acid L-cysteine. NAC is a precursor of glutathione, and glutathione eliminates the toxic breakdown products of the overdose.

Further investigation revealed that glutathione plays an important role in normal liver function and that concentrations of glutathione in the liver are greater than in any other tissue in the body. Not surprisingly, aging and any type of liver disease result in dramatic reductions in this critically important compound. What to do? As I have mentioned, taking glutathione pills will provide little antiaging benefit, but there are ways to raise glutathione levels in the liver. Precursors (building blocks that the body uses to make glutathione) include NAC; the amino acids glutamine, glycine, and L-cysteine; melatonin; and bioactive whey proteins. In addition, a number of natural products—

including DHEA, lipoic acid, and selenium—support glutathione production and metabolism.

CONCLUSION

Chapter 1 presented two quality-of-life charts. The first chart included decades of catabolic deterioration, otherwise known as pain and suffering, ending in death at the life expectancy point of 76.7 years. The second chart depicted an "extended" quality of life that avoids this degeneration and decrepitude, in which prime of life lasts fifty or sixty years and death comes much later (maybe at the age of 120). I didn't invent this new model. James Fries of Stanford University was the pioneer who saw this possibility more than twenty years ago, developing what he termed the "compression of morbidity."[65] He saw this as a necessity if we as an aging society were to avoid bankrupting our health care system and creating massive levels of suffering.

We now know that reducing catabolic damage and restoring youthful anabolic repair can dramatically improve the way we age. But if there's one thing that can dash our hopes for a long, healthy and vibrant life, it's stress.

FOUR

Stress and the Aging Process

If a microbe is in or around us all the time and yet causes no disease until we are exposed to stress, what is the cause of the illness, the microbe or the stress?

—Dr. Hans Selye, The Stress of Life

The topic of stress has come up quite a few times so far. I explained how stimulants like caffeine raise stress hormone levels, suggested that the way we think about time and aging is inherently stressful, and described stress as a catabolic turbocharger. Indeed, stress is the invisible saboteur. It silently weakens your immune system, accelerates aging, and can in a very real sense take you out of the game. Everyone knows this. We all know how we feel and behave when we're stressed. We know that tension constricts blood vessels, cutting off oxygen to billions of cells throughout the body and brain. We know that stress interferes with deep sleep and sets us up for a vicious cycle of fatigue, illness, and more stress.

This hit me one day in pathology class. My instructor was presenting a landmark study in which researchers from Ohio State University College of Medicine evaluated the effects of stress on immunity. Graduate students had been divided (based on the results of a questionnaire) into two groups: those who were experiencing college as an enjoyable challenge and those who were buckling under the strain. Comprehensive immune testing revealed that the stressed-out students had significant immune defects, including very low levels of a specific cell that is our primary anticancer defense.

"Wait a minute," I protested, "those students needed *greater* immunity, not less. Why wouldn't their immune systems help them out?"

"Mr. Cherniske," the professor began, "you are forgetting the name of the game." "No," I countered, "survival is the game, which is why I can't see the lesson here." The professor replied, "The lesson eludes you because you think survival refers to *your* survival, when, in fact, nature couldn't care less about you or me. It is the *species* that must survive."

"You mean . . . ?"

"Precisely, Mr. Cherniske. Those stressed-out students were in the process of being cut from the team. If you can't handle pressure, nature hands you a pink slip. Nothing personal. Weakness is just not good for the gene pool."

Since that day, I've paid special attention to this thing called stress. I spent years in a yoga ashram, went on to study biofeedback, hypnotherapy, and neurobiology. The more I learn, the more I understand the game. At first, it may seem cold and cruel, but the sports analogy is revealing. Remember that Mother Nature is the coach of this *Homo sapiens* team, and she's got new players showing up all the time— roughly 260,000 every day—so she has to have a way to cut some players to make room for the new talent. Immune failure leading to fatal disease is the perfect solution (not everyone can be struck by lightning). The good news is that a championship team requires the perfect blend of energetic rookies and experienced veterans. In other words, if you can show the coach that you have what it takes to win, she'll keep you on the team.

In Chapter 2, we saw that muscle mass is one mark of a winner. Another is the ability to excel under pressure. Together, these qualities are called longevity signals. And the proof of this scenario lies in the fact that in the graduate student experiment, stress-management training for the burnout group restored their immune competence in about ninety days.

THE ANATOMY OF STRESS

The human brain is an astounding survival tool. Normal experience (that is, occurrences similar to those the brain has already cataloged) is handled by an area of the brain known as the reticular formations (part of the thalamus). But when new sensory data is received, or anything that portends possible danger, a part of the brain known as the hypothalamus is instantly activated. The hypothalamus has a panic button and uses it often (motto: "Better safe than sorry"). This stimulates release of adrenocorticotrophic hormone (ACTH) from the pituitary, which, in turn, acts upon the adrenals to produce stress hormones, primarily epinephrine (adrenaline) and cortisol. These hormones flood the body, enabling us to respond to the danger at hand: the well-known fight-or-flight response.

Major Effects of Stress Hormones: The Fight-or-Flight Response

- The pupils dilate to sharpen vision.

- Heart rate and blood pressure increase to accelerate delivery of oxygen and fuel to the muscles and critical organs.

- Blood flow is diverted from noncritical areas such as the gastrointestinal tract to critical areas such as the heart, skeletal muscles, and liver.

- The liver releases glucose and fatty acids into the bloodstream. Glucose is for immediate energy, fat in case the fight or flight takes longer than expected.

- Bronchial tubes dilate to maximize exchange of oxygen in and carbon dioxide out.

Episodic Versus Chronic Stress

The nature of stress has changed a great deal since the fight-or-flight response was developed over 3 million years ago. You see, stress used to be *episodic*. Everything was peachy, and then, all of a sudden, there was a saber-toothed tiger to deal with. The stress response worked perfectly for that kind of challenge because ancient men and women needed that heart-pumping adrenaline rush. Whether they fought or fled, they used up every gram of glucose and fat that was poured into their bloodstream by the liver. When the stress was over, it was over. But today, for the most part, stress is chronic (long-lasting), and this same adrenal response is killing us.

Say you work hard on a project that is unfairly criticized by your boss. Suddenly, your face flushes, your heart pounds, and you want to scream. But screaming is frowned upon in most offices, so you stuff the feelings of anger and frustration. In fact, sitting at your desk, your body is going through exactly the same response that your ancestors experienced when faced with the tiger. The only difference is, you have nowhere to run and nothing to fight. Later that day, you find yourself stuck in rush-hour traffic. Under normal circumstances, you'd turn on the radio and cope, but you find yourself on edge. Pretty soon, you're cursing at other drivers and triggering another fight-or-flight episode.

Most people today have lives punctuated by similar experiences. In each case—whether it's traffic, a pink slip, an abusive spouse, a missed flight, or a jam-packed schedule—the one common denominator is that no immediate action is available to relieve the stress. Over time, here's what happens:

Effects of Chronic Stress

1. Your blood pressure rises. Depending on how many similar situations you have to endure, it may stay elevated, thus damaging the incredibly sensitive tubules of your kidneys. Ultimately, kidney function is compromised, which raises blood pressure even more, which contributes to further kidney damage, which raises blood pressure . . .

2. Because the stress response pretty much shuts down your gastrointestinal tract, your lunch turns into a mass of fermented and putrefying toxins. Over a period of time, this distress contributes significantly to several disorders, including ulcers, irritable bowel syndrome, colitis, constipation, diverticulosis, food allergy, yeast overgrowth, malnutrition, and colon cancer.

3. The glucose that is dumped into your blood goes unused, so the body has to produce an enormous amount of insulin to handle it. In time, this produces wild fluctuations in blood sugar. Elevated glucose accelerates glycation of vital proteins. Elevated insulin causes insulin resistance and ultimately diabetes. Because your muscles are not busy running or fighting, and therefore require no glucose, much of the glucose is converted to fat.

4. The fat that is dumped into your blood also goes unused, so it starts to clog your arteries.

5. Your adrenals become weakened and then exhausted. Because the adrenals contribute to the production and metabolism of some 150 hormones, you can imagine the downward spiral. Your blood pressure, brain and nervous system, energy metabolism, ability to manage stress, and immunity all suffer. There is not a cell in your body that is not affected.

And Now the Bad News . . .

The stress response causes the adrenals to decrease production of DHEA in favor of cortisol. We know that the immune suppression experienced by the graduate students in the Ohio State experiment was to a great extent caused by elevated cortisol and lowered DHEA. Declining DHEA is one trigger of the catabolic downward spiral, and we now know that it can begin a lot earlier than anyone previously thought.[1] Unfortunately, you can't continue to live a stress-filled life and simply compensate with a DHEA pill. That's like trying to fill a bucket with holes in it. Better patch the holes by dealing constructively with stress.

A COMPREHENSIVE RESPONSE TO STRESS

Although much of the information in this chapter has been stress-inducing, I'm just getting to the really good news—and it's *extraordinarily* good news. It confirms what researchers have suspected, which is that stress management confers direct, powerful, and measurable benefits in a fairly short period of time. Moreover, these benefits are cumulative, contributing to an upward anabolic spiral that can enrich your life in countless ways.

No, you don't have to sit in a cave and meditate (unless you want to); research has identified a wide range of effective techniques for any personality or lifestyle. The goal of stress management is not to eliminate stress but rather to transform it. Stress itself is not bad, especially when it leads to greater enjoyment of life or a more intense relationship with life. The people to whom I'm attracted incorporate a great deal of stress in their lives and use it to heighten their experience and expression of passion and vitality.

I like to think in terms of transforming stress into something positive: maximizing creativity, love, and joy. If you had a script and hated the ending, you'd revise it. Well, if you're not enjoying the script of your life, you have to understand that it can be revised, too. Please don't think I am trivializing the pressures and tragedies that life throws at us. I'm not saying that it's easy or simple to change your life. Sometimes, it's incredibly difficult, but it can be done—you just need the tools.

Change Without Stress

I think you'll agree that the primary stress trigger is *change*. Budget cuts, visits from in-laws, canceled flights, illness, the stock market, a new boss, teething babies, unexpected news of any type . . . Change is what pulls us out of our comfort zone. Thus, we have two choices when trying to reduce stress in our lives—either we stop change or we widen our comfort zones. Obviously, the first option is impossible. In fact, I think it's safe to say that change in our world will only continue to accelerate.

Widening our comfort zone is the same as saying *becoming more resilient*. And to give you a hint as to the most effective solution, let me ask you a question. Have you ever noticed that when grandparents came to visit, any slight change in plans was stressful to them, even though you were able to adapt and adjust quite easily? It's one of the most common causes of conflict when generations get together because older individuals are not nearly as resilient as young people. Grandma's ride to the airport is late. You tell her to relax because there's a later flight, but Grandma is falling apart. Why? Because she is experiencing the event in a completely different way. To you, it's an inconvenience. To her, it's a catastrophe.

Now, do you see that mental and emotional resilence is determined to a great degree by metabolism? In the early 1990s, researchers found that in dogs, low IGF-1 (that is, low anabolic metabolism) was associated with anxiety and panic (low emotional resilience).[2] Early researchers looking at DHEA were surprised to find extraordinarily high levels of the hormone in the brain and later discovered that the brain *manufactures* DHEA. Not surprisingly, they also learned that levels of this critical brain biochemical decline sharply with advancing years.

That led to experiments looking at the effects of restoring DHEA levels, and to some very surprising results. Working with an animal model, researchers discovered that DHEA had powerful anxiety-reducing effects, and the assumption was that it acted as a sedative, similar to Valium. Subsequent research, however, showed that DHEA was not a sedative at all—that the anxiety reduction was accompanied by improvements in mental acuity, decision making, memory, and learning ability.[3] Human studies have now confirmed the anxiety-reducing benefits of restored DHEA, and specific receptors in the brain have been identified.[4]

Turns out this is related to a well-known interaction between DHEA and the catabolic stress hormone known as cortisol. These two metabolic influences are always in a seesaw relationship, and scientists believe this is the crux of the age related decline of emotional and mental resilience. As we know, DHEA levels in the body and brain plummet as we age, while levels of cortisol tend to increase. This results in a dramatic shift in the cortisol-to-DHEA ratio, leading to a raft of maladies, including:

- *Poor sleep:* This is more than insomnia. People with an elevated cortisol/DHEA ratio can often get to sleep but either wake up often or, more important, are unable to get into deep (stage 4) sleep, which is where true healing and rejuvenation take place.

- *Fatigue:* This is not only related to poor sleep. Over time, elevations in cortisol result in lower metabolic efficiency. That means less energy being produced by trillions of cells throughout the body.

- *Memory loss:* Stress hormones, including cortisol, produce alterations in brain biochemistry in healthy people and especially those with Alzheimer's disease.[5] In Alzheimer's patients, those with higher levels of DHEA or lower cortisol performed better on memory and functioning tests.[6] Patients with depression showed improvements in memory as well as mood after raising their DHEA levels.[7]

- *Short-fuse syndrome:* Things that didn't bother you before are now irritating. Things that used to be irritating are now major stresses. This syndrome may include increased hostility.

- *Body aches; lower pain threshold.*

- *Excessive worry/anxiety.*

- *Depression.*

If this rings true for you—if you're finding the symptoms listed above increasing as the years go by—you now know there is a well-defined biochemical reason for it. This doesn't mean taking DHEA alone will make everything rosy, but it's a rational, safe, and critically important step that has been proved effective in well-controlled scientific studies.[8] Recently, a twenty-five-page analysis of animal and human research (with 308 references) was published in *Brain Research Reviews*.[9] It documented the ability of DHEA to:

- Enhance memory

- Reduce anxiety

- Improve feelings of well-being

- Improve mood

- Help protect against brain degeneration

The Evidence Mounts

This seesaw tipping to the catabolic side is accelerated by chronic fatigue syndrome, fibromyalgia, and adrenal insufficiency. All three conditions are associated with low levels of DHEA and other anabolic hormones.[10] In adrenal insufficiency, the adrenal glands simply cannot manufacture sufficient DHEA, and the cortisol/DHEA ratio of a forty-year-old patient might very well resemble that of a seventy-year-old. In 1999, an important paper was published in the prestigious *New England Journal of Medicine* showing that women with adrenal insufficiency experienced dramatic improvements when given DHEA.[11] Comprehensive psychological testing revealed that the women had less anxiety, better mood, fewer episodes of depression, and markedly improved feelings of well-being. What's more, these benefits led to precisely what you would imagine: higher sex drive, more frequent sex, and greater sexual satisfaction.

The issue here that is so often overlooked is that you don't have to wait for a diagnosis of adrenal insufficiency, chronic fatigue, or fibromyalgia before you take action to restore anabolic metabolism. You don't have to suffer with low emotional resilience and the spiral of self-doubt and distress. It's accurate to say that anyone over forty years of age has *some* degree of adrenal insufficiency.

DHEA has recently been shown to have physiological properties . . . which are associated with such psychophysiological phenomena as memory, stress, anxiety, sleep and depression. Therefore, the deficiency of DHEA might be related to the neuropsychiatric symptoms in patients with chronic fatigue syndrome.
          —H. Kuratsune et al., *"Dehydroepiandrosterone Sulfate*
          Deficiency in Chronic Fatigue Syndrome,"
          International Journal of Molecular Medicine

What About Depression?

Depression is one area in which enormous strides have been achieved, primarily due to the work of Dr. Owen Wolkowitz and his team of researchers at the Center for Neurobiology at the University of California in San Francisco. This group has performed double-blind, placebo-controlled clinical trials with DHEA and found it to be an effective antidepressant.[12] What makes this so promising, of course, is that Dr. Wolkowitz and his colleagues are simply restoring a natural hormone to the level that the body once produced. Interestingly, it appears again that the issue is not only the age-related decline in DHEA but the disruption in the anabolic/catabolic balance.[13] DHEA, in other words, may be the link between stress and depression. C. Norman Shealy, M.D., Ph.D., states, "We have never seen a depressed patient with optimal levels of DHEA. And no one we've seen with optimal levels of DHEA is depressed."[14]

The Stunning Reality of Age-Related Changes in the Balance of Cortisol (Catabolic) and DHEA (Anabolic) Metabolism

In men at age 70, the mean basal cortisol to DHEA ratio is increased about 10-fold over that of young men. There is a 40-fold increase in the mean cortisol to DHEA ratio of women age 70, relative to young

women. . . . Young and middle-aged individuals who have elevated cortisol to DHEA ratios, in the same range as the elderly, are likewise predicted to be at high risk for developing age-related disease.
        —O. Hechter, A. Grossman, and R. T. Chatterton Jr.,
        "Relationship of Dehydroepiandrosterone and Cortisol in Disease,"
                                    Medical Hypotheses

The Anabolic Spiral

I've described the upward spiral in which increased energy translates to more activity, greater muscle mass, and a renewed sense of confidence and power. Reading the medical literature, you might think this is a rather low-key series of events, because it's typically recorded as improvements in "well-being." That's because biomedical reviewers would edit out phrases like "awesome," "life-transforming," or "*I can't believe it.* I worked hard all day, went home, but instead of collapsing on the couch, I played with the kids and mowed the lawn. Then, that night, I made love with my wife for two hours and woke up feeling better than I have since I threw the winning touchdown in the game against Roosevelt High."

If that restoration of confidence and power sounds attractive to you right now, imagine what it will feel like for your parents and grandparents. Can you see that the decline in emotional and mental resilience associated with aging is very much related to a loss of physical strength, memory, and the ability to understand, analyze, and act on new information? Restoring anabolic metabolism can make a tremendous difference, and if we are in fact going to achieve life spans of 100-plus years, we'd better start thinking about this critical task.

The Other Side of the Coin

In looking at the catabolic/anabolic balance (that is, the ratio of cortisol to DHEA), I have been focusing on raising the anabolic side by restoring DHEA to youthful levels. But the other strategy—lowering the catabolic side of the equation—is equally effective. Stress-management counseling with AIDS patients has been shown to profoundly improve the cortisol/DHEA ratio and slow the progression of the disease.[15]

There are hundreds of organizations today that teach relaxation techniques, including biofeedback, self-hypnosis, creative visualization, breathing exercises, and more. One that stands out is the Institute of

HeartMath (IHM) in Boulder Creek, California. This nonprofit organization conducts a considerable amount of research, much of which has been published in national and international medical journals. IHM offers an array of books and tapes and also conducts resident programs in stress management. Its innovative technique, practiced for only one month, resulted in an average 100 percent increase in DHEA and a 23 percent decrease in cortisol.

This is very encouraging. IHM was not the first to document improvements in the DHEA/cortisol ratio after stress management, but these are certainly the best results obtained so far. Just think: by reducing the number of stress hormones coursing through the bloodstream, a person naturally starts producing more DHEA. More DHEA means greater energy, enhanced mental and emotional health, and a cascade of positive effects throughout the body.

The Pace of Change

Life in the twenty-first century is just too fast-paced and stressful. We all need proactive tools to manage change. We all need support from friends, family, and community. We need quiet time. Although I've focused a lot of attention on strength and action, I don't mean to give the impression that depression, anxiety, and fear can be easily banished by a sufficient amount of activity. This is not a "Hey, snap out of it!" approach, and while exercise, walking, biking, and other activities can do much to "change the channels of the mind," there is also a need for stillness. Fortunately, there are many ways to experience the centering we all need in a chaotic world. Virtually all religious traditions incorporate some form of alignment with the holy, be it silent or sung, in which worshipers tap into a power that transcends human limitations. This is a critical exercise—and one that has been shown to be profoundly strengthening, in terms of both wellness and longevity.[16]

Speaking of Lowering Stress Hormones

Did you know that millions of people intentionally raise their stress hormone levels every day, sometimes multiple times a day? Were you aware that there is an entire industry dedicated to ensuring that you go speeding down the catabolic highway as fast as possible? This is, of course, the caffeine industry, which spends hundreds of millions in advertising dollars every year to convince you to drink soft drinks and coffee as a way to "refresh yourself." Nothing could be further from the truth.

The principal myth, of course, is that caffeine gives you energy. In truth, caffeine gives you stress, which *feels* like energy when you're tired. The reason for this confusion has to do with another of those ancient survival mechanisms that still function in our twenty-first-century bodies—this one being that stress intensifies sensory perception.

This neurological wiring was very handy thirty thousand years ago. Danger appeared, stress hormones shot through the body, and the brain filed everything associated with that event with a red sticker that said: *Don't forget this. You almost got killed.* Today, there are very few club-wielding foes trying to do us in, so instead, we get the same increased alertness by drinking caffeine. The problem is that long-term, this stress will harm you. Please look at the damaging effects presented in the "Effects of Chronic Stress" list earlier in this chapter. Every one of those things happens when you drink coffee or slam your adrenals with soft drinks.

Of course, it's all dose-related. A little caffeine is a little catabolic. A lot of caffeine can potentially cancel out every advantage of the Metabolic Plan. The trouble is that no one can tell you what's safe. A 160-pound man drinking a sixteen-ounce cup of coffee at breakfast may be able to detoxify the caffeine by lunch and clear the excess cortisol out of his bloodstream by dinner. He sleeps like a rock, while his 110-pound wife lies beside him tossing and turning. She had the same cup of coffee for breakfast, but women detoxify caffeine much more slowly than men (primarily due to a smaller liver). Thus, her second cup at midmorning and her soft drink with lunch had a cumulative effect, sufficient to cause an alteration in her personality. Of course, all her friends just assume that she's "naturally" high-strung, and she herself has no idea that the creeping anxiety that gnaws at her in the middle of the night is not a sign of neurosis—it's caffeine.

The pervasive effect of caffeine is no joking matter. One client who kicked the habit told me, "It's as though a cloud has been lifted from my body and mind. I had no idea that I was such an angry and frustrated person." That's what I call the *long-burn* effect of cortisol. It's subtle but serious, and reducing or eliminating caffeine has been shown to greatly improve the success rate of a variety of therapeutic and stress-management programs.[17]

How to Get Off the Bean

You may have tried to quit caffeine already but experienced a pounding headache that quickly drove you back to your coffee cup. Perhaps you didn't know that the headache is due to increased circulation to the brain, something we all need. Caffeine, you see, tightly constricts blood vessels in the brain (part of the stress response). When you stop drinking coffee or soft drinks, normal circulation is restored, producing a temporary but excruciating headache.

To avoid the headache, fatigue, and depression associated with caffeine withdrawal, simply go slow. Wean yourself off caffeine so that your brain gets used to its normal flow of oxygen. You may also need help in restoring natural energy production or dealing with rebound constipation. These are not difficult to overcome as long as you know what's happening.

Remember, the reason for limiting caffeine is to restore anabolic metabolism and live a longer, healthier life. If you've been consuming a lot of caffeine for a decade or more, your body will need to undergo a significant amount of repair. Fortunately, it's never too late to begin. You'll read in Chapter 7 about an exciting group of substances known as bioenergetic nutrients. They can help restore your body's production of energy because they provide the raw materials your body needs to maximize metabolic efficiency. I highly recommend that you begin using these energizing nutrients *while* you're weaning yourself off caffeine.

There are basically two ways to get off caffeine:

1. *Cold turkey:* This is a mistake. Don't do it.

2. *Weaning—the no-headache, no-hassle method:* This works great when more than one person is trying to get off the bean, because everyone can drink from the same pot. Here you simply brew or mix your coffee with small amounts of decaf or herbal coffee (caffeine-free blends made with a variety of healthful herbs) and continue drinking the same number of cups. Over a two-week period, you gradually increase the amount of decaf or herbal coffee until you're drinking zero caffeine. Because there is no dramatic decrease in blood caffeine levels, you'll be decaffeinated and headache-free.

   Importantly, this method enables you to get used to new tastes, and if you're using herbal coffee (see Appendix A), these tastes will be surprisingly rich and enjoyable. If you use instant coffee, you can also blend it with an instant coffee *substitute* following the same technique. These grain-based beverages are sold in your natural foods store or supermarket.

Just Want to Cut Back?

I know. The idea of *quitting* caffeine might be daunting. Here are some tips that can help you reduce caffeine intake to a safer level:

- *Get a smaller coffee mug.* Over time, the body becomes accustomed to the influence of caffeine, so to get the same "jolt," we have to increase the dose—thus, the convenience-store thirty-two-ounce mugs with vented lids. That's not a cup of coffee; it's five cups in one container. Well, this can also work in reverse. Start decreasing the size of your cup until you get down to a reasonable ten to twelve ounces. That'll deliver about 165 milligrams of caffeine, which still might be too much for some people, but it's a step in the right direction.

- *Make your coffee weaker.* Whether you brew your coffee or use instant, you can decrease the amount that you use.

- *Add more milk.* If you already take milk with your coffee, simply add more. If this is not your habit, give it a try. Adding low-fat milk reduces the amount of coffee in the cup and decreases your caffeine intake. Plus the milk provides a valuable source of calcium and protein.

Cola Drinkers

Your task is to reduce both your caffeine intake and your sugar or aspartame consumption. For the first week, alternate each can of your normal soft drink with a juice–mineral water combination that has under 10 grams of sugar. Try some of the herb tea and juice blends found in health food stores. In week 2, start substituting caffeine-free colas for some of your cans of caffeinated cola.

By week 3, you can be off soda altogether and enjoying healthful beverages while you continue to get used to less and less sugar. After a month of being soda-free, if you've successfully reduced your sugar intake, too, you won't even like the overly sweet taste of colas anymore.

Important: No matter what method you use to decrease caffeine intake, you will need to make a concerted effort to *drink more water*. We'll discuss this in detail in Chapter 9, but right now, make sure always to have a container of water handy and drink small amounts throughout the day. Don't forget, thirst is what often drives us to the coffee pot or soda machine. If you stay hydrated, you can eliminate this trigger.

Brain-Defogging Aids

In the first stages of recovery from caffeine abuse, you may find that you can't organize your thoughts as effectively as you did when you were on caffeine. Caffeine creates a highly alert phase, and although this is followed by fatigue a few hours later, most caffeine users simply have more caffeine. This is the essential characteristic of addiction. Nevertheless, when you first get off caffeine, you may benefit from some nutritional support to overcome adrenal exhaustion. The following substances have proved helpful.

- *Ginkgo biloba:* Ginkgo improves cerebral circulation, dilates peripheral blood vessels throughout the body, and increases memory retention and concentration.[18] As such, ginkgo's effects on the body are essentially the reverse of caffeine's. Moreover, the herb protects brain neurons against free-radical damage, and evidence suggests that it may even be helpful in the prevention and treatment of Alzheimer's disease.[19] I recommend that everyone quitting coffee begin taking ginkgo extract, 24 percent standardized concentrate, in dosages of 50 milligrams to 100 milligrams daily during the first two weeks of withdrawal.

- *Gotu kola:* Gotu kola can help rebuild mental stamina, increase mental ability, and improve memory and learning retention.[20] It can also help you overcome the negative effects of stress and fatigue. The herb has been used in India for centuries, where it is reputed to be a "rejuvenator." Gotu kola doesn't contain caffeine, although it is often confused with kola nut, which does contain caffeine.

- *Berry concentrates:* Animal research published in the *Journal of Neuroscience* showing that blueberry concentrate can restore brain function has set off a flurry of articles about the mental-clarity benefits of berries. A number of compounds found in blueberries, including antioxidants and flavonoids, have nervous system–modulating activity (see Chapter 3), but don't expect to get a buzz from blueberry jam. There's not enough fruit and far too much sugar to benefit brain function. Instead, look for high-potency, sugar-free berry concentrates. I have found that one or two ounces can dramatically improve mental clarity, especially when the midafternoon "fog" rolls in.

SUMMARY: BEATING THE STRESS EPIDEMIC

Can there be any doubt that stress had reached epidemic proportions in this country? Health experts tell us that roughly 80 percent of all doctor visits are for stress-related disorders. We know the effects of stress on the body, mind, and emotions, but sometimes it seems as if we're caught on a treadmill like mice in a cage.

The treadmill analogy is not far off. While you're on it, there doesn't seem to be any escape from stress, and it's precisely that feeling of help-lessness that creates the damage. How many times have you looked back at a stressful situation and seen with perfect clarity what would have been the ideal course of action? But while you were in the thick of it, all you could feel was intense anger or fear. It's those thirty-thousand-year-old genes again. The dangers you are wired to deal with were episodes of immediate peril in which every ounce of energy and attention had to be mobilized to fight or flee. And here we are in the time-warp present, in which stress is entirely different. It's a kettle of soup ready to boil over at any moment.

Proactive Responses to Stress

The solution is hidden in the above paragraph. First of all, turn down the heat under the kettle. That means eliminating as much of the back-ground stress as you can. Reduce your intake of caffeine. Turn off the television set. Get together with your family, friends, or church and develop better support systems. Trade baby-sitting with a neighbor. Reach out for help, and help others whenever you can. We're all in this together.

Second, take some of the soup out of the kettle. That means simplifying your life as much as you can. If you're working an extra job so you can afford a boat, ask yourself if the cost to your health and the time away from your family are worth it. If you're going crazy driving your kids all over town, ask yourself if they really need to be enrolled in twenty different activities every day of the week. Think about community. For millennia, we lived in tribal organizations in which all tasks were shared. Tribal societies today illustrate this tremendous advantage in terms of both sharing responsibilities and creating more free time.

I believe we can gain a great deal through cooperative efforts. Not just logistical endeavors like car pools but meal sharing, walking clubs, block parties, potluck dinners, and discussion and reading groups. We tend to come together when there is a disaster. How about coming together to *prevent* disasters?

Closer Than Community

An intimate relationship with a significant other is also a powerful health and longevity factor. Close relationships provide a safe harbor amid the storms of life.[21] And it's not only that there is someone there to "lean on." Research shows that intimate relationships bring out the best in us. We maintain a sense of emotional resilience, dealing with the vicissitudes of life with more patience, understanding, and creativity.

Food for Thought

Eating right is obviously very important, but what's right? There are many conflicting theories (which tends to be stressful), but the issue boils down to a simple question: What is the human body *designed* to eat? The answer, backed by a great deal of excellent research, is the hunting-and-gathering diet: frequent small meals consisting mainly of plant foods, supplemented with a variety of protein sources and whole grains.

The stress-management benefits of this style of eating derive from what it omits (sugar and highly processed and chemicalized food) as well as what it includes (a wide variety of fruits and vegetables). New research shows that many of the flavonoids found in fresh fruits and vegetables have potent stress-management effects. Many of these compounds actually bind to the same brain receptors to which Valium binds. The result is a calming effect, but *without* the sedation and addictive potential of drug tranquilizers.[22] It's amazing what a natural foods diet provides in addition to vitamins and minerals.

To Sleep, Perchance to Rejuvenate

One of the first things people notice on the Metabolic Plan is that they're sleeping better—getting to sleep faster, staying asleep, achieving a deeper level of sleep, and consequently waking up more alert and rested. This has enormous antiaging benefits that cannot be obtained from any hormone, vitamin, pill, or potion. That's because your body uses the deepest level of sleep (known as stage 4) as an opportunity to shift into high-gear rejuvenation. The immune system accelerates healing, the nervous system repairs itself, and billions of cells are replaced or repaired every time you go into stage 4 sleep.

The importance of deep and restful sleep cannot be overstated. Everyone knows what it feels like to be truly rested. But most of us cheat on our sleep hours because of the pressure and deadlines we're under. If you presently do not sleep soundly or awake feeling tired, you may find that simply reducing your caffeine intake solves your problem. If you need additional help, try the following suggestions to help produce a deep, restful, rejuvenating sleep.

- *Regular exercise is a key factor.* When you enter the first level of sleep (stage 1), the brain queries the muscles to find out how much rest the body needs. If the muscles say, "Gee, boss, we haven't moved all day," the brain will set the sleep cycle differently than if the muscles are tired. Now, you don't have to be exhausted to get a good night's sleep, but well-exercised muscles send a message to the brain so that you enter a deeply restoring level of sleep.

  Note: It is best *not* to exercise strenuously right before bed, as the increased metabolic activity can impair your ability to fall asleep.

- *Develop regular sleep habits.* Researchers from the Department of Psychiatry at the University of Arizona have demonstrated that going to bed at the same time each night can significantly enhance sleep quality even in healthy people who are not sleep-deprived.[23] In their study, two groups of students were asked to sleep at least 7.5 hours each night, but one group was instructed to keep a regular sleep schedule, while the other group varied their bedtime from 10:00 P.M. to midnight. Compared with the sleep-only group, subjects in the regularity group demonstrated:

> Decreased daytime fatigue
> Greater and longer-lasting improvements in alertness
> Greater sleep efficiency (they fell asleep faster and stayed asleep through the night)

These benefits were realized after only four weeks.

- *Take the TV out of the bedroom.* In addition to giving you a reason to stay up late, watching television before bed can—depending on what you watch—bring the mind into a highly vigilant state, exactly when you want it to relax.

- *Reset your internal clock.* Eight hours of sleep beginning at 10:00 P.M. is more restful than eight hours starting after midnight. In other words, if you sleep from 10:00 P.M. to 6:00 A.M., you'll have more energy and vitality than if you slept from 1:00 A.M. to 9:00 A.M. You'll also get more done in the early morning than you will late at night after an exhausting day.

- *Eliminate ambient noise.* A HEPA (high-efficiency particulate air) filter can double as a white-noise machine, effectively covering up the disruptive noise of traffic, barking dogs, and the neighbor's stereo. Heavy drapes are also a sound investment, reducing both noise and light.

- *Don't use alcohol to wind down at the end of the day.* One glass of wine with dinner is normally fine, but excess alcohol will disturb your sleep cycle. Typically, you'll fall asleep easily but awaken in the night and have trouble getting back to sleep.

- *Take a bath before bed.* The water should be relaxingly warm but not overly hot. Add your favorite bath oil, gel, or bath salts and soak your cares away.

- *Use a deep relaxation technique or audiotape.* Tapes are available that combine soothing music or nature sounds with an effective guided relaxation voice-over (see Appendix A).

- *Herbs and nutrients.* Try one or more of the following just before bed to help induce sleep:

  Melatonin: This is a natural hormone produced by your brain that sets your sleep/wake cycle. Start with a very low dose (0.25 milligrams) in a sublingual (held under the tongue) tablet ten to fifteen minutes before bed.

  Sedative herbal extracts: Valerian, kava, chamomile, and a Chinese herb known as *Ziziphus spinosa* can all be effective in a capsule, tincture, or tea.

  Calcium citrate: Take 200 to 500 milligrams.

  Magnesium citrate: Take 200 to 400 milligrams.

  A mug of herbal tea with milk.

  A mug of warm milk and honey: The calcium helps you relax, and the honey is soothing.

CONCLUSION

As you've probably noticed, this book has a lot to do with understanding how we are programmed by millions of years of evolution. This long view provides all sorts of important clues for winning nature's game. You realize that we are, in every respect, natural creatures tied to nature in profound and powerful ways.

The fact that we have invented electric lights does not mean that sleep is no longer important for health and wellness. The fact that we have invented automobiles, television, and computers doesn't mean that we can become sedentary and not suffer terribly at some point. Sure, we have invented sugar, hydrogenated fat, caffeine, artificial colors, white flour, modified food starch, margarine, and a long list of pseudofoods, but that does not mean that these things are harmless when consumed day after day.

For millions of years, we ate nothing but whole, natural foods. We drank nothing but pure, clean water. We slept all night and kept active through most of the day. Those are the conditions for which we are designed, and to a great extent, our efforts to manage stress and enjoy optimal health come down to duplicating these simple behaviors as closely as possible. The good news, of course, is that with exercise technology, nutrition science, and brain research, we have incredible tools that our ancestors never had. The secret is to take advantage of what can truly be *the best of both worlds.*

What Do You *Really* Want?

And now for a different view you may not have considered. I'd like to suggest that there are different *levels* of stress, all the way from the obvious (traffic tickets, a fight with your spouse) to the partially hidden (caffeine addiction) to a level that is entirely hidden and quite subtle.

The subtle level of stress may be hard to see, but it is no less important. It involves a deep frustration that we all experience having to do with the way we define happiness. Now, stay with me here. This is not an abstract philosophical discussion. It's something I think you'll enjoy exploring. We'll start with a simple question: What is everyone's bottom-line core desire?

Answer: "To be happy." Correct? And although people define happiness in vastly different ways, all of these boil down to . . . what?

Answer: "Happiness is getting what I want."

I would like you to consider that this way of seeing the world sets one up for a deep level of stress, for the simple reason that the universe is not designed to provide you with everything you want. In fact, you've probably noticed that two things happen with frustrating regularity:

1. You don't get what you want.

2. You get what you don't want.

Thus, if you try to set up your life so that you experience all joy and no sorrow, life will be very stressful. This condition saps our energy and creates a great deal of unhappiness. Dealing effectively with this level of stress first requires us to recognize and accept the concept of *balance* in life. Life is not and cannot be an unbroken succession of good things. We are complex beings who experience life on several interrelated levels—physical, mental, emotional, and spiritual. Total absence of all pain, loss, and stress—be it from death, illness, job pressures, or family discord—might be experienced as pure pleasure on one level, but it would also ensure a lack of growth on others. It is through dealing with stress that we find opportunities to grow as human beings, to examine our lives—our hearts, minds, and spirits—and to mature in our appreciation for all aspects of the miraculous experience of life.

Life is not about avoiding stress at all costs. It is not about fleeing from anything that might make you sad in order to maintain the impossible illusion of constant happiness. Serenity is not found by hiding in a cave but in meeting the challenges of life in creative and effective ways.

I believe that happiness is not something you can get or manipulate or buy at any price. Happiness is something that happens when you create the right conditions. Like sleep. Can you make yourself fall asleep? No, but you can create the conditions wherein sleep happens. You turn off the lights, pull down the shades, fluff up your pillow, and close your eyes.

In fact, I'm of the opinion that nothing really precious or important happens because we *make* it happen. All the precious things in life are gifts. You don't decide to fall in love or to cry with joy at the sight of your child in her first school play. You don't try to enjoy a sunset or thrill to the sound of a symphony. But these things happen when you behave in certain ways, when you are open to life—not as you would narrowly define it, but life as it is.

I'm certainly not the first one to consider such things. You'll find a list of excellent books in Appendix A that can provide valuable insights into this modern dilemma. Some, like *The Art of Happiness: A Handbook for Living,* by the Dalai Lama and Howard Culter, provide specific exercises designed to expand your sense of appreciation for the totality of life. One could call this an unconditioned awareness, in that it frees us from all of the conditions that we place upon our happiness.

A valuable question to ask yourself is, "What is preventing me from being blissfully happy at this very moment?" Most people have a subconscious list of conditions that must be met before they can be happy. They have to finish school, have financial security, find the perfect mate, or live in the perfect house. I would like to suggest that such lists are never-ending and that experiencing true happiness necessitates dispensing with such conditions.

That doesn't mean that you stop looking for a life-mate or the perfect house, only that these blessings are no longer *requirements* for your happiness. Instead, they become an *expression* of your joy at being fully alive.

FIVE

How Good Do You Want to Look and Feel?

LOOKING YOUNG

Recently, I was presenting the metabolic model of aging at a conference for health care professionals. The audience included a wide range of practitioners, evenly divided between men and women, and the predominant age range was forty to sixty. In other words, they were mostly baby boomers. I was supposed to make a summary statement and, departing from the scientific format, decided to put the whole thing into perspective by asking a personal question.

"Imagine," I said, "that you are single and actively looking for a mate. You're at the stage in life where flings are not so attractive. You've gained a lot of wisdom and experience, and you're looking for a life-mate with matching interests and energy. Which would you prefer, a thirty-year-old who looks and performs like a fifty-year-old or a fifty-year-old who looks and performs like a thirty-year-old?"

The question got a lot of smiles because it took the whole concept of biological versus chronological age out of the realm of theory and into real life. Almost everyone said they would prefer the youthful fifty-year-old. "Good," I said. "Now I *know* you understand the metabolic model of aging."

The point, of course, is that chronological age is now irrelevant. It no longer matters what year you were born. The only thing that matters is how you look, feel, and perform. That determines your quality of life, including your attractiveness to potential mates.

For a television interview program, I was asked to bring a "success story"—someone who had followed the Metabolic Plan and achieved good results. I asked Susan G. to join me, and she made quite an impression. When she announced that she was almost fifty, the audience gasped, because she looked like a fit thirty-year-old. After the host verified this by examining her driver's license, he suggested that she probably spent a lot of time in health clubs and spas, implying that she had a leisurely life. "Actually, no," replied Susan. "I'm a single mom and teach elementary English and reading." Taken aback, he suggested that she must have good genes. She replied that she was a polio survivor and had struggled with additional health problems—such as insomnia, fatigue, and headaches—all her life.

Only then did he understand that Susan had accomplished something remarkable. She described how she now sleeps like a rock, how she lost weight, vastly improved her energy, and gained not only muscle but a renewed sense of confidence and inner strength. I said very little on this show because Susan personified every one of the points I would have talked about.

How to Look Good in Your Genes

We are all born with a genetic "package" that determines to some extent how we look. The genetic influence, however, is not as significant as you might think. Certainly, genes determine hair and eye color and general characteristics. Male-pattern baldness is purely genetic, as are diseases such as cystic fibrosis, sickle-cell disease, and Down's syndrome. There are also genes that increase our risk for diseases such as heart disease, breast and colon cancer, and Alzheimer's. Obesity certainly has a genetic component, but the prevailing view right now is that appearance is pretty much a do-it-yourself endeavor.

Metabolism and Your Skin

Of all the skin care products sold in the world, two account for more than 80 percent of sales: moisturizers and alpha-hydroxy/glycolic acids. The most common medical cosmetic procedure is collagen injections. What do all three have in common? They're only necessary as your metabolism becomes more catabolic. In fact, using these treatments is another form of symptom stomping: none of them deals with the underlying cause of wrinkles, lines, and sagging jawlines.

Moisturizers

It is said that we're born grapes and turn into raisins. The loss of moisture in the skin is reflective of a systemic dehydration that is part and parcel of the aging process. We all learned in school that the human body is 70 percent water, but that's only true if you're highly anabolic. The hydration level of most adults is 50 to 60 percent, and the reasons for this have a lot to do with loss of muscle (which holds water), accumulation of fat (which displaces water), and a raft of absurd habits, including the consumption of dehydrating beverages like soft drinks, coffee, tea, and alcohol. I'll cover this in detail in Chapter 9, but it's accurate to say that most American adults are perpetually dehydrated.

Nothing could be worse for your appearance. Water is the fountain of life for hundreds of billions of skin cells, which are growing, migrating to the surface, and sloughing off to make room for new cells. The biology of your skin involves water at every level. Every biochemical reaction, from the synthesis of collagen to the healing of microscopic wounds to the generation of new cells and the tone, strength, and appearance of every square inch of your skin depends entirely on the availability of adequate water.

Of course, that's not the only problem. Health-conscious people who drink plenty of water still get wrinkly. That's the metabolic side of dehydration. As we age, changes take place in the skin that allow water to evaporate from within and between the cells. I'm not talking about perspiration, which is temporary. This type of water loss is called *insensible:* you can't feel it, but it leaves you looking dry and old. So you turn to moisturizers, which work not by adding moisture to your skin but simply by forming an occlusive barrier to prevent the evaporation of water that's already there.

What if you could do the same thing, not by slathering your skin with expensive oils but by restoring the *natural* barrier mechanism of the top layer of skin known as the stratum corneum? That's the true metabolic solution, and it has nothing to do with water, even though the end result is that the water content of your skin will greatly improve. It has to do with an oily substance that keeps water in—a combination of cholesterol, ceramides, and fatty acids produced by the skin.

Importantly, this oil layer also plays a critical role in *keeping out* substances that might be injurious to the skin, such as chemicals, external toxins, and microbes. It even offers protection against ultraviolet radiation and injury from heat or cold.[1] The sad part is that you start producing less of this protective, beautifying, moisture-retaining fluid at about age twenty-eight.

• **Getting Back That Youthful Glow** Remember the oily skin problems you had as a teenager? The good news is that you don't have to go that far back. One of the hormones that had you running for the medicated cleansing pads when you were sixteen is DHEA, and restoring just a fraction of that in your later years can make a tremendous difference. Research shows that men and women (but especially women) taking DHEA experience significant improvements in the moisture, thickness, oil production, and overall appearance of their skin.[2]

Alpha-Hydroxy and Glycolic Acids

If you ask the salespeople at cosmetics counters what alpha-hydroxy and glycolic acids do, they'll say that they help slough off old dead skin cells so that new and (presumably) healthier cells can rise to the surface. That's half correct. What they don't tell you (what they generally don't even know) is that these acids kill millions of skin cells, and *then* you slough them off with a brisk rub with a towel. And that's OK. In fact, that's a good thing because we now know that one of the problems associated with old skin cells is that they don't die when they're supposed to. That's one reason why old skin looks old. It stops renewing itself.

The question is, why would old skin cells lose their ability to die and be replaced? Basically, it's an energy-saving feature of your amazing body. As you enter the catabolic, over-the-hill phase, the brain starts looking for ways to economize. The accumulation of fat represents such economy. Compared to muscle, fat is much easier to make and requires very little energy to maintain. Likewise, replacing what amounts to trillions of skin cells every year is quite a job. If you're over-the-hill, the body says, "Why bother?" and increases a biochemical known as alpha-fetoprotein (AFP). AFP interferes with programmed cell death, or apoptosis, and thus, the old, dry, and inflexible skin remains.

• **_Beating AFP from the Inside_** Dr. Marian Laderoute, a pathologist in Ontario, Canada, discovered this exciting connection. She found that the level of alpha-fetoprotein in the skin increases with advancing age. She also knew that DHEA inhibits AFP and was the first to propose that the appearance of wrinkles, lines, and old-looking skin is significantly caused by declining DHEA.

At this point, you may be wondering if it's better to take DHEA in tablet form or as a topical cream; the answer is, probably both. At the moment, though, no one has a reliable DHEA facial cream, but I'd imagine they are on the drawing boards of many skin care and cosmetics labs.

A NOTE ON ESSENTIAL FATS

Essential fatty acids, or EFAs (sometimes called vitamin F), are critically important to the health of your entire body, but especially your skin. DHEA sends an anabolic rebuild-repair-restore signal, but your body cannot follow this instruction without raw materials.

Today, the majority of Americans are consuming inadequate levels of EFAs. That may surprise you, knowing that, as a nation, we consume almost 40 percent of our total calories from fat. But the fat we consume in such prodigious quantities is, for the most part, nonessential. A better descriptor would be artery-clogging, cell membrane–destabilizing, cancer- and heart disease–promoting fats.

You get the picture. Essential fats are just that—essential. You cannot succeed in an antiaging or optimum health program without them. Nonessential fats will put you in an early grave.

How to Tell the Difference

Essential fats come from vegetables, grains, nuts, beans, and fish. Nonessential fats come from animals. Wasn't that easy? It gets a bit more complicated when you learn that food processors take essential fats (from soybeans, for example) and convert them to nonessential fats by hydrogenating them. So in addition to limiting your intake of fats from pigs, cows, and chickens, it's a good idea to avoid processed fats like hydrogenated and partially hydrogenated oils.

On the plus side, look to increase your intake of essential fats from vegetables (such as avocados), whole grains, unprocessed nuts and seeds, and oils from cold-water fish, olives, flax seeds, and the seeds of evening primrose, borage, and black currant. More information on essential fats is available in Chapter 8 (in the section entitled "Metabolic Factor 4: Longevity Foods").

Collagen Injections: Banking on Catabolic Customers

When people notice that the strong lines of the jaw, eyes, and cheeks are starting to sag, they often run to the plastic surgeon. Some get a face-lift, but many start with collagen injections. These injections add definition to the face, thicken the lips, and create a more youthful appearance. Unfortunately, if you are highly catabolic, your body will start breaking down this collagen with an enzyme known as *collagenase* before your credit card is back in your purse. End result: you'll be back for more injections in six or eight weeks.

The real solution is to make your own collagen by restoring anabolic metabolism, and put the brakes on catabolic collagenase. Then, even if you feel that you need injections, at least they will last a great deal longer.

• ***More Collagen Education*** Fibroblasts are important cells that predominate in the skin. They float in a sea of collagen and act as microscopic repair kits. When the skin is injured by stress, puncture, cut, or ultraviolet light, the fibroblasts produce collagen to mend and repair the damage. This new collagen keeps the skin healthy, thick, and smooth. The health of your skin depends to a great extent on the ability of fibroblasts to clone and multiply as the years march on.

But as we age, fibroblasts start producing a lot more collagenase than collagen, thus contributing to the breakdown of the vital elastic material that keeps skin soft and flexible. Just another piece of the catabolic puzzle. You already know from Chapter 3 that aloe vera (topical or ingested) has the remarkable ability to stimulate fibroblast collagen production, and so does DHEA. A study published in the *Journal of Dermatological Science* illustrates that DHEA increases collagen levels (anabolic restoration) and at the same time provides significant anti-catabolic benefits by reducing production of collagenase. The researchers conclude that DHEA plays a key role in skin aging by regulating the synthesis and breakdown of this important protein.[3]

• ***Glutathione (Again)*** Certainly, one of the most damaging factors in skin health is exposure to the sun. Even without getting a sunburn, our skin is damaged when ultraviolet radiation (UVA and UVB) stimulates the production of hydroxyl radicals. And what's the body's first line of defense against hydroxyl radicals? You guessed it, glutathione. In cases in which the skin is reddened by exposure, the massive free-radical production can overwhelm glutathione resources and compound the damage. Conversely, by optimizing glutathione production in the skin, free-radical damage can be prevented.[4]

• ***Repairing Old Damage*** In addition to free-radical damage, UV radiation alters the skin's immune response, which makes you more vulnerable to subsequent infection and even increases your risk for skin cancer many years later. Conventional wisdom holds that you cannot reverse the changes in deep levels of the skin resulting from UV damage, but that's why it's called conventional. Researchers at Unigen Pharmaceuticals in Broomfield, Colorado, have created an aloe vera extract with remarkable restorative power, and preliminary data shows that immunity may be restored even years after the damage is done.[5]

Metabolism and Body Composition

Health and self-image have a great deal to do with the ratio of muscle to fat, and it makes no sense to talk about one without the other. I know that diet promoters have done it for half a century—talked about losing fat without mentioning anything about muscle—and that's why diets don't work.

Catabolism = Defeat and Failure

Diets *don't* work—and by diets, I mean the conventional low-calorie approach—because they're inherently catabolic. You lose weight by starvation, which sends metabolism in the *wrong direction*. Remember that nature's game is *survival*. Remember that your genes haven't changed in thirty thousand years. These genes don't know that there's a refrigerator in the next room chock-full of calories. All they know is that when caloric intake is reduced (when you go on a diet), it means trouble, possibly death by starvation. And so the ancient DNA response is an alarm that says, "Emergency. Dramatic reduction in food intake. Lower metabolic rate to survival mode, decrease all unnecessary metabolic functions, store every gram of food as fat. This is an emergency. Lower metabolic rate . . ."

I am not exaggerating. The decrease in metabolic rate (calorie burning) for people on weight-loss diets can be as much as 30 percent. Even worse, the body cranks out lipoprotein lipase (LLP), an enzyme that increases the conversion of food (any food) to fat. Both of these effects are long-lasting. Thus, when hapless dieters go back to normal eating, they are primed to gain an enormous amount of weight.

Never think in terms of *weight* loss—think of *fat* loss. The term *weight loss* should be banned, because anytime you lose muscle, you have harmed yourself. You have lost highly anabolic tissue that's essential for maintaining ideal weight. Virtually all conventional diets cause the loss of muscle and are therefore catabolic. You may lose weight, but you accelerate aging. The most catabolic diets are those employing stimulants such as caffeine and the herbs ma huang (ephedra), kola nut, bissy nut, and guarana. These are not only catabolic; they're dangerous. (Imagine friends and relatives peering into the coffin . . . "My, wasn't she slim!")

The Metabolic Solution

There were no overweight cavepeople. Overweight people are a new development in the human experience, the result of two fundamental alterations of environment and behavior. First, of course, is the availability of limitless calories. For 3.5 million years, we had to work for our food. Hunters and gatherers expended approximately 2,000 calories in order to obtain 4,000 calories, for a net gain of 2,000 calories per day, which kept them both alive and fit. Today, one can easily consume 1,200 calories (a thick shake) and burn only 7 calories in the process of lifting the thirty-two-ounce cup of saturated fat and sugar to one's lips.

Then there's exercise. For millions of years, exercise was a part of life. Getting enough rest was the problem. Today, we face the opposite problem and wonder why the United States is the fattest nation in the history of the world. I'm not going to beat you over the head with statistics or give you a long list of diseases associated with obesity. I want to give you the secret to real and long-lasting fat loss. You've probably guessed it already. It's the anabolic key, the thing that will enable you never to diet again, ever. It's called muscle mass.

Of course, it's easy to say, "Gain muscle and let the muscle burn the fat." But for people in the catabolic stage of life, gaining muscle is difficult—thus, the dismal failure of exercise programs for overweight people. As we saw in Chapter 2, you first have to restore anabolic metabolism to improve metabolic efficiency. This results in greater energy, which you then use for exercise, and lo and behold, you get results. Assuming you have a sensible diet, the increased muscle burns plenty of fat.

I know. You think that's too long a process. You have a class reunion coming up in six weeks, and you want to lose twenty-five pounds. Sorry, I can't help you there. But if you're interested in getting off the diet roller coaster, Mother Nature offers an ideal weight plan with an unbeatable success rate (3.5 million years). And even if you're not over-fat (yet), the plan still works wonders. Why? Because muscle makes you look and feel great.

I'm not talking about Ahnold-type muscles. For men, looking young requires only a modicum of definition in the chest and arms and a relatively flat abdomen. For women, a small increase in muscle mass can be life-changing. It increases feelings of confidence and power. It improves energy and immunity. The problem, once again, is metabolism. As we'll discuss in Chapter 7, you cannot hope to succeed if you are highly catabolic. You won't gain muscle, and the effort is likely to result in injury. Everything hinges on restoring anabolic metabolism and gaining muscle. Then you let the muscle work magic in your life.

Yoga is a wonderful practice that can increase energy, stamina, and with the right metabolism, muscle mass. At the same time, it's also one of the best stress-management techniques. There are different styles of yoga that vary in focus—everything from gentle stretching to super-strenuous workouts. I suggest that you interview a prospective instructor to communicate your goals and learn as much as you can about the style he or she teaches. Then "sample" a number of classes until you find one that's right for you.

For thirty years, I've practiced (and often teach) a style of yoga known as Integral Yoga, which provides an extraordinary range of benefits. One of my yoga students was a slightly built woman in her mid-fifties named Dorothy. She came up one day after class and said that her whole life had changed. "How did that happen?" I asked. "It happened," she replied, "when I opened a door." Thinking that she was speaking metaphorically, I smiled and asked what kind of door. "A big, heavy door in the hallway at the university," she said. Dorothy went on to explain that she was a college instructor and that every day for ten years, she had stood in front of this heavy door, clutching her books and waiting for someone to open it for her. After hearing my presentation on anabolic metabolism, Dorothy started on the Metabolic Plan. About two months later, without even thinking, she reached the hallway door, slung a pile of books under one arm, and with her free hand, opened the door and walked through.

From that moment, she was a new woman. She realized that she had accepted many limitations in life based upon feelings of weakness and frailty. As she added muscle, she gained confidence and a sense of personal power. She had been wrestling with indecision regarding pursuing her Ph.D. but now eagerly launched into the program. She had turned down opportunities to travel yet was now busy making plans to spend a semester in Europe. I mention this story to illustrate that even relatively small changes can produce enormous results if those changes involve a restoration of anabolic metabolism.

A survey was conducted in which women rated the attractiveness of men by looking at a series of photographs. When the photographs showed only the men's faces, attractiveness was determined primarily by four features: eyes, nose, jaw, and symmetry (whether the right side of the face matched the left side).

When the photographs showed more of the men's bodies, however, facial features faded into second place as determinants of attractiveness. What mattered more? The guy's build. It didn't matter whether the women were twenty, thirty, or sixty—muscles ruled.

FEELING YOUNG

Energy is the currency of life. A lot of people think they need more money to live life to its fullest. Not true. You show me two people, one with a lot of money and the other with a lot of energy, and we'll see who's happier. The energetic person can always go out and make money, whereas the person with the money and no energy . . . what can he buy that will give him the passion, the intensity, the *juice* of life we all desire so deeply?

The best example of this I've ever heard came from my dear friend John Powell. John is a remarkable guy, one of a handful of people in the world who has competed on four consecutive Olympic teams. Can you imagine the dedication, endurance, and incredible strength it took to train intensely—and continuously—for twenty-six years? I helped John train for his last Olympic competition in 1984. That year, he silenced critics who thought he was too old by setting a world record in the discus. But fifteen years later, long after the stadium lights were turned off, the sound of the cheering crowds had faded, and a decade and a half of dust covered the medals and trophies, he found that it would take him an hour to get out of bed in the morning. No, it wasn't due to injury. He just couldn't think of a good reason to get up.

You see, champion athletes represent the pinnacle of anabolic power. For John and thousands like him, the downward spiral of catabolic metabolism was almost too painful to endure. So in 1999, we started working together again, this time for what might be called the Life Olympics. At age fifty-three, many would have been content with playing a little golf and watching TV, but not John. He understood that that was giving up, becoming a mere spectator in the game of life. So he applied himself with Olympic determination to the Metabolic Plan, and in ninety days, he called me up with the following message—one that I wrote down and look at every day, because it's universal, something we'd all like to say:

I had it, I lost it, . . . and I've got it back.

What John got back was more than energy. He got passion, intensity, and optimism—all the things that go with anabolic metabolism. In the chapters that follow, we'll look at all the ways that this plays out. We'll explore how anabolic hormones influence body and mind, how something as simple as sleeping better can profoundly affect how you feel all day, and how greater energy creates an upward spiral that can change everything about how you look and feel and experience life.

The operative word is *experience*. When was the last time you put off an important project, an exciting adventure, or a hot night with your honey because you just didn't have the energy? If you buy into the mind-set that 50 is over the hill, 60 is breakdown, and 76.7 is the end, that's what you will experience. To break free from that toxic mind-set, you need one thing more than anything else. You need energy.

The Energy Story

Walk into any convenience store and you'd think that energy was the easiest thing in the world to obtain. In the refrigerator case, you'll find little eight-ounce cans of colalike products with names like Greased Lightning. If you don't have time for a drink, right by the checkout stand, you'll find blister packs of tablets—products with names like Zow, Zip, and Slam. The implication, of course, is that you'll feel energized the minute you swallow these products. And of course, you will feel *something*, but it won't be energy. That's because the active ingredient in these products, as in the diet products mentioned earlier, is caffeine or another stimulant drug known as ephedrine. Manufacturers often hide this by using herbal sources of these drugs. Instead of caffeine, they'll list guarana, yerba maté, bissy nut, or kola nut on the label. Instead of ephedrine, you'll see ingredients like ma huang or Chinese ephedra. Bottom line: you're still just getting stress, which is a far cry from real energy.

You're Not Tired Because of a Caffeine Deficiency

If there's one take-home message from this section, it is this: Stimulant drugs do not, cannot, and never will give you real energy. They give you *stress*. Your body may interpret this jolt as something worthwhile because it provides a temporary increase in mental clarity, but to put that into perspective, let me ask you a question. If you were walking to work one morning not paying attention and stepped in front of a city bus and narrowly escaped getting flattened, you would become very alert. But would you say, "Gee, I think I'll do that every morning?"

Because caffeine raises stress hormone levels, we get a slap in the face that may seem harmless. Eventually, you get used to the increased heart rate and cold fingertips resulting from constriction of blood vessels. Over time, however, your health will suffer. Adrenals and nervous system are damaged. In the extreme, the mechanism is illustrated in post-traumatic stress syndrome, in which people are able to cope during the crisis but afterward fall apart from the accumulated stress.

Today, millions of Americans are falling apart because of the accumulated stress of a busy schedule, the unpredictability of life, and their caffeine addiction. I have counseled more than nine thousand clients, nearly all of whom believed they couldn't get through the day without caffeine. I explained that they got this bizarre idea from the people who advertise coffee and soft drinks. I told them to look at the facts. Forget the schmaltzy pictures of two women having a special moment over coffee and understand that consuming excess caffeine increases a woman's risk for heart disease, osteoporosis, anemia, PMS, panic attacks, fibrocystic breast disease, and certain types of cancer. For men and women, excess caffeine accelerates aging in three ways: it dehydrates the body, increases stress hormone levels (thereby suppressing immunity), and disturbs restful sleep.

The bottom line is this: Anything that raises stress hormone levels is a catabolic influence, and this influence is dose-related. A little caffeine is a little catabolic. A lot of caffeine (more than twenty-four ounces per day) can seriously impair your progress on the Metabolic Plan.

The good news, of course, is that improving anabolic metabolism and putting the brakes on catabolic activity will result in more energy than you've had in decades. And it will be energy that your body naturally produces, not stress from a coffee mug. Details are provided in Chapter 7.

Core Desires

But you want more than energy. And if energy is the currency, what can it buy? A ticket back into life as a *participant*. The intensity of *experience*. I laugh whenever I walk by a newsstand because it illustrates how deeply we all understand this core desire. Look at all the magazine covers and what do you see? Open the magazines and scan the full-page, four-color ads. Sure, there are a lot of sexy images, but what's behind the sex? What are all these sexy women and men doing? They're running, jumping, dancing, laughing, skydiving, in-line skating, and experiencing the joy of *movement*. I have never seen an ad portraying beautiful people watching television.

Metabolic Insurance

My job is to show you a new possibility called living life to its fullest. But when you take the white-water raft trip, backpack, ride a horse, or play tennis, you're going to need some metabolic insurance. As an emergency room aide, I saw what happens when people try to increase activity without tending to metabolism. The majority of Thanksgiving injuries were guys in their forties and fifties who thought they could play football again.

The last time they had played, they were in their anabolic twenties, but falling on the hard November ground under a pile of overweight, catabolic boomers is a completely different game. In their anabolic twenties, they had lots of muscle, which protected their bones and joints. Twenty-five years later, muscle mass was much lower, and the impact of a tackle or a fall was far greater. The impact was also increased by the extra weight they'd gained as well as by the decreased flexibility of tendons, ligaments, and joints. The net result of these changes was a huge number of sprains, tears, dislocations, fractures, pulls, and hernias. Even more unfortunate was the erroneous take-home message from all this pain. Because these guys didn't understand the metabolic model of aging, they concluded that they were just "too old" for that kind of activity. In reality, what they should have been saying to themselves was, "I'm too catabolic." They needed to make better cells and more muscle, essentially a "younger" body they were quite capable of building—if they only knew how.

Now We Know

Restoring anabolic metabolism enables you to restore flexibility to the connective tissue. That includes joints, tendons, ligaments, and even bones. It also means faster wound healing if you do get hurt. All of this translates into decreased vulnerability, which is important to all of us—not just weekend warriors. In a survey of people over seventy, their number one concern was fear of injury. Stairs, icy sidewalks, crowded elevators, and any moving vehicle represents a significant threat. The prospect of living an additional thirty or forty years with that level of vulnerability is certainly not very attractive. The Metabolic Plan is the only practical solution. Increased muscle creates metabolic armor. More flexibility and thicker skin mean fewer injuries. And most of all, stronger bones mean less risk for fractures.

Immunity

Illness also makes us vulnerable. I'll present a new view of illness and disease in the next chapter, but for now, I want to give you another key: you have a great deal more control over illness than you think. Television advertisers would like you to believe it's just a matter of fate. Someone sneezes and you get the flu. All children get middle-ear infections. Every spring, everyone has allergies. After age sixty, everyone develops arthritis and rheumatism. These messages—all of them absurd—are drummed into your head until you start to believe them. Why? So that you'll buy the products that treat the myriad symptoms of illness. Here's some refreshing news. You can prevent most of these conditions if you maintain peak immunity. Anabolic metabolism builds immunity, enhances the barrier mechanism of the skin and mucous membranes, improves organ function, and basically makes your body very inhospitable to microbes. Feeling powerful again includes having the confidence to go out without worrying about every cough, sneeze, and sniffle.

I have two major sources of immune stress: my kids, who continually bring home germs that my immune system has *never* seen, and frequent air travel. As I wait to board a 747, I often find myself listening to the hacks and coughs of the passengers with whom I will be sharing air for the next five hours. Fortunately, my immune system is about as vigilant and powerful as a twenty-year-old's, and I intend to keep it that way.

THINKING YOUNG

You think this section is going to be one of those "You're only as old as you feel" raps. No, there will be no rah-rah, go-get-'em-Tiger pep talks. Thinking young does not mean I want you to run out and buy a red convertible or act like a teenager. I want you to go much younger than that—somewhere between ages three and seven. Because your thinking back then about time and aging was probably very healthy and sane. There was an immediacy of experience that included a remarkable openness to new ideas. As an adult, the way you think about these critical facets of life is colored by years of anxiety about the future and remorse or reverie concerning the past. The result is that many people can hardly focus at all on the most important thing: the present.

This struck me after returning from a year in Asia and the South Pacific. Everyone experiences a period of reentry when coming back from foreign travel, but it usually passes after a few days or a week, and we get back into the American "swing" of things. This time, there was no getting back. For weeks, all I could do was walk around in disbelief because every conversation, every song on the radio, every magazine and newspaper was focused either on the past (witness the proliferation of oldies radio stations) or on the future. Again, the things that chain us to the past are guilt and remorse concerning the bad things and reverie for the good. The things that drag us ahead are speculation—plans to be happy somewhere in the future—and anxiety.

Watch yourself as you go through the day and see how much of your attention is firmly fixed in these areas. I would suggest that this reduces quality of life in subtle but significant ways, because it is only in the present that you can be truly alive. To demonstrate this, I recommend a simple exercise. Remember what a day was like when you were a child, how it stretched across what seems now to be an eternity of activity, play, adventure, meals, and then (forestalled as much as possible) bedtime. A day then was the same twenty-four hours, and yet today, those twenty-four hours seem to fly by in a flash. I believe the difference is *mindfulness*. As children, we were intensely present for almost every activity and event in which we were involved. Part of this intensity was the utter newness of experience; part was the lack of anxiety about the future. And then there was the fact that our lives (at least until we entered school) were not regimented into a clock-oriented schedule. We enjoyed a very primitive relationship with time.

Mindfulness is the practice of being present. We can regain the intense joy and exuberance of youth because it's always there. Mindfulness requires some getting used to. It involves becoming acutely present to every experience. When eating, this means being aware of every mouthful, the subtle nuances of taste and aroma; when showering, this means feeling the caress of hot water, the richness of soap, the nap of the towel. You are wholly engaged in life, with what you have and where you are, as opposed to running on autopilot toward some imagined happiness and fulfillment in the future.

With mindfulness, even unpleasant experiences are felt fully and completely. In this way, they are robbed of the power they often hold in our consciousness. After all, much of the pain of unpleasant experience is tied to the incredible amount of energy and attention we spend in preevent anxiety and postevent regret. Being mindful involves understanding that we cannot "unhappen" things that happen. "Go with the flow" is good advice, but it makes sense only when you have seen and deeply felt this flow in your life. The practice of mindfulness can reveal the flow in a powerful and life-altering way, enabling you to experience a "slowing down" of time, a shift in your relationship to the people, events, and priorities in your life.

Modern attempts at time management (planners, alarm watches, overnight and same-day mail delivery, faxes, cell phones, E-mail, 24/7 goods and services) cannot give us the freedom and sense of ease for which we yearn if we are not mindful. Genuine life experience, in other words, is not just a vibrantly healthy body but a vibrantly healthy life, which includes peace of mind. Creating (or at least contemplating) a shift in our relationship to time is an important step.

Tools for the Journey

Research has shown that yoga and meditation can lower blood pressure, relieve anxiety, enhance overall health, accelerate weight loss, improve sleep, and increase blood levels of DHEA. One of the most positive things I have done in my life is yoga. The movements, like Tai Chi, are centering, relaxing, strengthening, and stimulating all at the same time. With the right teacher, you can experience a sense of clear awareness and peace starting with the very first class. And it just gets better with practice.

Meditation: It's Not What You Think

People often imagine that meditation is an escape from worldly cares and concerns, a kind of cosmic cocoon. But that's the stereotype. Meditation is a very proactive practice. It will not bury or hide anything. On the contrary, it brings everything up for review. This review, however, is entirely different from your normal obsessing and fear. It is objective and calm, and there is a piercing clarity to the process that quickly brings priorities into focus.

And isn't that what we all want? We want to know what is *really* important, because life is short, and we don't want to waste time obsessing about stuff that is meaningless in the long run.

Meditation, of course, does more than help you sort things out. Remember that the mind, more than anything else, desires peace. Meditation provides that experience and helps to synchronize your actions with this core desire. The mind responds by creating the insights and awareness you need in order to remove stress from your life. "Hey, trading commodities is giving me an ulcer. I think I'd rather be a landscape engineer."

Meditation may also help your heart by decreasing risk for cardiovascular disease. A recent study compared a group of subjects with high blood pressure who completed a meditation program with another hypertensive group that took part in a health education course. The people who meditated for twenty minutes twice a day over the seven-month study period experienced a significant reduction in the thickening of their artery walls, indicating a reduction of risk for stroke and heart attack. Those in the health education group experienced an *increase* in artery wall plaque buildup. The researchers propose that meditation triggered anabolic repair mechanisms that helped clear fatty deposits from the blood vessels.[6]

Are you more likely to enjoy listening to soothing music or deep relaxation tapes? These are available from a number of sources listed in Appendix A. Special neuroacoustic tapes are also available, which use specific auditory cues to bring the mind into the alpha, or relaxed-awareness, state. Interestingly, many of these tapes use primordial sounds like ocean waves, a running stream, crickets, or the wind to help soothe and relax a frenzied mind.

Then and Now

We've discussed the biomarkers of aging, such as muscle mass, reaction time, hormone levels, and immune strength. There are equally valid *psychomarkers* to describe our mind-set or attitudes regarding time and aging. The essential point here is that we have a choice regarding how we think about things. If you study primitive societies that have no clocks or calendars—which, in fact, have no concept of time as we (mis)understand it—you find that their view of aging is positive, whereas ours is inherently negative. Those who study present-day hunters and gatherers, for example, are astounded at how different their conceptions of time are from ours. Hunter-gatherers do not measure age in years. To my hopelessly Western question "How old are you?" they would answer (through a translator), "Fine, wonderful." When I persisted in trying to find out when one of their elders was born, he indicated a tiny baby. In other words, he was born when he was very small.

Primitive peoples experience no pressure or anxiety related to time or aging. It never occurs to them to fear death. Death is something that happens in the course of events, like rain. The Western mind-set is baffling to them primarily because it focuses so much attention on the past and the future. For the most part, hunters and gatherers are connected deeply to the immediacy (and the intensity) of the present in a way that few of us are able to achieve. In regards to aging, they view it as an accumulation of experience and wisdom.

Here are the words we commonly use to describe people more than sixty-five years old. The most innocuous is *senior,* but the others all connote value judgments:

Aged
Elderly
Grizzled
Old
Gray

Here are the adjectives most commonly used by a tribe of hunters and gatherers when relating to their elders:

Wise
Respected
Venerable
Beloved
Experienced

Now, the sociologist might say, "Of course, primitive people have a different view of time. They have nothing to worry about. For them, nothing changes but the seasons. For modern man, the world is changing at a dizzying rate, and this alone is the cause of tremendous anxiety."

Excuse me, but when you and I get hungry, all we have to do is reach for the refrigerator door. When our children get sick, there's a hospital around the corner. We have insurance to insulate us from every conceivable misfortune. Primitive people had (and have) extreme challenges that you and I never face. It's just that they face these challenges in a very different way . . . together.

In primitive societies (the way we lived for millions of years), the individual is an integral and valued member of society, playing a *cooperative* role in virtually every activity, from building shelter to finding and preparing food. On the other hand, our present society (barely a few centuries old) is oriented around *competition* for goods and material assets. The illusion is that we are self-sufficient, but in fact, we are not. Few of us could survive if we had to gather our own food. Some believe as I do that much of modern angst is our alienation from nature and the increasing dependency on others for survival.

Then there is the ceaseless media drumbeat telling you that your body is not thin enough, your lips not fat enough, your car not fast enough, and your whites not white enough. To the degree that we buy into this, we will run out and buy clothes, automobiles, fragrances, and other consumer goods—chasing the promise that owning such things will make us complete and whole. We become blind to what really matters, but as the saying goes, the best things in life are not things.

So what do we do? We can't go back to a tribal society, but we can become more cooperative. We all need tools to manage change, and the best tool is the care and concern of friends. Support from friends, family, and community has been shown to reduce feelings of isolation and produce significant increases in anabolic biomarkers. Individuals who enjoy a deep sense of community—either religious, ethnic, or merely geographic—have decreased risk for heart disease and cancer. Community builds immunity.

What does all this mean to you? Perhaps it suggests the need for a shift in your relationship to time, from the frantic, time-is-running-out consciousness that prevails in today's society to a more relaxed experience of life. Remember taking the SAT exam? The pressure was *tremendous*, not only because the results would determine our college choices but because there was a time limit. We were trying to beat the clock. Well, put yourself back in that pressure-cooker experience and imagine the test monitor's making an announcement ten minutes before the buzzer. "Attention, students. If you need more time, feel free to take another hour to give it your best effort."

That's what *The Metabolic Plan* is all about: giving you more time so that you can get the most from—and contribute the most to—life. In this new model, there are limitless possibilities. In one lifetime, you could have three or more careers. Because the buzzer is not going to go off at 76.7, you can avoid the frenzy and anxiety of trying to cram everything in before age fifty. You can expect to be active, healthy, and free of chronic pain through your seventies and eighties and most likely far longer. You can create a reality in which vitality, joy, and meaning are *built into* your life, not something you slave for and hope to enjoy at some point in the future.

An Action Plan for Thinking Young

1. Affirm that *life expectancy* is irrelevant. A great deal of the aging process is under your control.

2. Think in terms of *life potential,* which at the moment is 120 years. Know that even this is likely to increase within the next decade. (*Note:* Every day in America, thirty-nine people turn 100.)

3. Enjoy the practice of mindfulness, which radically alters your perception of time and priorities.

4. Become aware of time spent spinning your wheels in anxiety, guilt, and speculation. Don't beat yourself up about such times (which will lead to more guilt); instead, place your attention on something immediate that is in front of you: the warmth of the sun, a good book, the smile of a child, or the remarkable fact that with every beat, your heart pumps life-giving oxygen and glucose to 100 trillion cells from the top of your head to the tips of your toes.

5. Practice a simple form of meditation that requires no training or special technique. Simply take twenty minutes every day to sit quietly and do nothing. No notepad to write down the logistics of the day, no music, no napping. Just the stillness of being.

THINKING LONG

Life extension is great, but the thought of living long but losing your memory, your ability to recognize the people you love, and ultimately forgetting how to sit and stand is a painful prospect indeed. Thus, it is foolish to talk about restoring the body without focusing an equal amount of attention on maintaining optimal brain function.

This is another area in which there is good news. Most of the current advances stem from a better understanding of brain biochemistry, some of which was covered in Chapter 3. You'll remember that the primary catabolic factors are oxidation and glycation. This means that the brain is terribly vulnerable to catabolic degeneration for three reasons:

1. More than 50 percent of the dry weight of your brain is lipid (fat) tissue, which is subject to oxidation.

2. The brain uses tremendous amounts of oxygen (25 percent of every breath you take), thus producing massive levels of free radicals.

3. Unlike your muscles—which can use glucose, fat, and in a pinch, even protein for fuel—the brain can use only glucose. Thus, although it accounts for only 2 percent of your weight, it uses nearly 30 percent of the glucose that you burn. This makes it highly vulnerable to glycation.

No wonder conventional wisdom says that if you live long enough, you'll get Alzheimer's disease. Of course, by studying centenarians, we now know that this isn't true, and the reason some people are protected may lie in their ability to produce greater brain levels of antioxidants. If you have not inherited this wonderful trait, what can you do? Follow the anticatabolic strategy outlined in Chapter 3 and remember the research I've mentioned regarding berries. It's worth reviewing because it represents such a significant antiaging breakthrough.

Researchers from Tufts University and the U.S. Department of Agriculture's Human Nutrition Research Center on Aging were intrigued by the ability of fruit and vegetable extracts to halt free-radical activity. They found that the onset of age-related brain degeneration could be delayed if young animals were supplemented with vitamin E and extracts of spinach and strawberry.[7] Unfortunately, not many of us started supplementing with antioxidants when we were children, so Dr. James Joseph and his team then tried treating older rats that were already demonstrating significant deficits in motor, memory, and learning skills. They tried a number of extracts but hit the jackpot with blueberries. Feeding blueberry extract restored all three brain functions. That's right: the blueberry-fed rats regained the youthful functioning of their brains, even though they were the human equivalent of seventy-year-olds.[8]

Look Before You Leap to Conclusions

With dramatic research like this, scientists scramble to find the active ingredient responsible for the observed benefit. In the case of berries, *antioxidant* activity was a top candidate. After all, researchers at Tufts University tested the antioxidant capacity of forty fruits and vegetables and found blueberries to be the most powerful. But as the USDA researchers pointed out, there are likely a number of active ingredients—perhaps hundreds—responsible for these extraordinary benefits, including a class of antioxidants known as anthocyanins and a larger group of nutrients collectively known as flavonoids.

We're learning that flavonoids enhance the integrity of the blood-brain barrier (BBB), and this is critically important for brain health. This barrier protects the brain from the multitude of toxins, chemicals, and biochemicals that gain access to the bloodstream, allowing only specific molecules—such as oxygen, glucose, and vital nutrients—to enter. In 2001 alone, more than five hundred studies were published relating to the role of the blood-brain barrier in brain injury, aging, and degeneration. The inability of this barrier to keep out aluminum, for example, is an important risk factor in Alzheimer's disease and other dementias. Aluminum is a neurotoxin that tends to accumulate in the brain and is associated with brain degeneration.[9]

It is important to understand that the blood-brain barrier is not an actual wall between blood vessels and your brain. It is an extraordinary modification of normal capillary tissue barely a few cells thick (less than one ten-thousandth of an inch). Researchers at the Cell Biology Laboratory at the University of Paris have been studying this barrier for more than twenty years and conclude that flavonoids play a critical role in maintaining its structural integrity.[10] This means that to achieve the brain-protecting and brain-restoring advantages illustrated in this research, you need to eat the fruit or a whole food concentrate. How much? Extrapolating from the animal data, health experts have recommended eating one to two cups of berries and/or cherries a day. Importantly, these fruits provide a host of additional benefits, including reducing risk for heart disease, cancer, and (if you include cranberries) lower risk for urinary tract infections and gum disease as well. Be sure that the berries or berry products you consume are certified pesticide-free.

Exercise Your Brain

You can take this two ways, and they're both going to help. First, research shows that if you exercise your brain by doing crossword puzzles, writing or playing music, playing chess, or even reading a good book, you will keep your brain functioning at a higher level. People who watch a lot of television, on the other hand, show earlier and more significant brain degeneration. The theory is that multitasking keeps the brain active and sharp, while TV locks the brain into a static and passive level of activity. This is also reflected biochemically. Watching television lowers metabolism to the level of deep sleep.

Second, we now know that exercising your muscles also improves brain function. This is another intriguing facet of the anabolic rebuild-repair-restore story. Researchers at the University of Illinois found that people who did *regular aerobic exercise* were able to improve short-term memory. With only thirty to sixty minutes of brisk walking per day, subjects achieved significant improvements in recall and reaction time. What's more, they experienced a greater ability to manage complex information. The authors of the study believe that increased oxygen delivery was responsible for these remarkable benefits, with only a 5 percent increase in oxygen supply to the lungs being sufficient for improved memory and learning skills. Other researchers at the Washington University School of Medicine and the University of British Columbia have confirmed that physical fitness and mental "fitness" are closely related.[11]

SEX

Looking and feeling great ought to have *some* influence on one's sex life, and in fact, the Metabolic Plan can produce dramatic results. Notice I didn't say XYZ tablets or capsules, but a *program* that restores youthful vigor and enjoyment.

The Irony of Aging

As we get older, sex becomes more satisfying. Women typically reach their sexual peak in their mid- to late thirties, in terms of both desire and enjoyment. Let's face it, we all need time to learn what works, how to ask for what we want, how to be optimally sexual. But for many women, a few short years later, they start to experience vaginal dryness and then a sort of atrophy. It's as if Mother Nature finally gives you the key to great sex and then changes the lock. Sexual intercourse often becomes uncomfortable or actually painful. Vaginal lubricants can help, but they don't alter the changes in vaginal tissue that accompany aging: the loss of moisture, smoothness, and suppleness. For that, you need the metabolic assistance of hormone replacement.

And what about men? Talk about a cruel joke. We remember being youthful studs, able to perform at the drop of a hat (or shorts) but having the sexual stamina of gerbils. Then, we get into our forties, and although erections do not appear as quickly, they last a lot longer. Everything finally appears to be working out. But soon after, erections start to fade, first in terms of hardness and then in terms of actually being able to achieve an erection at all.

Certainly, modern science has jumped (with more than $3.7 billion of collective research) to shore up men's flagging sexual performance. Everything from vacuum pumps to the surgical insertion of actual air pumps to penile injections (ouch!) and finally a tablet (whew!). Problem is that the tablets have a few side effects, which in more than a few cases have included death. (Man to Saint Peter: "I said I was dying to have sex, but you shouldn't have taken it literally.")

Why Is Sex So Powerful?

To understand the power of the Metabolic Plan to revitalize your sex life, you just have to remember that nature's game is survival. Your sex drive, in other words, exists only because it motivates you to perform an act that will result in procreation. Once you are past reproductive age, nature has absolutely no reason to maintain this drive, and this is reflected in the dramatic decline in DHEA starting at age thirty. By age forty, the desire for sex and the ability to enjoy sex start to diminish. Although some people see these developments as an inevitable part of life, others miss the intensity and excitement of sexual activity.

If you want to stay sexually active, I have good news. After raising DHEA levels, men often find that their sexual performance improves. Many report that erections become stronger, and ejaculatory volume and force are increased. Clinical reports show that women taking DHEA notice increases in libido even more frequently than males.[12] This might be explained by the fact that DHEA supplementation appears to raise testosterone levels in women more than in men.

The Anabolic Pleasure Principle

For the first time in the history of mankind, it appears that we can extend our life span and at the same time extend our number of sexually active years. That way, we not only get to enjoy the pleasures of sex, but at the same time, we send longevity signals to our cells that may postpone senescence and death.

Once again, the idea is to convince our cellular DNA that we are capable of reproducing. As long as that is a possibility, research with animals suggests we may be able to extend life span by 20 percent to 50 percent. As the saying goes, "Use it or lose it."

Of course, it's not simply a matter of taking a DHEA pill. DHEA will not instantly turn a middle-aged man or woman into a sex machine; but as an integral part of your Metabolic Plan, DHEA can make a difference. Additionally, I suggest you track hormone levels with a yearly comprehensive blood test starting at age forty and consult with your doctor about augmenting estrogen and progesterone (for women) or testosterone (men and women).

The Big Picture

Libido is powerful and tremendously important for the experience of certain pleasures. But life is a balance, and sex drive is not the be-all and end-all. There are times when other motivations and behaviors are more compelling and even more urgent. I spent six years in a yoga ashram (1972–1978) as a monastic student because there were lessons that I needed to learn that libido could not teach.

The good news is that we now have a choice and the tools to explore the further unfolding of libido into our fifties, sixties, and beyond. The sex drive is not an on-off switch but a continuum of feelings, emotions, and behaviors that affect every aspect of our lives. If we do nothing about metabolism, aging will slowly rob us of our energy and vitality. The Metabolic Plan can help us regain that lost fortune, and I believe we should celebrate and make good use of those gifts. With or without hormone replacement, restoring anabolic drive will increase feelings of youthfulness and vitality, helping you to fulfill your genetic potential for life.

The image has been used many times, but it is perfectly accurate: life is a symphony of experience, not one note played over and over. If we fall into that mind-set, growing old will be terrifying. Libido provides the bass notes, if you will, but a truly successful life requires the added harmony of wisdom, creativity, and compassion. The tragedy has always been that we run out of time and/or energy just when we have gained that wisdom. By restoring anabolic metabolism, you get not only energy and vitality but something else far more important—you get more time.

No Magic Bullets

I'll say it again to make sure nobody forgets: this is not a "magic-bullet" approach. You have to understand that no matter how attractive the instant-results mentality might be, *it has never worked*. Life is complex, and we are naturally attracted to simple solutions—one pill that will do it all. But whenever researchers have tried to find the magic bullet, they have failed.

The most popular drugs in America right now are a group of antidepressants classified as selective serotonin reuptake inhibitors (SSRIs). More than 50 million prescriptions have been filled, and a common side effect is sexual dysfunction: decreased libido, delayed orgasm, or inability to achieve orgasm.

While many people do benefit tremendously from antidepressants, it's important to look at the big picture. It's not a single hormone or drug. It's not anything that you can buy but rather what you do and how you live. An important new study found that sexual activity in older men and women was related more to physical activity and social interaction than to any hormone level. In other words, take a close look at your life. Are you an active participant, or have you fallen into the trap of being a spectator?

The entire Metabolic Plan is geared toward getting you passionately and intensely involved with life. If you are fifty years old, your chances of living to one hundred are not only good—they're excellent. But if you want those years to be active and vibrant, you have to take action now. Don't wait another twenty years, hoping for a miracle drug. It's time to wake up and start using the incredible resources we have available right now.

Illness, Immunity, and Metabolism

So far, we've been looking at the forces of anabolic repair and catabolic damage. But there's a third force that can take you out of the game at any time, and that's disease. This chapter looks at the importance of peak immunity as an antiaging strategy. After all, what good is an anti-aging program to someone who dies of a heart attack or cancer at the age of fifty-six? My job as a health educator, then, is to help you minimize your risk of disease. You won't be surprised to find that it has a great deal to do with metabolism.

For the most part, young people don't get cancer. Young people don't generally die from pneumonia, bronchitis, lupus, hepatitis, kidney disease, diabetes, tuberculosis, or the flu. These are the things that people over fifty die from. Now, at first, this sounds simplistic. Of course, old people die from these diseases. The question is why.

The standard medical response is that their immune systems fail. If you're satisfied with that answer, you haven't been paying attention. Conventional wisdom, in other words, simply *assumes* that failing immunity is an inevitable consequence of aging. But it's considered inevitable only because it's common.

The fact is, not *everyone's* immune system starts failing after age fifty, and while it's tempting to ascribe this strength to "good genes," studies with identical twins illustrate that only about 35 percent of aging is genetic.[1] One leading research group states simply, "Human longevity is moderately inherited."[2] What, then, are the other factors that determine immune competence?

Poor nutrition (a.k.a. the standard American diet) impairs immunity. A sedentary lifestyle impairs immunity. I've described how stress impairs immunity, and the connection between metabolism and immunity is undeniable. As anabolic drive declines, so does immune strength.

Do you see the message here? It is as if Mother Nature uses the immune system to reward or penalize us for our behaviors and habits. To the extent that we contribute to our own survival—by staying fit, handling stress, eating right—we are rewarded with a competent immune system. And for every transgression—obesity, a sedentary lifestyle, poor diet, unmanaged stress, cigarette smoking, alcohol abuse—our immune system is weakened, for the purpose of getting us off the team to make room for a more intelligent and motivated player.

Understanding nature's game also involves a change in the way you look at illness. Over the years, I have asked thousands of clients and students, "Is illness a bad thing?" They always look at me as if I were crazy. "Of course, it's a bad thing." And this is a trap—a limitation of thinking that obscures an important facet of nature's game.

Once again, we have been conditioned to ignore the essential balance of life. We define happiness as "getting what we want" and suffer for the times when the universe has other plans. In the same way, we believe that we should have perfect health unmarred by illness. In truth, *illness is part of the game.*

ILLNESS

The parallels between the distorted views of illness and happiness are striking. Even though we know deep in our hearts that "things" don't make us happy, we still fill our houses, garages, and even auxiliary rental units with stuff. In the same way, we have an instant fix for every sniffle, cough, or tummy ache. Advertisements for these products bombard us from television screens, billboards, and magazines, telling us that illness is abnormal, an impairment in your otherwise perfect life that should, at the very first symptom, send you *running* to the drugstore for help.

And so our relationship to illness is completely one-sided,

unbalanced, and this gets us into trouble. Nature created illness for a reason, and you'll never understand this if you view it as something to flee from, cover up, or suppress.

Now, I don't mean you should ignore preventive self-care. Don't go out and *try* to get sick. But when illness comes, consider that there is a reason for it at that moment. Usually, it is stress-related. You were working too hard, sleeping too little, eating poorly—the trap into which we all fall now and again. Since such behavior is clearly contrary to long-term survival (nature's prime directive), she has a tool known as illness that puts us out of commission for a while.

But since we believe that we know better, we reach for one or more over-the-counter remedies and go right back to our hectic, high-stress schedule. If you're like most Americans, you have a medicine cabinet filled to overflowing with these products: half-consumed bottles of cold medicines, decongestants, laxatives, antacids, nasal sprays, eyedrops, eardrops, painkillers, anti-inflammatories, and hemorrhoid creams. Last year, U.S. sales of such remedies topped $39 billion.

We just don't get it. Illness is a signal to slow down, get more rest, and rebuild your immune system with pure water, good food, and nutritional support. But here is something brand-new that has to do with the core message of this book. Illness is also critical for longevity.

What?

I got the first glimpse of this remarkable truth in high school and college, where wrestling was my best sport. I loved the challenge of competition, the endless strategy of moves and countermoves. And of course, the only way to advance in this or any sport is to continually face tougher and tougher competitors. Virtually all sports have a play-off structure that looks like this:

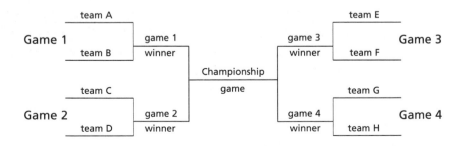

The purpose of this structure, of course, is to produce a champion—the individual or team that is the best, that has faced each level of challenge and prevailed. Are you seeing the similarity to nature's game of survival?

For me, this was a remarkable breakthrough. I was taking courses in biology and chemistry and then taking off my lab coat and going to the gym, where I would change into my wrestling gear. In the lab, I was looking at microbes and immune cells. On the mat, I was looking at a fellow from another school who thought he was a better wrestler. I realized that illness is a necessary part of the game and, furthermore, that running from illness with prescription and over-the-counter drugs would be like walking away from a tough competitor, saying to the coach that I refused to fight.

Here's a case in point. Nature has equipped us with a number of extraordinary immune weapons, most notably the ability to generate a tremendous amount of heat, known as fever. The inherent intelligence involved in this phenomenon is extraordinary, because you don't get a fever every time you get a cold. Fever is a weapon that is used only when necessary. It was developed millions of years ago to kill bacteria and viruses, and instead of acknowledging the astounding beauty of this immune tool, what do we do? We run to the drugstore to buy a medicine that will eliminate the fever. Far be it from modern man to endure *discomfort*. But what if I told you that every time you have a fever, your immune system learns an important lesson—a lesson recorded by antibodies and memory cells that cannot be learned if the fever is suppressed?

Illness is not a bad thing. I always wonder when someone boasts that he or she never gets sick. I assume that this person doesn't have children or travel very much, because exposure to new microbes is part of an active life, and the ensuing fight (if handled properly) makes us strong. But for someone to get sick a few times a year and recover quickly—now *that's* something to be proud of.

DISEASE

Disease is not the same as illness. It's what you get when your immune system has not been trained and strengthened. Let me give you another sports analogy. Someone who wants to be a champion boxer will work his way up the ladder of competition, knowing that at each rung, he will face a more skilled competitor, a competitor whose sole motivation is to hurt him as badly as possible while wearing padded gloves.

So training, for a boxer, is basically getting beaten up. What if the aspiring boxer were unwilling to endure this? What if he stayed home, lifted weights, and shadowboxed in front of his mirror . . . and then decided to take on the heavyweight champion of the world? You get the picture. Illness is the cuts and bruises of immune training. Disease is the knockout. Illness is a cold, stuffy nose, sore throat, earache, gastrointestinal virus. Disease is cancer, heart disease, stroke, pneumonia, tuberculosis, kidney disease, chronic obstructive pulmonary disease, and hepatitis.

HOW TO TRAIN AND MAINTAIN YOUR IMMUNE SYSTEM

We've discussed the idea of avoiding the hundreds of over-the-counter drugs that only suppress the symptoms of illness. The next phase is to actually strengthen your immune system to withstand the pummels and punches of disease. And forgive the combat-oriented imagery, but this aspect of antiaging is, in very real terms, a battle—and you're fighting for your life.

As we grow older:

- The population of powerful and vigilant natural killer (NK) cells declines. The NK cells that are produced are less active. NK cells are your best defense against cancer and viruses. You're the general. It's as if all of your special forces just left.

- The thymus gland—which for decades served as the military academy for your immune system, taking normal white blood cells and turning them into mighty T cells and nearly invincible NK cells—shrivels up. The thymus gland in the average sixty-five-year-old is no longer functioning . . . at all.

- The cytokine communication network that coordinates the immune system's defense strategy starts to break down. The intricate balance that prevents the immune system from attacking healthy tissue starts to fail. More and more damage from "friendly fire" is suffered in your joints, thyroid gland, and connective tissue.

- Memory cells that, over your lifetime, have retained the characteristics of every disease-causing microbe that you've encountered
die. That's normal. But for the first time, *they're not replaced.* Gradually, we lose our B-cell antibody defense system. Memory T cells
also disappear. We lose immunity to literally thousands of
pathogens and find ourselves facing a hostile environment with
fewer NK cells, fading T cells, and dwindling antibodies.

Hang on; reinforcements are available.

There are practical and effective steps you can take to build and
maintain peak immunity. These include diet, lifestyle, nutritional supplements, and metabolism. As you might guess, metabolism is the factor that makes good food, regular exercise, and vitamin supplements
really effective. In most people, for example, the immune system starts
to go "out of whack" starting at age forty. Powerful immune factors like
interleukin-2 (IL-2) begin to decline, while other interleukins that dys-
regulate immunity (like IL-6) start to increase. Scientists have even
found that levels of IL-6 predict longevity, with mortality (the likehood
of death) being associated with higher levels of IL-6.[3] What is the best
way to lower IL-6? Restoring anabolic metabolism with regular exercise
and DHEA.[4]

THE THYMUS FACTOR

The fact that the thymus of mice and rats also atrophies with age—just
as ours does—allowed researchers to look at the influence of metabolic
hormones on this critical immune process. They found that administration of catabolic hormones (cortisol or dexamethasone) accelerated
the shrinking or atrophy of the thymus, whereas DHEA *prevented* that
degeneration.[5] There is even extraordinary evidence that administration
of DHEA restored critical immune functions in animals after the thymus had been entirely removed.[6]

"Big deal," say the skeptics. "DHEA produces healthy rodents. Who's
to say that the same thing can be accomplished with humans?" Well,
three top endocrinologists from the University of California, San Diego
School of Medicine. This research team gave DHEA to a group of elderly men. In two weeks, remarkable immune improvements were
noted, and in twenty weeks, the results were astounding. The study,
published in a leading gerontology journal, is entitled "Activation of

Immune Function by Dehydroepiandrosterone (DHEA) in Age-Advanced Men."[7] The following list summarizes the anabolic benefits of DHEA supplementation revealed in the study.

Benefits Achieved

- IGF-1 (the body's major repair and rebuild biochemical) increased significantly.

- The unbound (biologically active) fraction of IGF-1 increased even more.

- There was a profound restoration of immune function:

    Increased monocyte production—the workhorse cell of the immune system
    Increased B-cell production—meaning enhanced antibody defense
    Very significant increase in B-cell response to foreign invaders
    Very significant increase in T-cell response to foreign invaders
    Increased interleukin-2 production, leading to improved cytokine balance
    Increased NK cell production
    Increased NK cell activity

Look at the list of immune benefits, most related to thymus function. Getting beyond the med talk, this is like putting more police on the street, giving them faster cars, bulletproof vests, binoculars, night vision, more ammunition, and a better communication system. Once again, here's the model:

1. Aging is a metabolic process.

2. Metabolism is significantly determined by hormones.

3. Restoring anabolic hormones helps maintain peak immunity.

4. Peak immunity extends life, in terms of both years and quality.

Of course, it's more than DHEA. A collaborative research group from Tufts University, the University of Florida College of Medicine, and the

Veterans Affairs Medical Center in Gainesville, Florida, created an animal model of age-related immune dysfunction. They noted that, just like people, old mice infected with influenza fare worse than young mice, due to a loss of T-cell defenses. Not only that, the old mice (just like humans) start to produce biochemicals that *impair* the production of antiviral defenders such as interferon and interleukin-2 (IL-2).

In their experiment, however, they introduced a single variable—some vitamin E in the diet of one group of mice. Over the next eight weeks, the vitamin E–supplemented group fared remarkably better than the control group. Vitamin E strengthened the animals' antiviral defense, lowered the level of infection in their lungs, and increased the production of IL-2 and interferon.[8] That's antiaging.

The same level of scientific support exists for each of the immune-boosting agents that follow. But you can't just run to the health food store and grab every product on the shelf that's labeled "immune support." Remember, this is warfare. You don't use a cruise missile to kill a gnat, and you certainly don't reach for the flyswatter when you're fighting a grizzly bear. This is a strategic endeavor in which you use the appropriate agent for the job at hand. I divide the plan into four stages.

THE METABOLIC PEAK IMMUNITY PLAN

Nutritional Supplements

Stage 1: Readiness Drill

- *When:* Immune maintenance: five to seven times a week.

- *Purpose:* Immune wake-up. Get the troops organized and ready to fight.

- *Weapons* (all doses are daily unless otherwise noted):

    Low doses (100–300 milligrams per day) of the following herbs:
    Schizandra
    Astragalus
    Ganoderma (reishi mushroom)
    Siberian ginseng

Green drink (for example, a powdered combination of wheat grass, oat grass, barley grass, spirulina): two teaspoonfuls in sixteen ounces of water

Garlic (Use in cooking or take one capsule per day.)

Cayenne (Use in cooking, salsa, hot sauce.)

Multivitamin with minerals, preferably one taken with two or three meals

Vitamin E: 200 international units

DHEA: 10–25 milligrams

7-Keto: 25–50 milligrams

Alpha lipoic acid: 100 milligrams

Aloe vera (preferably a 2:1 liquid concentrate): one to two fluid ounces

If you are very active, L-glutamine 500–1,000 milligrams after a strenuous workout has been shown to reduce illness and infections.[9]

Stage 2: Yellow Alert

- *When:* At the first sign of illness.

- *Purpose:* To win the skirmish before it becomes a battle.

- *Consult with:* Nutrition-oriented physician (optional).

- *Weapons:*

    In addition to stage 1 agents (adjust quantities as shown below or add):
        Moderate doses (300–500 milligrams) of the following herbs:
            Schizandra
            Astragalus
            Ganoderma (reishi)
    In addition to multivitamin:
        Vitamin C with bioflavonoids: 250–1,000 milligrams
        Vitamin E: 400 international units
        Coenzyme Q-10: 60 milligrams
        Selenium: 100 micrograms
        Garlic capsules: one capsule twice a day

Cayenne
Zinc lozenges (three per day)
Alpha lipoic acid: 100 milligrams twice a day
N-acetyl-cysteine (NAC): 500 milligrams
Aloe vera (preferably a 2:1 liquid concentrate): two to four fluid ounces

Stage 3: Red Alert

- *When:* If illness deepens or becomes chronic.

- *Purpose:* To win the battle before it becomes a war.

- *Consult with:* Nutrition-oriented physician (mandatory).

- *Weapons:*

  In addition to stage 2 agents (adjust quantities as shown below or add):
  High doses (500–1,000 milligrams) of the following herbs:
  Schizandra
  Astragalus
  Ganoderma (reishi)
  Echinacea extract
  Cordyceps extract
  In addition to multivitamin:
  Vitamin C with bioflavonoids: 500 milligrams three times per day
  Vitamin E: 800 international units
  Glutamine:[10] 500–1,000 milligrams per day
  RNA/DNA: 500–800 milligrams (Do not use if you have a tendency to develop gout.)
  Coenzyme Q-10: 150 milligrams
  NAC: 500 milligrams twice a day
  Aloe vera (preferably a 2:1 liquid concentrate): Four to six fluid ounces
  Arabinogalactan (a polysaccharide-rich extract from larch trees): 500 milligrams

Stage 4: All-Out Massive Action

- *When:* When the course of illness becomes critical.

- *Purpose:* To win the war.

- *Consult with:* Nutrition-oriented physician specializing in your specific condition.

- *Weapons:*

    In addition to stage 3 agents (adjust quantities as shown below or add):
        Coenzyme Q-10: 150 milligrams twice a day
        IP-6 (derived from rice bran): 1,000–2,000 milligrams
        NAC: 500 milligrams three times a day

The Exercise Factor

Scientists have long observed that people who exercise regularly live longer. This is due to cardiovascular fitness leading to better circulation. Exercise also makes the bones stronger and maintains greater oxygen delivery (via deep breathing), especially important in later years. But what explains the fact that exercisers experience less illness throughout life? That turns out to be associated with something that happens every time we are strenuously active. We give ourselves a "fever." It is this temporary but significant elevation in core body temperature that destroys significant numbers of bacteria and viruses. Immunity: Use it or lose it.

Range-of-Motion (ROM) Exercise

You have more lymphatic fluid in your body than blood. Lymph bathes every cell, playing an important role in immunity and detoxification (removing toxins and metabolic debris). To circulate blood, you have a fantastic pump in your chest. Your lymphatic system has no pump. How does lymph circulate?

It circulates through *movement*, especially movement that involves muscles and joints going through their full range of motion. Sounds like yoga, and sure enough, yoga is great for improving lymphatic circulation. The inverted poses (such as shoulder stand) are especially beneficial. Of course, you don't have to practice yoga to get a good lymphatic "workout." Dancing, rock climbing, bouncing on a trampoline, basketball, swimming, Tai Chi, and martial arts are all wonderfully effective.

The Iron Factor

In Chapter 3, I described the critical importance of maintaining optimum iron levels, in that both a deficiency and an excess of iron can accelerate aging. It is well known that iron deficiency anemia impairs immunity and anabolic repair, but we are now learning that even a moderate excess of iron accelerates catabolic damage and increases risk for cardiovascular disease and cancer. High iron levels accelerate brain degeneration and liver disease (including hepatitis C). So you have to ask the question, why do we tend to accumulate iron? Why would nature create such a dilemma?

Evolutionary biologists point out that in early adulthood, iron loss is a critical factor. Menstruating women lose iron every month. For millions of years, men lost iron through blood loss associated with survival-related injuries. Thus, we developed an extraordinarily efficient way to absorb, store, and recycle iron so that virtually none of the mineral is lost through sweat, urine, or the intestinal tract. This worked just fine for the first 3 million years of human history, when the goal, once again, was to assure procreation. After all, anemic women become infertile. Anemic men have low sperm counts.

But here we are in the twenty-first century, living into our eighties. Women are living nearly half of their lives after menopause; men only lose blood if they nick themselves shaving; we eat enormous quantities of iron-rich meat, and thus many accumulate toxic levels of iron. How do you deal with this dilemma? You monitor tissue levels of iron with a serum ferritin test (see the section in Chapter 3 entitled "How to Measure Iron Status Accurately"), and if it rises above 180, you give blood. If the blood bank doesn't want your blood (for example, because you have hepatitis or another risk factor), your doctor will drain a pint and dispose of it. If you just can't stand needles, there is another way:

- Adopt a low-iron diet, including little or no red meat. Do not use iron cookware.

- Remove iron with substances that bind with free iron, facilitating its removal through the kidneys or gastrointestinal tract. These substances—known as iron chelators—include:

  Malic acid (found in apples, apple juice, and aloe vera)
  Garlic and onions, including garlic capsules
  Beans
  Fiber, especially insoluble fiber found in whole grains
  Calcium disodium EDTA (Use under the direction of a physician.)
  IP-6 (inosine hexaphosphate, found in whole grains and some nutritional formulations)

Lead and Mercury

Lead and mercury are highly toxic metals that can profoundly suppress immunity. They pose a significant health risk for adults but are particularly dangerous for children and are cumulative over the course of a lifetime. Now that lead has been removed from paint and gasoline (the major sources of exposure), most people assume that the lead problem has been eliminated, but nothing could be further from the truth. First of all, lead in the environment didn't evaporate in 1973 when automakers switched to unleaded gasoline. U.S. soils still contain an estimated 5 million metric tons of lead that accumulated before that date. This lead gets taken up in the food chain; delivered to your dinner plate via fish, animal, or vegetable; and accumulates in your body.

Lead is such a common industrial material that it shows up in factory smoke and the contaminated soil, water, and air around battery factories, metal shops, auto body shops, and dozens of industries. Surprisingly, one of the biggest sources of lead in your life (assuming you're not a plumber or stained-glass artist) may be your nutritional supplements. Lead contamination in calcium supplements remains a significant problem, even though an FDA warning on this issue was published in 1981. Since then, studies have confirmed that many forms of calcium still contain lead in amounts that exceed EPA safety guidelines.

Since millions of Americans (including many children) are supplementing with large doses of calcium, this is an issue that cannot be

ignored. In 1993, researchers tested seventy brands of calcium supplements and found high levels in a significant percentage.[11] One
product contained 25 milligrams of lead per 800-milligram dose of
calcium! Taken over a period of time, this product alone could result
in diagnosable lead poisoning (defined as blood lead levels greater
than 10 micrograms per deciliter). As you might expect, the products
derived from bonemeal contained the highest concentrations of lead,
simply because cows (like humans) accumulate lead in their bones.
But soil and shell sources of calcium (dolomite and unrefined calcium
carbonate) also contained considerable amounts of lead. Bottom line:
Request a certified heavy-metal assay from your nutritional supplement manufacturer. If it doesn't have such an assay, switch to a company that does.

Do your children play with or suck on your car keys? Keys contain
lead. Even handling your keys and eating finger food can deliver a significant amount of lead into your mouth.

And speaking of your mouth, did you know that somewhere between 30 and 40 percent of the "silver" filling in your teeth is mercury?
That's a significant source of this toxin for most of us, followed by shell-
fish, other fish, fungicides, and pesticides. No one uses Mercurochrome
or Merthiolate anymore, but boomers will remember putting liberal
amounts of these stings-less-than-iodine, mercury-containing medicines on scratches and cuts. Well, guess what? The mercury you absorbed directly into the cut is still with you—primarily in your bones
and brain.

Lead and Mercury Detoxification Action Plan

All of the iron-binding agents listed in the previous subsection will help
eliminate lead and mercury to some degree, but you may need professional help to do a complete job. How do you know? A prevention-
oriented physician will be able to screen your hair, urine, and blood for
lead and mercury. Laboratories that specialize in these valuable tests are
listed in Appendix A. Do not rely on a hair test alone. Hair can be contaminated with environmental lead and mercury, giving you a falsely elevated reading.

If you have toxic levels of lead and mercury, discuss with your doctor a detox program that will include the following:

- Oral, and possibly intravenous, EDTA

- NAC (N-acetyl-cysteine), sometimes in high doses, to raise glutathione levels

- Lipoic acid

- Pectin (found in apples, pears, and citrus fruits)

Avoid mercury amalgam fillings. There are a number of practical, better-bonding, longer-lasting materials available. What about the fillings already in your mouth? This has been a huge debate for twenty years, and positions range all the way from "They're no problem" to "They'll kill you." Even the research on the release of mercury from amalgam fillings is confusing, but here's one thing on which every dental professional agrees. If you choose to have your amalgam fillings removed, do it sensibly.

Before you start, consult with a prevention-oriented physician to have a twenty-four-hour urine test for lead and mercury. He or she will administer a lead- and mercury-binding agent intravenously, and you'll collect your urine for an entire day. The lab will measure how much of these toxic metals your urine contains. This gives you important baseline information that your dentist can use to develop a prudent and safe replacement strategy. Follow-up testing will verify that the mercury burden on your body and brain has been reduced.

The Resident Infection Factor

No discussion of aging and immunity would be complete without looking at how we tend to accumulate resident or chronic infections along the way. Obviously, the most serious is HIV, with nearly a million Americans presently infected. There are also more than 11 million Americans with hepatitis and 40 million with herpes. Another chronic infection that is often overlooked is parasites; an estimated 30 million Americans are harboring one or more organisms.

HIV

HIV is so often fatal because it is not just a drain on immunity. It attacks the immune system directly, infecting a group of T cells known as helper/inducer cells (also known as CD-4 cells).

Decreased production of anabolic hormones, especially DHEA, is associated with impaired immunity. When DHEA levels were measured in a group of HIV-positive men, not only were their DHEA levels lower than in healthy men, but the level was directly proportional to the severity of their disease. As DHEA levels rose, so did the CD-4 count.[12]

While this gives us no conclusive picture, it strongly supports other evidence that anabolic metabolism is critical for optimal immune function and that low DHEA levels contribute to the advancement of disease. What everyone is wondering at the moment is whether supplemental DHEA will be effective in the treatment of AIDS. That remains to be seen. But let's look at another intriguing piece of the puzzle that we discussed in the last chapter: the ratio of catabolic to anabolic metabolism as reflected in cortisol and DHEA.

DHEA levels are normally inversely related to cortisol: as cortisol increases, DHEA declines. Apparently, when the body is under chronic stress, the adrenals shift activity from DHEA to cortisol. Some experts believe that this may be the single most important mechanism to explain the well-known stress-induced impairment of immunity. But how would that affect the progression of AIDS?

Researchers have found that DHEA is a "modest inhibitor" of HIV replication, meaning that DHEA doesn't stop the virus from duplicating, but it slows the virus down.[13] Even more important is the fact that cortisol, the body's primary catabolic hormone, accelerates HIV replication. There appears to be a tug-of-war in the bodies of HIV-positive individuals between cortisol and DHEA. To the degree that cortisol wins, the disease progresses. In support of this hypothesis, a report was published entitled "HIV and the Cortisol Connection: A Feasible Concept of the Process of AIDS."[14]

Certainly, anyone infected with the human immunodeficiency virus should pay careful attention to anabolic and catabolic metabolism. Good evidence suggests that maintaining a high anabolic status will help prolong life, and that right now is the name of the game. A cure for this disease *will* be found. You just want to be around to receive the treatment.

Herpes

The herpes family of viruses includes herpes simplex I and II, herpes zoster (also known as shingles), Epstein-Barr virus, cytomegalovirus, and chicken pox. All appear to be incurable but controllable. Thus, treatment focuses on keeping the virus in remission. Evidence is growing that DHEA and its metabolites can strengthen the body's antiviral defenses, resulting in fewer herpes outbreaks.[15] It stands to reason: a powerful immune system is quite capable of keeping the lid on herpes infections, and lowering stress hormones is also an effective preventive strategy. The Metabolic Plan is designed to accomplish both of these important tasks.

Parasites

The class of disease-causing organisms called parasites includes literally hundreds of species, ranging from microscopic one-cell protozoa to tapeworms sometimes measuring three feet in length. Parasites are carried by food, water, wind, and soil, as well as insects, animals, birds, and fish. Pets carry parasites, many of which can infect humans. Pets also carry fleas and ticks, which carry parasites. Amazing.

These organisms have been coevolving with us for millions of years, and like viruses and fungi, their presence in the body serves no useful purpose. Thus, infection with parasites taxes and suppresses immune function and may lead to serious illness and even death.

Most people think that parasites are rare in spanking-clean America. But there has *never* been a time when parasite infection was *not* a major cause of illness.[16] In fact, a number of factors have resulted in increased—not decreased—risk.

- *Widespread travel:* More and more Americans are traveling to parts of the world where the water, food, and soil may be contaminated with parasites. Importantly, symptoms may only start after the traveler has returned home, making diagnosis more difficult. In a recent outbreak of eosinophilic meningitis reported in the *New England Journal of Medicine,* the primary symptom (splitting headache) only appeared in some of the victims a month after their return from Jamaica.[17] Travelers can also carry parasites back home, where infection of family members is possible.

- *Modern international food distribution:* Today, food is flown to the United States from every corner of the globe. Testing for parasites is impossible because they are usually carried as eggs or cysts, not visible organisms. Proper handling and cooking, of course, reduce risk of infection, but problems still arise: food is often cooked "rare," and cutting boards and utensils can be infected.

- *Popularity of new ethnic foods:* Any meat, fish, or fowl that is not thoroughly cooked can carry parasites, but dishes containing semicooked meat may be safe if properly marinated or smoked. Sushi, on the other hand, is almost always served raw. Public health officials in the United States have noted an increased incidence of parasite infections with the rising popularity of sushi bars. Reports in the medical literature describe a wide range of symptoms from raw fish–transmitted parasites, from mild diarrhea to life-threatening infection with frightening organisms like *Anisakis,* which can penetrate the gastrointestinal tract and injure internal organs.[18]

- *The sexual revolution:* Individuals who have numerous sexual partners increase their risk for infection with *Trichomonas,* a venereal parasite that affects mainly women. Contrary to popular belief, however, men are often infected. The organism can cause chronic urethritis and prostatitis and may account for up to 20 percent of nongonorrhea venereal disease in men.[19] Men can also be asymptomatic carriers for many years, and even without symptoms, the infection exerts a suppressing effect on immunity. *Trichomonas* infection can be chronic or even lifelong in both sexes, and public health experts estimate that up to 25 percent of sexually active Americans may be infected.[20]

Myth: Parasite infections are rare.
Reality: Based on medical records and disease patterns, health experts claim that three out of every five Americans (60 percent) will experience parasitic infections in their lifetime.[21]

Myth: It is easy to tell if you have parasites because there are obvious signs.
Reality: Most individuals and even many doctors overlook this problem because parasites often do not cause the classic symptoms of gastric distress. The fact is, many parasites do not produce significant diarrhea at all,

and those that do only cause such symptoms at one stage of their life cycle.

Myth: Almost all parasite infections are cleared up after the organism completes one life cycle.
Reality: Many parasites can establish long-term infection states by evading or suppressing immune system control. In one study of chronic giardia, the mean duration of infection was found to be 3.3 years,[22] and infection with *Strongyloides,* an intestinal worm, can persist for 30 years or more.[23]

Myth: Detecting parasite infections is easy.
Reality: Spot stool analysis is still the most commonly prescribed test for parasites, even though it has been found to be inadequate in most cases.[24] At the very least, such tests should be conducted three to four times, five to seven days apart, in order to properly evaluate the presence of parasites. Even then, however, there are significant problems with this method of testing.

As I mentioned, many parasites spend much of their life cycle *outside* the intestine, and no number of stool tests will detect them. Ascaris worms, for example, have a pulmonary phase in which the parasite larvae reside in the lungs and later migrate through the bronchial tubes. During this time, as well as in the first two to three months in the intestinal stage, the organism produces no eggs and will not show up in stool tests.

Fortunately, more sensitive and comprehensive analytical methods have been developed in the last ten years. See Appendix A for a list of clinical laboratories specializing in comprehensive parasite testing. I must add that there are a number of questionable techniques now in common use for the detection of parasites. Live blood analysis, in which a drop of blood is examined under a microscope, is one widely used but unproven procedure.

• **Perspective** It is not my intention to paint a picture of imminent peril from parasitic infection. In the majority of cases, parasites are diagnosed and treated, or resolve through immune system surveillance.

The point is, however, that these removal processes may take weeks, months, or even years, and during that time, the parasite adds significantly to the burden on the body's immune system. This is in part because parasites produce toxins. In addition, parasitic damage to intestinal membranes is often severe, allowing for absorption of these endotoxins and other allergenic material into the bloodstream.[25]

Parasite Action Plan

- Have a separate wooden cutting board for meat. Wash and microwave the board after each use. I recommend using a *wooden* cutting board. Although it was commonly accepted that plastic would be a safer material, there is now proof that microbes can survive well on plastic surfaces, whereas they are absorbed into the cellular structure of wood and die there.

- Wash hands carefully when preparing chicken, fish, or meat.

- Wash vegetables carefully with a stiff-bristle brush.

- Don't let your kids play in fountains or other untreated surface water (such as fish ponds).

- Be careful with water when traveling abroad. Use bottled and preferably carbonated water or bring your own filter. Filter technology is awesome these days, a most welcome development from the "old days," in which hours a day were spent boiling water.

- When traveling abroad, carry a bottle of garlic capsules and cayenne. Use liberally. In addition, take two to three capsules of grapefruit seed extract per day.

- Comprehensive testing for parasites should be done if you have any chronic digestive or respiratory condition. Anyone who has traveled in Asia, Africa, Central America, or South America should be tested, even in the absence of symptoms. See Appendix A for specialty labs.

- Do not self-diagnose or self-treat. Parasitic infections are best treated by an infectious disease specialist.

Periodontal Disease

By far the most common resident infection is gum disease, a chronic immune stress experienced by three out of four adults over the age of thirty-five. In Chapter 3, I presented a comprehensive treatment approach, including daily flossing and brushing, semiannual professional cleaning, and supplementation with antioxidants and cranberry concentrate.

CARDIOVASCULAR DISEASE

Years ago, I was struck by a report showing that the quarter of the population that eats the fewest fruits and vegetables has more than *triple* the heart disease rate compared to the quarter with the highest intake. Cardiovascular disease, the cause of approximately 1 million deaths in 2001, is preventable. In fact, raising antioxidant levels in the blood is probably the single most important step you can take to prevent a stroke or heart attack.

That may surprise you. After all, your doctor only mentioned fruits and vegetables in passing, while he or she was nearly obsessed with your blood pressure and cholesterol. Now, don't get me wrong. It *is* important to deal with elevated cholesterol and blood pressure, but the truth is, your antioxidant status is actually more important. An enormous study conducted by the World Health Organization on thousands of men and women from sixteen nations illustrated that a low level of vitamin E in the blood was *more than twice as predictive* of a heart attack than either high cholesterol or high blood pressure.[26] Research published in the *American Journal of Clinical Nutrition* shows that blood levels of vitamin C are inversely related to blood pressure, meaning that as vitamin C levels in the blood increase, blood pressure decreases.[27] Researchers at Rockefeller University have shown that supplementation with N-acetyl-cysteine (NAC) lowered blood levels of the most dangerous cholesterol fraction, known as lipoprotein (a), by 70 percent![28]

Antioxidant nutriture (reducing catabolic metabolism, covered in Chapter 3) is only one of the facets of the Metabolic Plan that will dramatically reduce your risk of cardiovascular disease. The other important factor, of course, is restoring anabolic metabolism, and as you already know, the most comprehensive anabolic influence in the human body is DHEA. A study published in the *New England Journal of Medicine* reported that:

> A 100 micrograms per deciliter increase in DHEA sulfate concentration corresponded with a 48% reduction in mortality due to cardiovascular disease and a 36% reduction in mortality for any reason. The natural level of DHEA sulfate was measured and those individuals with higher DHEA sulfate levels lived longer and had a much lower risk of heart disease.[29]

Those dramatic observations were followed by years of subsequent research in which hundreds of scientific studies illustrated that raising DHEA was safe, effective, inexpensive, and easy. In May 2000, a report was published in the *Journal of Clinical Endocrinology and Metabolism* showing that levels of DHEA are universally low in people with heart failure. Not only that, but the relationship is linear, meaning that as DHEA levels decline, heart disease worsens.[30]

To really grasp the extraordinary opportunity we now have to reduce needless suffering and death, you have to understand that heart disease is a complex problem. It is not simply a cholesterol or blood pressure problem, although these factors play a role. You don't have clean arteries and then wake up one day with clogged arteries. Atherosclerosis proceeds along three well-understood stages, and *every one* of those stages is influenced by DHEA and antioxidants.

- *Stage 1:* Cholesterol is oxidized, producing free radicals, which damage the artery wall. The injury site collects cellular debris, calcium, protein, and ultimately cholesterol to form the plaque that blocks blood flow. Antioxidants prevent the oxidation of cholesterol so that the initial injury does not occur. Now *that's* prevention.

- *Stage 2:* In the lining of an artery, abnormal cell production contributes to the atherosclerotic process. DHEA prevents this excessive cell proliferation: this has been proved with tissue cultures, animals, and humans. In coronary patients, for example, those with artery blockage greater than 50 percent were found to have lower DHEA levels than those without such extensive blockage. In fact, as blood levels of DHEA increased, there was a corresponding drop in the number of diseased blood vessels and the extent of coronary blockage.[31]

To test this association further, researchers conducted a long-term study with patients who had undergone bypass surgery. Once again, DHEA levels predicted the relative success of the surgery. In patients with low levels of DHEA, abnormal cell proliferation caused rapid degeneration of their new arteries.

- *Stage 3:* As plaque accumulates in an artery, the result at first may be chest pain or ministrokes known as transient ischemic attacks (TIAs). Heart attacks and strokes are caused by a *complete* blockage that prevents oxygen from reaching the heart or brain, resulting in cell death. This blockage is usually caused by a clot that lodges in the narrowed artery, and these clots are commonly made up of blood cells called platelets.

Now stay with me here. This sounds complicated, but it's information that may very well save your life. Platelet aggregation is the rate at which platelets clump together. The natural adherence of platelets is critically important to normal clotting, but if they become too "sticky," they can form abnormal clots that greatly increase risk for heart attack and stroke. DHEA, flavonoids, fish oil, and antioxidants have all been shown to decrease abnormal platelet aggregation. Notice I said *abnormal* aggregation. Unlike more drastic drug therapy, these natural agents do not interfere with normal and necessary clotting and repairing mechanisms. In one study, human volunteers were given either DHEA or a placebo and then administered a clotting agent. Those taking the DHEA experienced a remarkable decrease in platelet aggregation, even to the point of *complete normalization,* while none in the placebo group experienced such benefits.[32]

In addition, recent research with human volunteers suggests another way in which DHEA may help prevent and even dissolve abnormal clots. After taking supplemental DHEA for only twelve days, a group of men showed enhanced ability to dissolve fibrin, a structural component of blood clots.[33]

A NEW VIEW OF CANCER

Cancer kills more than 500,000 Americans every year, and it is arguably the most feared of all disorders. There's a reason for this. One out of every three households will experience the pain and suffering associated with this devastating disease. I would like to present a new and more hopeful view of cancer, not by offering improbable or unproven cures but by explaining the latest findings on the cause and nature of cancer. Bottom line: Cancer is a metabolic disorder—one in which normal growth cycles go haywire and the body is destroyed by unbridled cell proliferation.

At first, this appears to be counter to the central argument of this book, which is that antiaging is accomplished by restoring and maintaining highly anabolic metabolism. It must be underscored, however, that cancer is not caused by anabolic metabolism but by a *disorder* of anabolic metabolism.

There is no evidence, clinical or experimental, to suggest that anabolic factors, including sensible intake of DHEA and 7-Keto, stimulate abnormal cell proliferation. In fact, the opposite is true. Maintaining optimal DHEA levels greatly enhances immunity and *reduces* abnormal cell growth. Cancer in fact is associated with *low* DHEA levels. Dr. Marian Laderoute, a pathologist for the Bureau of Infectious Diseases in Ontario, Canada, and contributor to numerous cancer journals, has stated that the specific mutations required for carcinogenesis can be traced to a failure of immunity and cell regulation that takes place as a consequence of falling levels of DHEA.

This does not mean that maintaining youthful levels of DHEA will prevent cancer. Perhaps that would have been possible before the industrial revolution, which began dumping into our air, water, and food what are by now more than nine thousand chemicals known to cause or contribute to cancer.

What Are They Thinking?

It amazes me that this onslaught of poisoning continues unabated, while the government pours billions of dollars into a "war on cancer," which we are clearly losing. If the people who are spending those billions would walk outside on any given day in any city in America and look at the polluted sky, they would see one reason that we are losing the war. Then, standing at the checkout counter of any supermarket, they will see two other reasons that we are losing the war on cancer. First, the grocery carts are filled with ultrasweet, chemicalized, high-fat, nutrient-poor, low-fiber, highly processed food. And 60 percent of the people pushing those carts are overweight.

The National Cancer Institute estimates that 80 percent of all cancers are preventable. And yet our society promotes not prevention but exactly the opposite: cancer-causing foods (such as nitrate-laden processed meats), cigarettes, and a sedentary lifestyle. If you truly want to reduce your risk for cancer—and reliable evidence suggests that the reduction can be dramatic—you will have to in some way break away from the hypnotic trance of pop-culture diet and lifestyle.

You will also have to keep a careful eye on your exposure to industrial pollutants that show up in your food, air, and water. This will not be easy. The incidence of cancer is accelerating in great part because of the poisoning of our planet. Over the last century, cancer has gone from the eighth leading cause of death (accounting for fewer than 4 percent of deaths) to the second leading cause (accounting for nearly 20 percent of deaths).

According to Dr. Samuel Epstein, a leading toxicologist, the reason for this epidemic is crystal clear. He points out that from 1940 to 1990, the total annual production of synthetic organic chemicals increased from 1 billion to more than 600 billion pounds. (Did you get that? In one year, 600,000,000,000 pounds—600 times the output of just fifty years earlier.) In his landmark book *The Politics of Cancer* (Sierra Club Books, 1978), Dr. Epstein explains how this chemical contamination pervades our air, water, food, and ultimately, our bodies.

As long as the industrial giants can convince you that cancer is *your* fault, they're off the hook in terms of having to curb their poisoning of the environment. Part of that propaganda effort is the concept that cancer is inevitable—that it's just a matter of time before normal genetic error produces cancer.

In reality, however, scientists cannot produce cancer by random mutation. No lab tech has ever sat and watched cell division in a test tube or cell culture that ultimately became cancer. Lab techs always have to *do* something to those cells to induce *the specific mutation* that produces cancer. And what do they commonly do? They expose the cell culture or animal to a concentrated dose of the same type of chemicals to which you and I are exposed every day in small doses. Or they expose them to high levels of radiation, virtually the same thing to which you and I are exposed every day in smaller amounts from the sun, nuclear power plants, X rays, and the back of computer screens. The message is clear: cancer risk can be reduced, but it will take more than a vitamin pill.

The Metabolic Anticancer Action Plan: What Will It Take?

Diligence

Consciously decrease your exposure to pesticides, herbicides, and industrial chemicals. Eat less pesticide- and hormone-laden, high-fat meat. Purchase or grow organic food whenever possible.

Teamwork

There are plenty of organizations dedicated to protecting the environment. Help them with your dollars and your time. Help the people you love stop smoking. Support efforts by the American Medical Association and other health organizations to ban smoking in public places, to ban all advertising for cigarettes, and to support smoking awareness efforts through the media.

Knowledge

Again, cancer is *not* a random mutation. A specific series of events must take place to enable the mutation to evade multiple defenses that every cell can employ against abnormal growth. This is not difficult to understand. In fact, it's downright inspiring, and knowing what causes cancer is critically important for anyone interested in longevity.

Picture the DNA molecule like a twisted ladder. You remember the drawing in your biology text. Stretched out, it would be nearly three feet long, but this astounding molecule is folded so tightly that every cell in your body contains an exact copy. In other words, every cell in your body contains all the instructions required for the development, growth, repair, and replication of a hundred trillion cells.

During cell division, the DNA molecule "unzips," and the rungs of the ladder (called bases) must be duplicated in order to create a copy for the new cell. In your body, this occurs hundreds of billions of times every day. Spend just a minute reflecting on the unfathomable magnitude of this process.

During cell division, however, DNA is exposed to a number of potentially damaging conditions. I described in Chapter 3 how the high-oxygen environment of the cell produces massive numbers of free radicals. In addition, cells are exposed to a raft of internal and external toxins as well as UV radiation from the sun. Because these factors cause or contribute to DNA damage, they are known as carcinogens (*carcin* = "cancer," *gen* = "generator").

Since error must occur, the cell has an intricate built-in quality-control (QC) system. When DNA is damaged, QC enzymes detect the error and fix it. One astounding enzyme, *DNA polymerase,* shuttles along the DNA ladder at lightning speed. Given the chance, there is no damage that DNA polymerase cannot repair: it's like an instant repairman with an infinite tool kit.

If an error is not detected or repaired in time, certain internal cell functions don't work right, and the second QC level is apoptosis, or suicide. A message is transmitted to another gene that says, "Replication error. Abort cell."

If this signal is not properly transmitted or received and the cell completes the replication cycle, you now have a defective cell. But in this case, *external* cell functions don't work right, and so such cells are usually killed by neighboring cells. If the defective cell escapes tissue-level QC (for example, by breaking free from neighboring cells), it is detected by the immune system and destroyed.

When I was learning this, it seemed as if the whole class was worried about the one in a billion error rate. But I was astounded at the *accuracy* rate. Imagine copying the entire *Encyclopaedia Britannica* and getting just a few letters wrong . . . and doing this billions of times every day for a hundred years. As I keep saying, the human body is miraculous.

Even so, cancer happens. And we come once again to the situation in which conventional medicine says, "Oh, well, that's just the way it is. Let's go out there and treat all those cancers." Whereas preventive medicine says, "Cancer is extremely rare in the young, and risk increases in direct proportion to advancing age. Fully 80 percent of all cancers occur after age sixty-five. What, then, is the condition enjoyed in youth that is diminished as we age that allows cancer to evade the body's intricate and powerful quality-control functions?"

The answer, of course is *anabolic metabolism*—the ability of the body to maintain optimal cell function, including peak production of intracellular antioxidant enzymes to neutralize free radicals before they can damage DNA, and DNA repair enzymes to fix any damage that does occur. For those errors that evade initial stages of cell quality control, high anabolic metabolism also promotes peak immunity, including restored levels of NK (natural killer) cells, which detect and destroy cancer cells long before they become a tumor. Bottom line: The age-related increase in cancer incidence is due primarily to deficits in DNA repair, cell signaling, and immunity. Anabolic metabolism has the potential to restore all three functions to more youthful levels.

This exciting aspect of metabolism and cancer is illustrated by experiments in which rampant cancer cells were injected into an early-stage mouse embryo and the resulting animal was entirely normal! Thinking that the cancer cells were somehow destroyed by the embryonic immune system, scientists then labeled the cancer cells to learn of their fate. Imagine their surprise to find that the cancer cells had been incorporated into the tissues of the mouse and were behaving quite well as normal cells.

The only explanation is that the cancer cells had been somehow "reprogrammed" by the powerful anabolic signals produced in early stages of life. We know that hormones create longevity signals, but I'm willing to bet that the cell-regulating influence of anabolic metabolism involves remarkable levels of cell communication that have not yet been identified.

Nature's Game Revisited

As you might guess, DNA polymerase levels decline with age, as do other repair enzymes like endonuclease. In addition, specific quality-control genes start to malfunction, including the tumor-suppressor gene and my favorite (and I am not making this up) the dihydrofolate housekeeping gene.

There is a familiar pattern here of Mother Nature's pulling the rug out from under the aging body. The question is, are these declining levels of DNA repair factors themselves repairable? Many biochemists, including myself, believe that they are and that natural products will be found that enhance gene expression for DNA repair enzymes, cell growth factors, anticancer immune cells, and other aspects of aging that were previously thought to be immutable. Already, there is promising evidence for an impressive number of natural compounds:

Nutritional Tools for Cancer Prevention

- *Polysaccharides from aloe vera:* These polysaccharides provide immune-stimulating and anticancer effects.[34] These benefits have been demonstrated in animals from both topical application and, to a significant degree, oral ingestion. A growing number of aloe extracts is becoming available in health food stores.

- *Alpha lipoic acid:* This substance enhances the synthesis of glutathione, a major cancer fighter within the cell. (See Chapter 3 for dose instructions.)

- *Inosine hexaphosphate (IP-6):* This substance has powerful anticancer activity, documented in more than a dozen studies. It is derived from whole grains or available as a concentrate.

- *N-acetyl-cysteine:* NAC enhances glutathione synthesis. (See Chapter 3 for dose instructions.)

- *Green tea:* Green tea contains powerful antioxidants known as polyphenols, more potent than vitamins C or E.[35] Most of the human studies with green tea have centered around its ability to prevent certain types of cancer, including cancer of the lung, breast, stomach, and small intestine.[36] The polyphenols in green tea appear to interrupt communication between cancer cells and the biochemical factors that promote their growth. Consuming green tea with meals can also help inhibit the formation of nitrosamines, which are cancer-causing chemicals formed from the nitrites found in cured meats like ham and bacon.[37]

- *Vitamin E and other antioxidants:* People who contract cancer generally have lower serum levels of vitamin E,[38] and vitamin E supplementation has been shown to reduce risk for certain types of cancer.[39]

- *Selenium:* Deficiencies of selenium have been associated with an increased cancer risk, and selenium supplementation has been shown to reduce the incidence of several kinds of cancer, including cancers of the lung, colon, prostate, and breast. Selenium is used by the body to produce a number of enzymes critical for optimum health. As an antioxidant and a glutathione precursor, selenium helps to prevent cancer, but recent research also suggests it may be effective in slowing the progression of the disease.[40]

- *Coriolus versicolor:* This common shelf mushroom has demonstrated significant anticancer activity and is used extensively in Japan along with chemotherapy and radiation. As with aloe, the active ingredient has been shown to be the polysaccharide fraction.[41] Extracts of coriolus are just starting to appear in health food stores, but I recommend using this powerful substance under the guidance of a health care professional.

- *Pomegranate extract:* This extract contains the highest concentration of *ellagic acid* of any fruit or vegetable. Ellagic acid exerts powerful anticancer activity by enhancing cellular detoxification and stimulating the production of glutathione enzymes.[42]

- *Sulforaphane and diindolylmethane (DIM):* are natural anticancer compounds found primarily in broccoli and broccoli sprouts. Sulforaphane has been shown to have remarkable cancer-prevention potential, and its uptake into cells is greatly enhanced by the presence of guess what—glutathione.[43]

- *Fats and oils:* Increase fish oil, an excellent source of the essential fatty acid EPA, shown to reduce risk for cancer.[44] Olive oil also shows promising evidence of cancer risk reduction.[45] Decrease polyunsaturated fatty acids (PUFAs), such as corn and safflower oil, as well as saturated fat.

- *Flavonoids and carotenoids:* These substances are found in berries and other fruits, vegetables, whole grains, and beans. In addition to a wide variety and multiple servings of such foods, consider supplementing with a flavonoid/carotenoid complex containing resveratrol, quercetin, silymarin, rutin, hesperiden, and curcumin. Berries are also a rich source of ellagic acid (see "Pomegranate extract" above).

Note 1: In the above list, quercetin, silymarin, green tea, fish oil, resveratrol, and curcumin all appear to work by inhibiting an inflammatory enzyme in the body known as cyclooxygenase-2, or COX-2. New research demonstrates that cancer cells use inflammation to survive and spread throughout the body. Conversely, dozens of clinical trials are currently under way to examine the cancer-preventive effects of natural and synthetic COX-2 inhibitors.[46]

Note 2: Cancer cells also thrive in a low-oxygen environment, which means that care should be taken to ensure that tissues throughout the body are receiving adequate oxygen. Since aging is associated with decreasing oxygen uptake by the lungs as well as declining oxygen delivery by the red blood cells, effective cancer prevention must include attention to these factors. A detailed discussion of iron nutriture was presented in Chapter 3, and we'll look at the importance of exercise, deep breathing, and respiratory efficiency in the next chapter.

It should also be noted that cancer patients are often iron deficient and conventional treatments (radiation, chemotherapy) can cause or contribute to anemia. Since studies show that cancer patients who are anemic have dramatically increased mortality,[47] treating anemia becomes a matter of life or death.

CONCLUSION

Immunity is obviously an important longevity factor, and regardless of how *long* you live, it also influences the *quality* of your life. After all, disease not only shortens life; it can also make life miserable.

I've described how immune competence depends to a great extent on our actions. If nature rewards us for behaviors that contribute to survival, it is important to understand that these instructions (to boost or weaken immunity) are not coming from an outside source but from the very DNA that governs all of our cells. It's the 3-million-year-old genetic code that was written to ensure that only the best genes got passed on to future generations.

Many of these influences are obvious. Smoking or overconsumption of alcohol are clearly not behaviors that will lead your DNA to send supportive signals to your immune system and brain. But other influences are very subtle and often overlooked, such as the value of kindness, compassion, and generosity.

It would be a mistake if people took *The Metabolic Plan* as a manual for living longer at others' expense. Instead, I would like to focus on the powerful immune and longevity benefits associated with altruism and community. People who enjoy a close network of friends and family have a lower risk for heart disease and cancer. What's more, if this group has a mission that is felt to be of benefit to others, the immune enhancement is even greater than if the group's activity is perceived as value-neutral. There are, in other words, two aspects to community: the supportive environment established by and directed toward the group members, and the sense of care and concern extended to the larger family of mankind. Knowing what you know about Mother Nature, does any of this surprise you? Once again, it comes down to behaviors that support the overarching goal of a stable and successful team.

Related to this, of course, are the well-established immune benefits of laughter. Happiness is good for the gene pool—as helpful as fitness and altruism. That's because joy is contagious, supportive, and beneficial for the overall mood of the group. How many times has humor defused a tense situation, eased some pain, or opened a door to understanding? Altruism, community, and laughter are longevity signals that ripple through the individual (microcosm) and the society (macrocosm) because they help lift us all to joy. In the next chapter, we'll explore how these feelings can be amplified by movement and exercise.

SEVEN

Energy, Exercise, and Metabolism

There is no drug in current or prospective use that holds as much promise for sustained health as a lifetime program of physical exercise.

—Journal of the American Medical Association

What if you went to a financial adviser, paid a handsome consulting fee, and were handed a slip of paper that said, "Buy low. Sell high." You'd be outraged. Or what if you were depressed and went to a therapist who smiled and said, "Just snap out of it." These are just a few examples of what I call useless advice, and every day we hear similar things about exercise from young, extremely fit people who think that exercise is the easiest thing in the world.

I'd like to begin this chapter by acknowledging that exercise is difficult and often frustrating. Difficult primarily because you don't always have the energy and frustrating because you don't always see results. Here's some good news: All of that can change. Your experience of exercise, the time it takes your body to recover, and the results you achieve are all dependent on your metabolism, and that's something over which you have a great deal of control.

Following are four scenarios that I have heard thousands of times in clinical practice. See if any of them describes your experience with exercise.

Janet was an energetic achiever. In college, she was active in sports, and even after starting her own business, she stayed in shape with regular workouts and tennis. When she turned thirty, she felt, as she says, a "shift." Her tennis game suffered, workouts were more difficult; still, she persevered. After marriage and a child, she started gaining six or eight pounds a year, so that when she looked in the mirror on her fortieth birthday, she was aghast.

Janet was smart. She knew diets didn't work, having watched every one of her dieting friends lose weight only to gain it all back—and then some—within a year. So, determined to lose forty pounds "the right way," she hired a personal trainer and started working out four times a week.

After three months of hard work, she had lost eighteen pounds, and her percentage of body fat had improved from 31 percent to 27 percent—significant, but far from her goal. Her trainer explained that she was at a plateau, and in order to lose more weight, she would have to increase both the duration and the intensity of her workouts. As she told me, "With two kids and a full-time career, the chances of that happening were about the same as winning the lottery."

Ben experienced a similar wake-up call when he turned fifty. Many of his friends were taking early retirement, but as Ben explained it, "I didn't feel old. I just *looked* old." He decided to get back in shape and enrolled in an exercise program at his local YMCA. After three months of hard work, he noticed very little improvement in muscle tone. Ben concluded that getting back in shape was simply not possible—that he was in fact over the hill and should stop trying.

Roberta and her husband Michael gave each other health club memberships for Christmas. Both started working out in earnest (along with millions of other Americans) right after New Year's. After two weeks, Roberta felt exhausted and decided to quit exercising "for a while." For a while turned out to be forever. "I just couldn't bring myself to go back into something that was making me feel bad," she explained.

Michael experienced some fatigue as well as muscle and joint pain, but his response was more "macho." Determined to work through it, he upped his workouts to four times a week; then he pulled a muscle in his upper back. Michael's doctor said he would have to stop exercising "for a while," and that also became forever. Looking back, Michael said that there were two factors that ended his exercise program: fear of reinjury and the fact that Roberta dropped out of their exercise pact.

These four examples represent the experience of millions of baby boomers, and in each case, the underlying problem was not willpower; it was *metabolism*. Janet was doing everything right, but the stress of raising children and balancing a career accelerated her downward metabolic spiral. She learned the hard way that effort does not equal success if you're on the catabolic side of life. On the Metabolic Plan, she lost fourteen pounds in ninety days, not something you'd see in sensational newspaper ads, but she was delighted. It was *real* weight loss, documented by a decrease in body fat to 22 percent. Best of all, she knew that if she stayed in the anabolic "zone," she'd never have to think of dieting.

Ben found that gaining muscle was nearly impossible at age fifty. I pointed out that his memories of lifting weights and seeing results were from his anabolic twenties. The good news, of course, was that he could restore that metabolic advantage. "No way," said Ben. "I'm not taking anabolic steroids." I laughed. "Of course not," I assured him. The prescription drugs abused by bodybuilders are high-potency synthetic analogs of testosterone. Their dangerous and sometimes even lifethreatening side effects are due to the fact that they elevate testosterone to levels ten to twenty times physiological normal.

"I'm talking about DHEA and an even safer metabolite known as 7-Keto," I explained. "The target dose is one that will bring your DHEA level to that of a thirty-year-old, and studies show that testosterone levels will be for the most part unchanged."

Thus assured, Ben then became curious. "If DHEA is such a great bodybuilding aid, why aren't all the muscleheads using it?" I explained that many bodybuilders were in fact using DHEA, but those looking for superhuman physiques often had to resort to anabolic steroids. Ben agreed that he was not out to win any contests. He just wanted his thirty-three-inch waist and fourteen-inch biceps back. On the Metabolic Plan, he got both in a little over three months.

And what about Roberta and Michael? They both realized that they had made mistakes. Deciding to exercise is easy, but finding the energy to fuel that exercise is something else altogether. And protecting fifty-year-old muscles, ligaments, and tendons is not something you can do overnight. They learned that anabolic metabolism must be restored before you can expect exercise to be enjoyable.

THE MISSING LINK IN AMERICA'S FITNESS PROGRAM

I went to a bookstore the other day and browsed through a dozen books on exercise. Most of what I found could be very helpful for people age eighteen to thirty-five, but for anyone over thirty-five, these books were next to worthless. They provide a great deal of information about *why* we should exercise, but most of us already know why. The problem is that when we try to "just do it," we feel as if we've been hit by a bus.

Please read the following sentence carefully:

If you are over forty, you can read any number of exercise books, watch all the exercise videos, and try to follow the programs— and you will *not* get results, you will *not* feel great, you will *not* succeed, and you will *not* want to try again . . . ever.

I'm sorry for the negativity. I believe in a positive approach to life and its problems, and I'm going to give you some wonderful positives in just a moment. But I need to make this one point crystal clear. Every program that expects you to "just do" something that scientific research proves your body can't "just do" is self-defeating.[1] If you want to achieve true fitness and vitality, you have to stop beating your head against the wall. You have to understand the rules of nature's game and learn how to bend them in your favor. It's not willpower; it's *metabolism*. It's not motivation; it's *biochemistry*. It's not your attitude; it's your *hormones*.

Once your body shifts into *catabolic* metabolism, exercise:

- Makes you feel exhausted, not invigorated

- Makes every muscle and joint in your body ache

- Produces minimal results

- Increases the likelihood of injury

The failure of the fitness movement to provide a solution to this indisputable biological fact explains why so few people past the age of forty are able to remain fit. It explains why fewer than 6 percent of women over forty can be considered "active" as defined by the performance of thirty minutes of moderate exercise three times a week. As these sobering statistics sink in, let me assure you that getting active and regaining fitness are not only possible; they've never been easier.

METABOLIC KEYS

If you are over forty and want to exercise to achieve greater vitality, the *only* way to succeed is to *change your metabolism!* When you restore youthful, anabolic metabolism (the rebuild-repair-restore metabolism, which normally lasts until about age thirty):

- Your body produces aerobic enzymes that escort fatty acids into the muscle to create energy. This means you will finish exercise with normal blood sugar and a feeling of invigoration.

- You will avoid the muscle and joint pain that exercise produces in the no-longer-young. Joints, bones, and connective tissues are strengthened by increased production of collagen and structural proteins such as glucosamine and chondroitin.

- You will see results in a short period of time.

- You will have better skin tone and muscle tone and, if desired, bigger, stronger muscles and less body fat.

- You will be safeguarded against injury by the heightened activity of anabolic repair metabolism. Muscle protects the vulnerable, less flexible ligaments, tendons, joints, and bones. Moreover, increased anabolic metabolism means greater flexibility.

The Energy Factor

If you won the lottery today, no one would have to tell you to go shopping. That's what people naturally do when they have a lot of money. In the same way, when you win the energy lottery, no one will have to beg, cajole, or in any way motivate you to exercise. You will do it naturally because that's what people do when they have an abundant supply of energy. The good news is that your chances of restoring youthful energy levels are a great deal better than your chances of winning any lottery. In fact, with the Metabolic Plan, it's a sure bet.

That's because every step you take builds on the last step. If you do it right, in other words, there'll be little pain and a lot of gain. This comes from the simple fact that your body craves exercise. Oh, you may not feel that way right now, but once you step on the path to fitness—marked "metabolism"—you'll be amazed. When you exercise, everything works better, and I mean *everything*.

David came to my office with the midlife blues. He was moody, overweight, had no energy and no real passion for life. As you can imagine, this was not great for his marriage. After a thorough physical exam, David's doctor gave him a clean bill of health and suggested psychological counseling. I believe that counseling is an extremely valuable practice, but in this case, I suggested that David put that on hold, and his doctor agreed to give the Metabolic Plan a test.

"Don't tell me to exercise," David said at our first meeting. "I've tried aerobics, exercycle, stair climbers, and rowing machines. I hated them all and only felt worse." "Oh, no," I replied, "I would *never* suggest such a thing. Sending you to a gym at this point would be like entering the Indianapolis 500 in a Ford Pinto."

Like most people, David didn't know where energy comes from. Like most, he believed that the men and women working out at the local health club were there because they had a lot of energy. "In reality," I explained, "they have a lot of energy because they're working out." I showed David a highly magnified photograph of a muscle cell from a sedentary person, pointing out the structures within the cell known as *mitochondria* that generate energy. Then I showed him a similar photo of a muscle cell from a fit person of the same age. "What do you see?" I asked. "A lot more of those mitochondria," he said. "In fact," I explained, "up to *ten times* more energy-producing mitochondria. Not only that," I continued, "the fit person's mitochondria are more dense and produce more energy compared to those of a sedentary person." "So if I got fit, I'd have *ten times* the energy I do right now?" David asked, in surprise. "More or less," I replied. "Think how that would feel."

Over the next 120 days, David climbed out of the sedentary hole into which he'd fallen by following the step-by-step approach described in the following pages. He experienced the use-it-or-lose-it phenomenon firsthand, as his body started to produce fat-burning enzymes, energy-storing enzymes, increased mitochondrial density, and greater respiratory efficiency. After a stunning 10 percent improvement in maximal oxygen uptake (a test known as VO₂ max), I explained that this indicated he was extracting a great deal more oxygen from every breath he took, not only during exercise but twenty-four hours a day.

In a very real sense, he souped up his Pinto body. Only then did he venture back to the gym, and by that time, just about everything in his life had improved. His enthusiasm and energy resulted in a promotion at work, he was sleeping better and waking up more refreshed. And his mood? He described it as a fifty-pound weight being lifted off his shoulders. His wife loved her "new" husband and gladly agreed to swap the cruise vacation they'd been planning for a bicycle trip through the rolling hills of California's wine country. David illustrated what I've been saying for decades. Even if the fitness parade passed you by, you now have an opportunity to catch up. *Everyone* can participate.

"OK," I can hear you asking. "If energy must come first, how do I get more energy?" I'm glad you asked.

Exercise, Aging, and the Downward Spiral

As we lose the anabolic metabolism of youth, we lose muscle mass. With decreased muscle, our bodies begin to interpret the amounts and types of exercise that we did in our youth as *stress*. This shift increases the production of the catabolic hormone cortisol, which actually lowers DHEA, suppresses immunity, and contributes to a number of degenerative problems. Clearly, this vicious cycle must be reversed.

DHEA Builds Energy and Muscle Mass

We have discussed how optimizing DHEA restores healthy anabolic metabolism. DHEA also raises levels of a repair biochemical known as insulinlike growth factor-1, or IGF-1. This can decrease your recovery time after a workout and dramatically improve muscle repair and synthesis. Gerontologists have known for decades that IGF-1 decreases as we age, but they accepted this decrease as an irreversible result of the aging process. We now know that declining IGF-1 can be reversed.

Researchers gave DHEA to a group of men in their late fifties. After only thirty days, they documented an astounding 90 percent increase in IGF-1. This translates into greater muscle growth for athletes over thirty and better muscle maintenance for anyone over fifty. Just as important as these anabolic benefits, increased IGF-1 also means decreased risk for heart disease. IGF-1 improves circulation and helps prevent the formation of abnormal clots.

Another benefit of DHEA supplementation is a marked improvement in muscle definition soon after beginning a strength-training program. An excellent study reported in the *Annals of the New York Academy of Sciences* concluded:

> DHEA in appropriate replacement doses appears to have remedial effects with respect to its ability to induce an anabolic growth factor, increase muscle strength and lean body mass, activate immune function, and enhance quality of life in aging men and women, with no significant adverse effects.[2]

DHEA isn't the only tool available to you as you begin an exercise program. You can improve your capacity for physical and mental activity *even further* through bioenergetics and connective tissue support. These two aspects of a full nutritional support program can increase your performance and your enjoyment of exercise, helping you realize your full potential for optimum health and longevity.

The Bioenergetic Boost

As an adviser to members of the 1984 U.S. Olympic track-and-field team, I was asked to develop a formulation of natural compounds to help our athletes reach and maintain peak performance. Stimulants like caffeine, ephedra, and guarana were out of the question, not only because they were banned but because they do not enhance speed, strength, or any aspect of athletic skill. Instead, my research focused on the specific nutritional requirements of cellular energy production— that biochemical assembly line within each cell known as the Krebs cycle. These unique and critically essential substances are known as rate-limiting *bioenergetic nutrients,* meaning that a shortage of any of them will reduce your ability to create energy.

Not surprisingly, these turned out to be many of the same nutrients that have been stripped out of the modern diet through soil depletion, processing, and cooking. We may like the taste and convenience of refined sugars, modified fats, and highly refined starches, but our bodies are designed for something quite different. In fact, extensive testing illustrated that I was working with athletes who, no matter how much they ate, were essentially malnourished.

We are thus faced with two choices: we can return to hunting and gathering, or we can restore bioenergetic nutrients to peak levels. The latter course of action resulted in significant improvements in performance for my Olympic athletes. Soon after, I realized that these specific nutrients could be used to improve the metabolic efficiency of *just about anyone*. The formulation that helped elite athletes shave a few minutes off their marathon time could help an unfit person walk around the block, eliminate the mood and energy slumps that many people experience during the day, and help restore youthful vitality. So much for the "inevitable" decline in energy production. In truth, there is no scientific basis for age-related fatigue, and I have hundreds of case histories to prove it.

Vital Bioenergetic Nutrients: The Super Seven

Each of the following nutrients is required for the efficient production of energy in your cells. When they are present at optimal levels, the body produces all the energy you need to work, play, and enjoy life. The seven nutrients needed to fuel the energy cycle are:

1. *Alpha ketoglutaric acid (AKG):* Although it sounds like something from a chemist's lab, AKG is an essential nutrient found in every cell of the human body. As a vital component of the energy-producing cycle, AKG levels help determine the body's metabolic efficiency. In a study with human volunteers, supplementation with AKG resulted in enhanced oxygen delivery and improved exercise tolerance.[3] AKG is also required for the optimal metabolism of carbohydrates, fats, and proteins.

Suggested daily dose: 300–500 milligrams.

2. *Vitamin B6:* Vitamin B6 is another key metabolic nutrient, necessary for both aerobic and anaerobic energy production. It is also a building block for numerous biochemicals, including the enzyme needed to produce DHEA, and it plays an important role in carbohydrate metabolism. Vitamin B6 is one of the nutrients most

likely to be destroyed by food processing or high-heat cooking, and insufficiency is common. The combination of vitamin B$_6$ and AKG has been shown to decrease the accumulation of lactic acid in working muscles. Since lactic acid contributes to the muscle soreness that causes many people to stop exercising, optimizing levels of these nutrients can make exercise easier and more enjoyable.

Suggested daily dose: 10–15 milligrams.

3. *Coenzyme Q10:* This essential nutrient is needed for cellular respiration. Every cell of your body—from the top of your head to the tips of your toes—breathes. Energy is produced when oxygen is combined with fuel derived from food. This biochemical "combustion" is sparked by coenzyme Q10.

   CoQ10 is normally obtained from a group of nutrients known as ubiquinones, which are often eliminated or destroyed in a highly processed diet What's more, CoQ10 levels tend to decrease rapidly with age. Sixty-five-year-olds have only about 20 percent of the CoQ10 they had in their prime.[4]

Suggested daily dose: 30–200 milligrams.

4. *Chromium:* Chromium's importance in bioenergetic nutrition stems primarily from the cofactor role it plays with the hormone insulin. Since insulin is required for the delivery of fuel to brain and muscles, insufficient chromium can contribute to fatigue and low metabolic efficiency. Research conducted by the U.S. Department of Agriculture found that 90 percent of the people studied were obtaining inadequate levels of chromium from their diet[5]

   Interestingly, there is a powerful DHEA/chromium connection. Both can help correct the metabolic defect known as *insulin resistance,* which contributes to diabetes and heart disease. Both have been shown to help lower blood cholesterol, and both can help reduce the incidence of atherosclerotic plaques.

   In fact, restoring optimum levels of chromium can help increase the amount of DHEA that is available to your body.

Hyperinsulinism, a condition of excessive insulin production, can often be eliminated by correcting a chromium deficiency.[6] That, in turn, will naturally raise DHEA levels.

Suggested daily dose: 200–300 micrograms.

5. *Acetyl-L-carnitine (ALC):* This bioenergetic nutrient does double duty by enhancing energy and improving mental clarity. It's a naturally occurring substance that carries fatty acids into the cell for conversion into energy. At the same time, the acetyl part of the molecule helps the brain produce an important neurotransmitter known as acetylcholine.

Suggested daily dose: 100–1,000 milligrams.

6. *Alpha lipoic acid:* I've described the breakthrough studies of Bruce Ames and others that documented the tremendous bioenergetic benefits of acetyl-L-carnitine and lipoic acid. It is believed that the ALC boosts energy production by mitochondrial oxidation and the lipoic acid neutralizes the free-radical by-products.

Suggested daily dose: 50–200 milligrams.

7. *Potassium and magnesium aspartate:* More than thirty years of research supports the use of potassium and magnesium aspartate as antifatigue agents.[7] Like AKG, these mineral/aspartic acid complexes appear to enhance vitality by improving the efficiency of the energy production cycle. They are also essential for cardiovascular health and muscle contraction.

Suggested daily dose: 300–500 milligrams.

Protecting Connective Tissue

Bioenergetics can help you regain lost energy, and restored anabolic metabolism can greatly enhance your ability to maintain high muscle mass. Neither, however, decreases your risk of injury. A forty-five-year-old who suddenly finds he can bench-press two hundred pounds again may forget that he is pushing that weight with middle-aged joints. And it's not just macho men; women also notice dramatic strength improvements on the Metabolic Plan and may push too far too fast. It's important, therefore, to go slowly when getting back in shape and develop an awareness of connective tissue health.

Your skeletal and muscle systems are designed to work together in perfect harmony, allowing your body to maintain just the right mix of flexibility and rigidity. Flexibility enables us to move, dance, run, and jump. Rigidity gives control to these movements so that we don't constantly injure ourselves. Flexibility and rigidity are regulated through the action of joints (which limit the movement of bones) along with ligaments and tendons (which hold joints together and attach muscle to bone).

As we grow older, our joints and connective tissue become dehydrated, much the way our skin does. Scientists have found a specialized group of compounds known as *proteoglycans*, which strengthen and hydrate the tendons, ligaments, and joints. Two well-known proteoglycans are chondroitin and glucosamine. These can be restored in two ways:

1. *Exercise:* In true metabolic-model-of-aging fashion, research shows that exercise stimulates the body to produce new collagen and higher levels of repair and rebuild proteoglycans.[8] This is stunning new data, illustrating one of the pitfalls of research. Physiology texts have always asserted that collagen is basically inert. It gets stiff, you get stiff, you die. Turns out this was true only for the people the researchers were studying, the vast majority of whom were *sedentary*. In people who remain active, collagen synthesis may take place at any age, and the strength of existing collagen can be improved.[9]

2. *Anticatabolic supplements for supple joints:* Chondroitin sulfate has been used as a therapeutic nutrient for centuries. It's a major ingredient in homemade chicken soup! At the health food store, chondroitin sulfate is usually derived from bovine or chicken cartilage. Also available are *glucosamine sulfate* and *N-acetylglucosamine*, which perform similar functions.

    Other important components of a connective tissue support

program include boron, silicon, vitamin C, vitamin D, calcium, magnesium, and manganese. These substances can sometimes be found in a single tablet or capsule.

The Upward Spiral

1. Optimal bioenergetic nutrients increase energy production.

2. Greater energy leads to easier and more enjoyable exercise.

3. Easier exercise leads to more consistent exercise.

4. Regular exercise enhances sleep quality (deeper, more rejuvenating sleep).

5. Deeper sleep increases production of DHEA and growth hormone.

6. Increased anabolic metabolism leads to enhanced protein synthesis, accelerated repair and rebuild activity throughout the body, increased muscle mass, and enhanced fat burning. Anabolic metabolism also contributes to increased production of aerobic enzymes that enable the body to burn fat and to increased glycogen (energy) storage in muscles. If two people the same age and weight start running, the one who begins the race with higher glycogen stores will win and feel better afterward.

7. Decreasing catabolic metabolism leads to reduced soreness and pain associated with exercise.

8. The visible results of this spiral are less fat and more muscle. The intangible results are feelings of invigoration and vitality leading to greater motivation. It is unlikely that anyone who experiences these changes will ever go back to a sedentary life.

HOW DO I START?

Now that you're giving your body the nutritional support it needs to get the most out of exercise, you're ready to start. I know you want to go climb those steps with Rocky, jump up and down, and raise your arms in victory; but remember, slow and steady takes the prize.

- *Avoid the "weekend warrior" syndrome.* Consistent, moderate exercise spread out over the entire week is more beneficial than intense activity concentrated in a day or two. Remember, it's not about "buns of steel" or Terminator biceps. If you're just beginning to exercise, follow these principles:

  Exercise should be moderate. Fatigue and exhaustion can actually slow your progress toward fitness and weight loss. Moderate exercise stimulates your metabolism without throwing your body into motivation-killing exhaustion.

  Consistency is more important than intensity. There's an "energy warehouse manager" in your brain that predicts your energy needs based upon past experience. If you lead a sedentary life, the warehouse manager knows that you don't need much energy, so he sends most of the excess calories into storage (to your thighs, for example). So sporadic exercise only confuses the manager. One day, he runs out of energy, and the next day, there's a surplus. The result is that your body experiences no real increase in metabolic efficiency or fat burning.

  But when you do consistent, moderate exercise, the message to your brain is this: "This body is now an active, dynamic body that requires a great deal more energy than before, so I need to stop storing so many calories as fat and keep more in ready reserve for all this activity." The good news is that this message can be loud and clear even without long, intense exercise sessions. The most important thing is consistency.

- *Use the metabolic point system.* When you first add exercise to your daily routine, you want to send as many "activity messages" as possible to the energy warehouse manager in your brain. You want the manager to get the message that your active body is going to require increasing levels of *energy.* Repeating the message consistently is the key.

  Studies show that any activity—such as gardening, housework, golf, bowling, shopping, or badminton—can contribute to improved fitness and greater metabolic efficiency. These fairly low-key activities are also excellent additions to more strenuous exercise. So get in the habit of taking "activity breaks" several times each day. I've developed a point system that can be helpful. From the accompanying table, you'll see that each suggested activity is associated with a number of points. Your goal is to accumulate points throughout the week so that your seven-day total is *at least* 100.

EXERCISE TABLE

Activity	Points
Walking briskly (3–4 miles per hour)	25 for over 45 minutes 15 for half an hour 5 for 15 minutes
Conditioning or calisthenics	25 for over 45 minutes 15 for half an hour 5 for 15 minutes
Home care, general cleaning	10 for over 45 minutes 5 for half an hour or less
Mowing the lawn	20 for over 45 minutes
Golf, carrying own clubs	10 for 18 holes 5 for 9 holes 3 for driving range
Home repair	25 for vigorous labor 15 for moderate labor 5 for general labor
Gardening	25 for vigorous labor 15 for moderate labor 5 for light gardening
Cycling moderately	20 for over 45 minutes 10 for half an hour 5 for leisure cycling
Dancing vigorously	25 for over 45 minutes 10 for half an hour

Actively playing with children	20 for over 45 minutes of
	    physical play
	10 for half an hour
	5 for carrying child
	    throughout the day

Singles tennis	20 per 3 matches
Doubles tennis	10 per 3 matches
Racquetball	25 per 2 matches
Squash	25 per 2 matches
Sex	25 for over 45 minutes 15 for half an hour 5 for 15 minutes
Walking the dog	10 for over a mile 5 for 1/2 mile
Bowling	10 for 20 frames 5 for 10 frames
Frisbee	25 for ultimate game 10 for over an hour of catch
Jogging, moderate effort	15 for over 3 miles 5 for less than 2 miles
Show shoveling	25 for over half an hour 10 for 15 minutes
Climbing stairs instead of taking elevator:	
1 Floor	3
2 Floors	6
3 Floors	9
4 Floors	12

Hint: The most efficient activity in the list is walking. Walking is easy, inexpensive (it requires only a good pair of walking shoes), and can be done almost anywhere. Bad weather? Walk in your local shopping mall. Walking provides the most points for the least effort and time. Start slow and gradually increase your pace so that you're able to cover two miles in thirty minutes. Then extend the duration to as long as you can. A good one-hour power walk will earn you 25 points. Do that four times a week and you've already reached your 100-point minimum metabolic goal.

Walking is such an efficient exercise because it uses the largest muscles of your body (front and back of your thighs). In fact, you may decide that you like walking so much that you can dispense with the point system altogether and simply purchase a digital pedometer. These wonderful devices are available in sporting goods stores and can make a world of difference in your fitness program. There's something about having a pedometer clipped on your belt that provides an effective, gentle reminder to move. Since the device registers every step you take (even pacing around the office while talking on the phone), the steps add up quickly, and research shows that logging ten thousand steps per day will take you far toward your fitness goals. The ten thousand–step target has also been shown to enhance just about any weight-loss program. You'll find yourself checking your pedometer midway through the day and adjusting your activity levels—almost automatically—to reach your ten thousand–step goal.

Hint: Duration is especially critical if fat burning is your goal. It takes about thirty minutes for your metabolism to switch from a carbohydrate-burning mode to a fat-burning mode. Therefore, every minute you exercise beyond the thirty-minute threshold burns fat![10]

THE NEXT LEVEL: STRENGTH TRAINING

In order to maximize the benefit of all the exercise you're getting, you need to increase your upper-body strength. Exercises like walking, jogging, tennis, basketball, and racquetball emphasize the major muscle groups in the legs and provide relatively little benefit to the upper body.

Sixty-five percent of your muscles are above the waist. Because these are probably your most underdeveloped muscles, your upper body is the easiest place to build muscle mass quickly. We're not talking about pumping-iron kind of muscles; rather, building muscle tone. Research shows that using light weights (three to five pounds to start) can effectively and efficiently strengthen arm, chest, back, and shoulder muscles. For best results, do your strength training on alternate days to give muscles time to recover.

Get Help

For years, I tried to write out careful instructions for weight training. I reviewed dozens of videos and recommended the best. Still, people went out and hurt themselves. I've concluded that it is *absolutely essential* to use the guidance of an exercise professional, at least for a few sessions. A certified expert will help you set realistic goals and, most important, show you safe techniques for each exercise. Whether you're using hand weights, machines, or a combination of both, there is simply no substitute for professional guidance. This technical assistance is often included with health club membership fees. If you have the financial means, you may want to sign up for personal training—in which case, a trainer will stay with you throughout your workout, watching, correcting, and guiding you through each phase of your program.

More Help

Please review the discussion of branched-chain amino acids (BCAAs) presented in Chapter 3. BCAA supplements (1,000–2,000 milligrams) are particularly valuable after a strenuous workout. They can accelerate strength gains, improve mood, and send you out the door feeling like a million bucks.

THE FINAL FRONTIER: MAXIMAL TRAINING

The term *maximal training* refers to a strength-training program that works your muscles *to the max*. With this advanced technique, you may do just ten repetitions per exercise, but you use so much weight and move the weight so slowly that the eleventh rep is impossible. Maximal training is the most efficient use of your time and energy, but you need to build up to it slowly with the supervision of a qualified fitness trainer. If you are over forty, the joint and tendon support nutrients described above are essential.

Men tend to get into maximal training more than women because of sheer testosterone. You can see it in the machine and free-weight area of any gym. All the guys are groaning like primates because that's what it takes to maximize a muscle's capability. Ask the fellow who's just finished a 250-pound bench press how he feels. He's had to gather every ounce of strength in his shoulders, arms, chest, and back to do it, and he feels *fantastic*.

On the other hand, women have not generally considered maximal weight training for two reasons. First, they didn't know they could, or they weren't given the option. Second, most women have an aversion to "bulking up." However, this fear is largely unfounded. Due to hormonal differences, it is very difficult for women to develop enormous muscles. Women bodybuilders require eight to ten years of intensive training to develop the prizewinning bodies we see on TV. Those muscles will never appear on an average woman who does a twenty-minute workout four times a week. But that twenty-minute strength-training session will have enormous benefits. Remember, increasing muscle tissue is the most reliable path to enhanced metabolism, greater energy, and effective weight management.

Women who are interested in strength training can especially benefit from taking DHEA. DHEA actually helps replicate the energy level, confidence, and assertiveness of youth so that women, with proper training, can enjoy maximal workout techniques.

THE FORGOTTEN FACTORS: STRETCHING AND RELAXATION

No matter what your level of exercise, stretching may be the missing link to your success. Daily stretching will make all the difference in keeping your muscles and tendons limber as they adapt to your new routine.

There are a number of reasons why people don't stretch. Many feel pressed for time and dive into a workout, sometimes with painful results from tight muscles used too much or too soon. Set aside a minimum of five to ten minutes per day for your stretching routine, which can consist of yoga postures or any other combination of stretches. The best time is right before exercise.

Rest is also an important component of fitness. To get the maximum benefit from your program, be sure to take at least one day off per week. A day of rest will give your muscles the opportunity to rebuild themselves and become even stronger. As the intensity of your workouts increases, you will need to take off two days per week—one in midweek and one on the weekend—to continue reaping the greatest benefits.

STRENGTHEN AND STRETCH WITH YOGA

Yoga may be the most advanced system of stretching and toning ever developed. Yoga postures have the added advantage of increasing your flexibility and range of motion and strengthening your muscles and tendons.

The nonforce movements of yoga are natural and safe. This five-thousand-year-old practice can be undertaken by just about anyone. It is self-paced, and no special equipment is needed. While it is possible to learn yoga from books or videos, I highly recommend attending at least a few classes with a qualified yoga instructor. Since there are different yoga styles, it's best to interview prospective teachers to get a sense of the style they teach. Some classes are quite vigorous, while others focus more on relaxation. You may want to sample a number of different classes to find the one that matches your fitness and flexibility goals.

SOME FINAL THOUGHTS

Your Fitness Goals

What are your fitness goals? Do you just want to feel better and have more energy? Are you trying to decrease body fat? Or are you ultimately interested in bodybuilding and maximal workouts?

Clearly defined goals are the key to keeping up your motivation and building on your success. Take a few minutes to write out your fitness goals. Think in small increments and make your goals attainable. One example of a realistic, attainable goal is "I will walk for thirty minutes four days a week."

"I want to lose thirty pounds" is probably too big to start with. If you have weight to lose, don't worry so much about the exact number of pounds. You'll drive yourself crazy and kill your motivation running to the bathroom scale every day. Just remember that there were no overweight cavemen or -women. The Metabolic Plan is designed to help you develop a youthful, powerful, energetic, and highly efficient body. As a result, your body weight will tend to normalize over time; that is, it will find the weight that is right for you, based on *your* body type, not a weight-chart reading derived from national averages. This approach to weight management may *seem* slow (one pound per week is optimal), but you'll be fitter than ever before, and you'll be more likely to keep the weight off. Remember, you'll be trading light-but-bulky fat tissue for dense muscle tissue, so the inches will come off far more quickly than the pounds.

METABOLIC PLAN WEIGHT MANAGEMENT BENEFITS

Research published in the July 2000 issue of *Current Therapeutic Research* illustrates that increasing intake of 7-Keto™ (7-oxo-DHEA) can significantly enhance weight (and fat) loss when combined with exercise and moderate calorie reduction. In this double-blind, placebo-controlled study, volunteers supplementing with 7-Keto lost 6.3 pounds in eight weeks; the placebo group lost only 2.1 pounds. Importantly, the 7-Keto group lost a mean of 2 percent of body fat, which was three times the fat loss experienced by the placebo group.[11]

Some people have a harder time reducing body fat than others simply because of genetics. If you want to lose weight, an important question to ask yourself is, "What is my genetic potential for that?" Set your goals accordingly. Strive to maximize your health, vitality, and fulfillment in life, with whatever genes you have inherited along the way. I encourage people to reject the popular notion that equates beauty with an almost scarecrow thinness. Healthy bodies come in all sizes.

Staying Motivated

The key to keeping your motivation up is to design an exercise program that suits you. In addition to setting realistic goals, ask yourself the following questions:

- What am I willing to do to achieve my fitness goals?

- In order to exercise, do I need to make an appointment with a trainer?

- Would I prefer to exercise alone?

- Would I prefer to exercise with a friend or in a class?

- What rewards can I give myself for sticking with my program (new walking shoes, tickets to a Broadway play, and so forth)?

Seeking Expert Advice

If you are carrying extra weight or have any medical condition that requires special attention (such as high blood pressure or diabetes), see your physician before beginning any exercise program. If at all possible, hire a certified fitness trainer, especially if you are new to exercise. Enlist the help of a physical therapist for problems that may require specially designed exercises. People with chronic back pain, for example, are often afraid to exercise, even though the right exercise taught by a professional might significantly improve their condition.

One of the beauties of exercise is that people who are just starting out see the greatest results in the shortest period of time. With a balanced natural foods diet and renewed anabolic metabolism, you will be set to enjoy a completely new experience of vitality and health.

EIGHT

Optimal Nutrition:
Building Blocks of the Metabolic Plan

*We are living in a world today where lemonade is made from artificial
flavors and furniture polish is made from real lemons.*

—*Alfred E. Newman*

METABOLIC FACTOR 1: THE FACTS ON FOOD

The Metabolic Plan—indeed, any effective antiaging strategy—depends
upon two things: supporting anabolic repair and reducing catabolic
damage. Nutrition plays a key role in *both* of these endeavors. Repair
obviously requires raw materials, which must come from the food we
eat. Remember that your body needs only about forty-two nutrients to
stay alive, but to optimize anabolic metabolism, you need literally hundreds of compounds. These include many nutrients that have been
stripped out of the American diet through food processing and selective breeding.[1] You create about 300 billion new cells each day. If critical materials are not available, your body will make do, but over time,
cellular integrity is compromised.

Likewise, suboptimal nutrition will cause catabolic damage. Dr.
Bruce Ames, one of the lead researchers who discovered the mitochondrial energy breakthrough discussed in Chapter 2, has identified eight
key nutrients that help to prevent DNA damage. Ames and his team
have published studies showing that fully half of the American population is deficient in one or more of these critical compounds.[2] The cause
of this serious problem is not money or lack of good food. It is confusion.

Are You Confused?

I have on my shelves no fewer than a hundred books that purport to lay out the ideal diet, and they range from the sensible to the absurd. Entire movements have been launched by charismatic leaders and supported by tens of thousands of true believers based on a diet of nothing but fruits and nuts, or a single "miracle food" such as blue-green algae or apple cider vinegar.

It's tempting to say that the health foods movement caused our confusion, but this pales in comparison to what the giant food corporations have foisted upon us. Cereal companies and bakers have defined what Americans eat for breakfast. Was this discussed among competent nutritionists and designed according to the needs of men, women, and children? Not at all. Whole grains were refined, sweetened, and packaged for scant pennies per serving. Bread was made to resemble pastry, and thus, breakfast became, within a few generations, an onslaught of refined carbohydrates.

And what of lunch? Today, more than 55 percent of Americans eat lunches consisting mainly of more refined carbohydrates combined with highly processed meat in the form of hamburgers and cold cuts. The only vegetable to be found in such fare is a leaf of wilted lettuce, some ketchup, or perhaps a highly salted slice of pickle.

How did we get into such a mess? Follow the money. There is no whole-grain, exercise, broccoli, blueberry, or carrot lobby. But the food giants—including the meat, candy, coffee, soft drink, cereal, and dairy industries—have been influencing public policy and dominating media advertising for almost a century. And today, we are the fattest society that has ever lived.

Like mice in a cage, we tend to eat what the food giants feed us. If there is one creative step you can take to improve your success on the Metabolic Plan, it is to leave the cage (it's not locked) and think for yourself. Aging is a metabolic process, and diet is a tremendous factor. Diet determines energy, blood sugar, and insulin. It determines to a great extent the amount of fat and muscle on your body. It influences your risk for disease. Julius Richmond, a former U.S. surgeon general, stated that if you do not drink excessively or smoke cigarettes, the single most important factor influencing your health (and therefore how long you live) is nutrition.

The results indicate, for the first time, that a semi-purified rodent diet designed to mimic the human Western diet can induce colonic tumors in normal mice without carcinogen exposure.
—H. L. Newmark et al., *"A Western-Style Diet Induces Cancer in the Colon of Normal Mice,"* Carcinogenesis

How to End the Confusion

You know what I'm going to say. After all, for seven chapters, I've been asking you to think and exercise like a hunter-gatherer. Now I want you to eat like one. I'm going to suggest that the ideal diet is the one humans ate for millions of years, before the invention of breakfast cereal, candy bars, fake fats, French fries, chicken tenders, soft drinks, coffee, doughnuts, potato chips, and burgers. It's the diet we were designed to eat.

Does that mean we should go out in the woods and gather roots, berries, and tender shoots?

No. I suggest that we identify the *characteristics* of a hunting-and-gathering diet and match those with food choices that are readily available. What are the characteristics of a hunting-and-gathering diet?

Eat Whole, Unrefined Foods

Refining and processing food removes critically important nutrients. Processing wheat into white flour, for example, eliminates 85 percent of the CoQ10, 90 percent of the vitamin E, and virtually all of the fiber. In all, nineteen nutrients are reduced or destroyed. The fact that manufacturers then add back thiamine, riboflavin, and niacin and call the product "enriched" is a joke.

Vitamin A and beta carotene may survive some food processing, but they are very sensitive to oxidation and are protected only by the presence of vitamin E. When vitamin E is removed or destroyed (a common event), subsequent loss of vitamin A and beta carotene may be as high as 90 percent.[3] When beta carotene is added to margarine, 40 percent of the vitamin is destroyed *while it is still being made.*[4] By the time the product is shipped, stored, and used, who knows if any of this nutrient is still available.

Virtually all essential nutrients are altered to some degree by food processing. Those that are most often depleted or destroyed include vitamins C, E, and B₆, folic acid, thiamine, riboflavin, zinc, copper, magnesium, manganese, selenium, and chromium.

Eating a highly processed diet, you run the risk of being undernourished no matter how much food you eat. And no vitamin pill can make up for that. There are nutritional factors in whole natural foods that have not been identified. A new mineral was discovered in 1995. New flavonoids are identified every year.

In June 2000, researchers at the University of Minnesota resolved a long-standing controversy. Many studies had shown that a high-fiber diet reduced risk for cancer and heart disease, but other studies found no such benefit. The University of Minnesota team found that the difference came from the fiber *source*. Reviewing the diet and medical records of more than eleven thousand women over a decade, they found that women who consumed fiber from whole, unrefined grains had a far lower mortality rate than women who ate the same amount of fiber, but from refined sources.[5] In other words, eating whole-grain bread is better than eating white bread to which manufacturers have added processed fiber. Eating an apple is better than eating apple pie.

Research clearly shows that intake of whole grains, fresh fruits, and vegetables is associated with decreased risk for cardiovascular disease, cancer, and diabetes. Together, these account for more than 75 percent of all deaths in America. Food selection is clearly at the very core of any antiaging strategy.

Eat a Wide Variety of Foods

With the impressive variety of foods available in our modern supermarkets, it may surprise you to learn that our hunter-gatherer ancestors ate a wider variety of foods than most modern men and women. This is true of the ten or so remaining hunter-gatherer groups on the planet, who consume around seventy-five different wild plants.

Variety is one of the most important principles of optimal nutrition—because whatever nourishment you don't get from one food, you can get from another. In America, we have plenty of food choices but not much variety. Surveys show that the average educated American eats no more than eleven types of food.[6]

How can that be? Most people believe they eat a varied diet. But when you ask someone to list what kinds of grains he eats, for example, a typical response includes bread, rolls, breakfast cereal, crackers, cookies, sandwiches, spaghetti, pasta, cakes, biscotti—all of which are simply different forms of wheat.

You get the idea. We tend to eat what our mothers prepared. We eat what we like. We get into food ruts that last a lifetime, until our awareness changes and we realize that we live on a planet with incredible diversity. There's a reason for diversity. It's not just for show. A varied diet ensures that we will be optimally nourished for a long and healthy lifetime.

HOW TO EAT MORE FRUITS AND VEGETABLES (EVEN YOUR KIDS WILL DO THIS!)

Can't get your kids to eat anything that doesn't come in a package? Try this: Buy a Vita-Mix blender. Believe me, I don't get anything from the Vita-Mix people. But I saw a demonstration at a medical conference, bought one, and instantly (and easily) doubled my consumption of fruits and vegetables. Better yet, my kids love whatever comes out of this amazing machine. This is going to sound like a TV jingle, but the Vita-Mix makes soup in seconds, creamy ice cream out of leftover fruit, smoothies that provide three servings of fruit *per glass*, and a hundred other delicious meals and snacks. See Appendix A.

Eat Uncooked Foods as Often as Possible

Between 1985 and 1999, more than eight thousand cookbooks were published in the United States. That's eight thousand more than were published in the first 3 million years of human existence. Cooking, in other words, although extremely popular, is a very new development, and one that destroys vital nutrients—most notably antioxidants—before they make it to our mouths.[7] That doesn't mean that you should never cook food. Cooking meat, fish, and poultry (the oldest form of cooking) is important for food safety (see the discussion of parasites in Chapter 6); cooking is also one of life's pleasures. However, it is wise to consume as much of your fruits and vegetables as possible in their raw, natural state.

Eat Mostly Plants

The hunting-and-gathering diet consisted of approximately 70 percent vegetables and fruits. This is precisely what leading experts arrive at when they calculate the ideal diet from nutrient tables. Research suggests that consuming high amounts of fruits and vegetables early in life confers significant anticancer benefits later on. Evidence is mounting, for example, that a woman's lifelong risk of breast cancer may be most significantly reduced by a high antioxidant intake during years fifteen to twenty-five.

Eat Smaller, More Frequent Meals

In 1981, I was sent to study the Kupoka, a tribe of hunter-gatherers in Papua New Guinea, and they studied me just as intently. They were most surprised by my habit of postponing hunger to preset times known as "meals." And they were aghast at the quantity of food I consumed at those events. Overall, they thought that this was both hilarious and stupid.

They, on the other hand, ate when they were hungry and stopped eating when their hunger was satisfied. This meant roughly 250 to 300 calories for an active tribesperson—the amount we civilized folks normally consume before the entrée. In reality, it takes a small quantity of food to satisfy hunger. If you don't believe this, try it yourself. Next time you're hungry, eat slowly and be sensitive to the point when your hunger is gone. Most people find it's somewhere between one-third and one-half of the meal.

There are two reasons for our tendency to eat beyond hunger satisfaction, the first being that we eat too fast. It takes about twenty minutes for your brain to get the message (via the hormone cholecystokinin) that hunger has been satisfied. So when you eat quickly, it is very easy to overeat. You may even feel hungry the entire time you are eating, so you consume more than you need. Eating in a slow and relaxed manner gives your brain time to receive the message that you're full.

We also tend to overeat because we know that our next meal is at least four to five hours away. Hunter-gatherers don't operate on this schedule. They will eat again in an hour if they get hungry. The hunter-gatherer style of eating, which could be called *grazing*, is without a doubt the most efficient way to eat. Studies show that people who consume two thousand calories a day via grazing tend to lose weight, while people eating the same number of calories at lunch and dinner (as 90 percent of Americans do) tend to gain weight. What's more, digestion, nutrient absorption, and metabolism all tend to improve with smaller, more frequent meals.

You can get in the habit of grazing by keeping healthful snacks in the office or around the house. Fresh vegetables and fruit are good choices, as are protein bars, whole-grain crackers, and other high-fiber grain products. I use a powdered "green drink" mixed in a glass of water at midmorning and midafternoon. My favorite contains a long list of organic, dehydrated high-nutrient vegetables, including wheat grass, barley grass, alfalfa, and spirulina. This not only satisfies my hunger but provides the phytonutrient equivalent of three or four bowls of salad.

Using this snacking or "grazing" strategy allows you to arrive home in the evening without the ravenous hunger that causes so much overeating at night. You'll find it easy to consume smaller portions because your body's energy needs have been satisfied consistently throughout the day. Your blood sugar levels will be stabilized, and as a result, your energy level will stay consistently high rather than swinging wildly up and down.

The Meat Issue

Our ancestors ate wild game freely and whenever they could. So do hunter-gatherers today. The difference, however, between this wild meat and domesticated beef is staggering. A study of fifteen species of African animals showed a fat content of just 3.9 percent. In contrast, thanks to modern breeding and feeding practices, beef today contains 25 percent to 35 percent fat.

Not only is this meat marbled with fat, but every gram of it is nonessential, artery-clogging fat. Compare that with wild game, which is low in total and saturated fat and relatively rich in polyunsaturated fatty acids. In fact, research shows that lean meat from wild game actually lowers cholesterol levels and contributes significant amounts of essential fats, iron, zinc, and vitamin B_{12}.[8]

Modern meat is also laced with antibiotics and hormones that are required to keep animals alive in fetid feedlot conditions. This has resulted in an astounding increase in diseased animals going to market.

In July 2000, news wires were abuzz over the U.S. Department of Agriculture's reclassifying as safe for human consumption animal carcasses with cancers and open sores. In the case of tumors, the new guidelines state, "Remove localized lesion(s) and pass unaffected carcass portions."[9] That means your next USDA-approved steak could come from a cow with cancer.

There are numerous reasons to decrease your intake of meat and to purchase meat that is raised organically. Recent studies with the elderly show a remarkable increase in mortality related to high meat consumption,[10] and the personal health issues are matched by problems of global ecology and world hunger. The resources (land, water, and feed) required to produce a single pound of beef could be used to produce sixty-five pounds of rice or beans. In his landmark book *Diet for a New America* (Stillpoint Publishing, 1987), John Robbins pointed out that if Americans reduced their intake of meat by a mere 10 percent and fed people with the grain that was saved, world hunger could be eradicated.

Chicken Is Not a Health Food

Sorry to burst your bubble. The idea that chicken is somehow better than beef is only true in the sense that certain cuts are lower in cholesterol and saturated fat. In terms of overall health, however, chicken is more dangerous. Consider that each year in the United States alone, contaminated chicken kills approximately one thousand people and sickens thousands more.[11] Recent studies have found that about 30 percent of chicken is contaminated with salmonella and over 60 percent with a related fecal bacteria known as campylobacter.[12] Since such startling statistics are related mostly to the factory farm method by which commercial chickens are raised, you can improve food safety significantly by purchasing organically raised poultry, handling it carefully, and cooking it properly.

Is a Strict Vegetarian Diet Best?

There are many arguments for a vegetarian diet, including ethical and religious beliefs. But the health arguments are usually based on faulty comparisons of vegetarians and meat eaters. They are faulty because they compare vegetarians, who are generally very health-conscious, with the general population, consisting mainly of sedentary people who eat large quantities of junk food and on average consume meat at two meals a day seven days a week.

Thus, all such comparisons are invalid. What is a valid comparison? Compare vegetarians to *health-conscious meat eaters*—people who consume fish two or three times a week, organically raised poultry maybe once a week, and red meat a few times a month. Or study the Mediterranean diet. The people of southern France and Italy have health statistics as good as any vegetarian group you can find.

The Mediterranean Diet

Eating as most Mediterraneans do is an excellent diet. The emphasis is on fresh vegetables, fruits, and whole grains, with moderate amounts of fish, chicken, and occasional red meat. Other components of the Mediterranean diet include heart-healthy and immune-stimulating foods such as olive oil (which actually helps to lower serum cholesterol), garlic (which decreases platelet aggregation, enhances immunity, and lowers blood pressure), tomatoes and tomato sauce (which contain high levels of lycopene, a potent anticancer carotenoid), and red wine (which contains medicinal compounds known as polyphenols and anthocyanins, known to decrease risk for heart disease).

No one knows what ingredients are most responsible for their excellent health, but surveys show that some Mediterranean cultures enjoy protection against heart disease equal to or better than American vegetarians. What's more, Mediterranean people are very social; as we have said, community builds immunity.

As in all things, the key is moderation. Stick to one glass of wine per day and go easy on the pasta. But above all, remember that eating can be one of the great pleasures in life.

What About Eggs?

Eggs are a great source of protein as long as they are not eaten raw or undercooked. Adequate cooking (no runny yolk) is necessary to kill potential salmonella organisms. On the other hand, eggs should not be overcooked or burned. You'll remember from our discussion of glycation in Chapter 3 that overcooked proteins such as meat and eggs can create toxins known as AGEs (advanced glycation end products). Avoid breakfast buffets at which the eggs have been heating (and glycating) for hours. In addition, I strongly recommend that you spend a little extra money on eggs from organically fed, cage-free chickens. Regarding cholesterol, moderate intake of eggs (three to five per week) has not been associated with increased cholesterol levels or any adverse health effects.

FLASH! DIET LOWERS BLOOD PRESSURE AS EFFECTIVELY AS DRUG THERAPY, AND YOU DON'T HAVE TO BECOME IMPOTENT!

One of the little-discussed side effects of blood pressure drugs is that they tend to make men impotent, which may help explain some studies showing that men treated with drugs to lower their blood pressure and cholesterol have increased mortality compared with men who are not treated with these drugs. In 1997, a group of researchers tested a dietary approach to hypertension and found that it produced results as good as drug therapy without the side effects.[13] Known as the *DASH* diet (Dietary Approaches to Stop Hypertension), the plan includes eight to ten servings a day of fruits and vegetables (about three times the national average). Sound familiar? This plan fits well with the metabolic concept of smaller, more frequent meals consisting primarily of vegetables and fruits, along with generous portions of low-fat protein. The DASH diet worked even though it did not limit sodium intake. This is good news indeed for 50 million Americans looking for a sensible approach to lowering their blood pressure. As an added benefit, the diet also decreases risk for diabetes and cancer.

METABOLIC FACTOR 2: DIGESTION

Think of your digestive system as a chemical "fire." Eating a large meal (especially one high in fat) is like throwing huge logs on a small fire. It doesn't work, and neither does your digestion after the kind of meal that most of us eat. Importantly, undigested food does not evaporate. It passes into the colon, where it is fermented by intestinal bacteria. This fermentation, and a related reaction known as putrefaction, produce a long list of toxins that can be absorbed into your body.

Here are a few important tips for optimizing digestion and reducing your risk for bloating, gas, abdominal pain, and intestinal disease:

Steps to Better Digestion

1. Eat small amounts. Many experts recommend four to five small meals rather than two or three large meals each day.

2. Chew your food well. This increases digestive efficiency, especially in the stomach, where food needs to be mixed well with gastric acids.[14]

3. Eat slowly. Remember that the premeal stomach is quite acidic, and the ingestion of food dilutes or buffers that acid. Effective digestion depends upon the stomach's ability to reacidify during a meal, and the slower you eat, the better. Adequate stomach acid activates gastric enzymes and initiates protein breakdown.

3. Don't wash your food down with a beverage, especially a soft drink. Your mother was right. Although beverages may provide the lubrication effect of saliva, they lack the amylase enzyme important for starch digestion. This does not mean we should avoid drinking water with meals. In fact, a glass of room-temperature water taken with a meal may enhance digestion. The point seems to be that the water and food should not be taken in the same mouthful (chew well and swallow first, *then* take a drink), and the water should not be ice-cold. Ice water can reduce the activity of enzymes in your saliva and stomach.

4. Last but not least is the essential factor of *relaxation*. So often, we are rushed and anxious about eating or face difficult stress in our lives. Proper digestion requires a relaxed state of mind and body. Anxiety alters the production of hydrochloric acid in the stomach and tightens abdominal muscles, interfering with normal peristaltic movement.

Classical or soft instrumental music tends to put people at ease when eating and results in a number of behavioral changes conducive to improved digestion. When volunteers were exposed to calming music, their pace of eating decreased dramatically, as did the size of the meals consumed. In fact, they took almost twice as long to eat fewer calories than when lively music was playing. They said that food tasted better, and they had fewer digestive complaints plus a greater feeling of satisfaction from the meal.[15] This makes perfect sense, as the longer we chew a food, the more pleasure we receive from the aroma (chewing forces air from the throat to the nose) and the taste (starches are broken down into simple sugars by the salivary enzymes).

By contrast, jazz and rock music have been shown to increase eating speed and impair digestion. Music *volume* also plays a significant role. Animal and human experiments both show that as music volume is increased, there is a significant increase in meal size and speed of eating.

METABOLIC FACTOR 3: ACID/ALKALINE BALANCE

It's no wonder people are confused about the issue of acid/alkaline balance. If you collect books, magazines, and health guides from health food stores, you'll find that they often contradict one another. The same foods will be called acid by one author and alkaline by another. Some devise entire charts based on invented terminology, such as subacid, acid, and acidifying. And while these well-meaning but misinformed authors are splitting hairs, they forget that these foods will be swallowed into a stomach that is hundreds of times more acidic than any food on their list.

Does that mean these lists are useless? Yes. If you have such a list on your refrigerator and you've been trying to reconcile the contradictions among different health gurus, you can now throw the list away and relax.

The simple truth is that the words *acid* and *alkaline* refer to the acid/base characteristics of any liquid. This is measured on a pH scale, with acid going from a pH of 6.9 (very mild acid) to pH 1.0 (very strong acid). Alkaline is measured from pH 7.1 (mildly alkaline) to pH 14 (extremely alkaline). Obviously, pH 7 is perfectly neutral.

When one speaks of the acid/alkaline *balance*, or the acid/alkaline equilibrium, it refers to the relative pH of the blood, which must be kept within a narrow range around 7.4 (slightly alkaline). This vital function is accomplished most efficiently by a number of mechanisms, including automatic buffer systems in the blood and the pH-regulating action of the lungs and kidneys.

In *acidosis*, or acidemia, the pH of the blood is too acid (less than 7.35). In this case, blood buffer systems will adjust toward alkaline, and the rate of breathing will increase to remove carbonic acid by exhaling carbon dioxide (CO_2). Next, the kidneys increase the acidity of the urine, and balance is quickly restored.

Note: Acidosis is *not* caused by eating acidic foods such as lemons and oranges. It is most often the result of a disease state such as in diabetes, kidney disease, or respiratory disorders that limit the release of CO_2 from the lungs.

Alkalosis, or alkalemia, is less common than acidosis but can result from hyperventilation (too rapid breathing), loss of stomach acid because of excessive vomiting, or overuse of antacids or ulcer medications. In this case, blood buffer systems adjust toward acid, and breathing becomes more shallow to conserve CO_2 and raise carbonic acid levels in the blood. Once again, the kidneys contribute to the balancing act by excreting more alkaline urine.

Measuring the pH of food as it exists outside the body is irrelevant. The intricate process of metabolism is the story of what happens to food *after it's consumed, digested, and absorbed.* In the final stages of energy production, most of the components of a food are oxidized except for the minerals (you can't burn rocks, right?). This therefore leaves a residue, or "ash," that is either alkaline, acid, or neutral, depending on the mix of minerals found in the food.

Sulfur, phosphorus, and iron form acid ions in the body. These minerals are found primarily in *proteins,* such as meat, fish, poultry, eggs, grains, and most nuts. These foods are therefore called *acid-forming foods.* Soft drinks, the bane of the American diet, contain no protein but lots of phosphate and carbonate, and thus are very acid-forming. Coffee is acid-forming because it stimulates gastric acid secretion; its metabolism involves the production of other acids, including uric acid, by the body; and it depletes alkaline minerals such as calcium and magnesium.

Sodium, potassium, calcium, and magnesium form alkaline reactions in the body. These minerals are found primarily in fruits and vegetables, and so these foods are called *alkaline-forming foods.*

As you can probably see, *acid* and *alkaline* are neutral terms. It's not that acid-forming foods are "bad" and alkaline-forming foods are "good." What nature provides and we tend to ignore is the essential *balance* that is required for optimal health and effective anabolic repair.

Moreover, as we age, it becomes more difficult for the body's buffer-ing systems to balance the highly acidic American diet. Remember that most people in our society drink more soft drinks (which are highly acid-forming) than they do water. In addition, most Americans con-sume far more meat and chicken than they do fruits and vegetables. And there is another factor that is as important as diet, and that is ex-ercise.

The primary buffering system of the body is *respiration*. If the pH of the blood starts to fall, your breathing rate increases to remove carbonic acid in the form of carbon dioxide. Neat. Works great. The problem is that people become sedentary, and the natural buffering activity of exercise-stimulated deep breathing simply doesn't happen. A sedentary person, in other words, will suffer from the double whammy of a highly acid diet and low respiratory function. The obvious solution is to exer-cise regularly to the point at which you notice your rate of breathing comfortably increase. In addition, deep-breathing techniques such as are taught in most yoga classes can do wonders for restoring alkaline balance.

The Bottom Line

Excess metabolic acid in the tissues and blood accelerates catabolic ac-tivity dramatically, whereas slightly alkaline conditions promote ana-bolic repair. Metabolic acidosis, in other words, is associated with accelerated aging.[16]

Interestingly, it works both ways. Increasing anabolic metabolism helps to restore acid/alkaline balance and decrease catabolic activity. Conversely, reducing metabolic acidosis by restoring alkaline pH can help the body shift into anabolic rebuild and repair metabolism.[17] Per-haps the best example of this is the effect of acid/alkaline factors on bone health.

We have long known that high-protein diets increase your risk for osteoporosis. Numerous theories have been proposed to explain this, but it now appears that a high intake of acid-forming foods (primarily meat, poultry, and eggs) over the course of a lifetime accelerates the loss of alkaline minerals (calcium, magnesium, and potassium) from the bones. In other words, the body depletes one system (the skeleton) in order to maintain balance in another, more sensitive system (the blood).

In support of this theory, the *New England Journal of Medicine* reported a study in which postmenopausal women were given an alkalinizing agent (potassium bicarbonate) to neutralize the acid produced by a high-protein diet. Researchers were able to see significant improvements in the bone retention of calcium and phosphorus in just two weeks.[18] Does this mean that we should all be taking potassium bicarbonate supplements? Not really. A more sensible conclusion is that we should *eat less meat and more fruits and vegetables*.

Acid/Alkaline Action Plan

Maintaining optimal alkaline balance is critical to the Metabolic Plan. This is accomplished not by referring to complex tables and "food-combining" charts but by:

- Exercising regularly

- Eating less meat, poultry, and eggs

- Eating more fruits and vegetables

- Reducing or eliminating coffee and completely eliminating soft drinks

- Drinking plenty of pure water (a minimum of eight glasses per day)

METABOLIC FACTOR 4: LONGEVITY FOODS

So far, we've discussed the hows and whys of the anabolic nutrition approach. The following is a list of specific foods that foster that goal. Some enhance anabolic metabolism, and others reduce risk for age-related disease. Either way, these foods can help you maximize both the quality and the quantity of your years ahead.

- *The Allium family of vegetables:* The Allium family includes garlic, garlic shoots, onions, leeks, shallots, chives, and scallions. There isn't another group of plants that has more extensive and impressive scientific support for remarkable health benefits. Include small amounts of alliums in your daily diet instead of loading up once or twice a week. Evidence gathered in the Iowa Women's Health Study suggests that one-third to one-half of a clove of garlic per day was sufficient to confer a whopping 50 percent reduction in risk for colon cancer.[19]

Intake of alliums has been associated with decreased risk for cancer of the skin, stomach, liver, lungs, and cervix. Major anti-aging components include more than seventy different sulfur compounds, which, among other things, foster the body's production of glutathione. Red onions also contain quercetin, a flavonoid with antioxidant and anticancer activity.

Allium vegetables can also reduce heart disease risk by helping to lower cholesterol and preventing the formation of abnormal clots. What's more, they're powerful immune stimulants with antibacterial and antiviral activity.

- *Whey protein:* In Chapter 2, I explained the critical role of protein in anabolic repair. Whey protein concentrates deserve special mention for a number of reasons:

  Digestibility

  Superior amino acid profile

  Rapid utilization by the body (highly bioavailable)

  Whey proteins are like express delivery of precut lumber to your building site. And in addition to their anabolic benefits, they also help to reduce catabolic damage by strengthening immunity, protecting the brain, and promoting the synthesis of glutathione (see Chapter 3).

- *Chili peppers:* Another immune stimulant, chili peppers (cayenne, capsicum) can help ward off a cold and may reduce your risk for other, more serious illnesses. Cayenne has been shown to help prevent cardiovascular disease, and the high flavonoid content may help prevent certain forms of cancer. Suggested use: Be careful! Some types of chili peppers are *extremely* hot. Sprinkle in soup, salad dressing, and Italian, Mexican, or Asian cuisine. For a morning pickup, mix a quarter teaspoonful of chili peppers in eggs or orange juice.

- *The cabbage-broccoli family (Brassica):* Cabbage, Brussels sprouts, kale, turnips, turnip greens, collard greens, broccoli, cauliflower, rutabaga, kohlrabi, and radishes all contain powerful anticancer compounds known as *indoles* and *isothiocyanates*, which boost immune protection against cancer and other diseases.

- *Carrots, sweet potatoes, and yams:* Research suggests that one medium carrot per day can cut your risk for lung cancer by over 40 percent. Two and a half carrots a day have been shown to decrease blood cholesterol an average of 11 percent. Carrots provide healthy amounts of beta carotene, vitamin C, calcium, magnesium, and fiber.

- *Nuts and seeds:* "Perhaps one of the most unexpected and novel findings in nutritional research in the past 5 years has been that nut consumption seems to protect against heart disease." So begins an excellent report in the *American Journal of Clinical Nutrition* showing that eating nuts reduces risk not only for heart disease but for all natural causes of death.[20] Seeds—especially sunflower and flax seeds—may provide even greater benefit owing to their rich supply of antioxidant phenolic acids, artery-friendly essential fats, vitamin E, selenium, and anticancer lignans.

- *Medicinal mushrooms:* Fresh shiitake mushrooms are available at most grocery stores and are also available dried in packages. Shiitake contain a powerful immune-stimulating polysaccharide known as *lentinan.* Other power-packed culinary mushrooms include maitake, coriolus, and reishi.

- *Comprehensive "green drinks":* Today, powdered green drinks are available that can dramatically increase anabolic repair by providing hundreds of critical repair nutrients in a single serving. Look for products that combine a variety of earth and sea vegetables and make sure all ingredients are organically grown. Importantly, even the best ingredients can suffer if they are processed with high heat. A new technology known as vacuum-assisted dehydration allows for the processing of such products at temperatures that do not exceed 80 degrees.

  Since green drinks tend to have a strong taste, manufacturers often "cut" the product with sweeteners and fillers. You want concentrated *greens,* not dextrose, maltodextrin, or lecithin. Read labels carefully.

- *Cold-water fish:* Mackerel, herring, Icelandic cod, salmon, and sardines all provide valuable omega-3 fatty acids (EPA and DHA), which can help prevent the formation of abnormal blood clots and decrease risk for heart disease. If you don't care for fish, 1,000 milligrams of fish oil in capsules will approximate the benefits of a three-ounce serving of fish.

Note: Consult with your physician if you are taking a blood-thinning medication such as coumadin, as the natural blood-thinning activity of fish oil may have an additive effect.

- *Olive oil:* Reduce your use of butter (which is high in saturated fat) and throw out the highly processed margarine made with hydrogenated oils. Forget the polyunsaturated corn and safflower oils. Instead, enjoy the rich and mellow flavor of first-press, virgin olive oil. Olive oil provides vitamin E and heart-healthy monounsaturated fats and can help lower cholesterol.

- *Berries:* Refer to Chapter 3 for a discussion of the brain-protecting, brain-restoring benefits of blueberries and other berries and cherries. Overall, a cup of blueberries per day can provide significant antioxidant and flavonoid benefits that may improve memory, mood, and cognition. Fortunately, sugar-free berry concentrate drinks are also available, which provide convenient high-potency nutrition for daily use.

- *Green peas:* There's a wonder food just waiting for you in the freezer section of your grocery store: frozen peas. Frozen green peas are picked and packaged so fast that they have virtually the same nutritional value as fresh peas. A three-quarter-cup serving contains 6 grams of protein, less than 1 gram of fat, 3.5 grams of fiber, and 35 milligrams of calcium. They're packed with folic acid and antioxidants such as vitamin C and lutein. Lunch-box tip: If you pack a salad, top it off with frozen peas. They will thaw by lunchtime and keep your salad fresh and cold in the meantime.

- *Bran cereals:* You've heard these cereals recommended for their fiber content, but that's not the half of it. Bran cereals like All-Bran, Bran Buds, and 100% Bran also contain high amounts of inositol hexaphosphate (phytic acid, or IP-6). This compound has been shown to stimulate the immune system and significantly reduce risk for heart disease and cancer.

- *Spices:* In Chapter 3, we discussed the remarkable antioxidant benefits of a group of spices, including cayene (chili pepper), garlic, turmeric, cumin, rosemary, oregano, and paprika. Some of these (most notably rosemary and turmeric) are also natural anti-inflammatory, COX-2 inhibitors.

- *Dark green, leafy vegetables:* The only leafy vegetable most people eat is lettuce, a nutritional lightweight. Try to include kale, chard, spinach, beet tops, and mustard greens in your diet. These longevity foods are packed with minerals, vitamins, carotenoids, flavonoids, and perhaps most important, folic acid.

Question: How can we have a list of longevity foods and not include soybeans? Answer: Because soybeans need a discussion all their own.

The Soy Story

Asians who eat a lot of soy have a lower incidence of certain cancers, most notably breast cancer and prostate cancer. But is there a *causative* relationship between soybeans and a lower incidence of cancer, or is it merely an association? In other words, I sing in the shower every morning and the sun rises. Does my singing cause the sun to rise, or do these events simply coincide? You get the picture.

Scientists first looked to see if there was a causative factor. And they found two components of soybeans with anticancer activity. The first are phytoestrogens, a group of compounds (for example, genistein and daidzein) that have estrogenlike activity in humans and animals.

The plant estrogens in soybeans have very weak activity in humans. But because they bind to estrogen receptors in a woman's breasts and reproductive organs, it is believed that they block the binding of more powerful estrogens that she may be producing, estrogens that promote cancer. In men, a similar benefit may be achieved in the reduction of prostate cancer, in which estrogen plays a contributing role.

Second, scientists found a group of *protease inhibitors* in soy and other beans. These biochemicals inhibit the digestion of protein by interfering with the activity of two important enzymes, trypsin and chymotrypsin. Protease inhibitors interfere with cell communication, protein metabolism, and cell growth.[21] This may contribute to anticancer defense in humans by interfering with the growth and spread (metastasis) of tumors.

So we now have a documented cause-and-effect relationship between soybeans and two anticancer biochemicals. What do we do with this valuable information?

- *Option 1:* We promote soy as the perfect food for all human beings, including infants.

- *Option 2:* We carefully evaluate the effect of phytoestrogens on pregnancy and fetal health. We evaluate the effects of phytoestrogens and protease inhibitors on the growth of children, and we look for possible side effects resulting from decreased estrogen binding. Estrogen, for example, plays an important role in the maintenance and repair of the brain.

Right now, unfortunately, many Americans are pursuing option 1 with wild abandon. Fueled by the burgeoning soybean industry and supported by thousands of health food enthusiasts (motto: Where's the next panacea?), the soy frenzy has extended to the mass marketing of soy milk, soy protein powder, soy cheese, soy burgers, soy candy bars, soy butter (to replace peanut butter), and soy-enriched cereal, bread, pasta, and chips. Concentrates of soy phytoestrogens are sold in capsules, and the FDA now allows manufacturers to claim heart-disease-prevention benefits for any product providing twenty-five grams of soy protein per day.

This could be a big problem.

Excessive soy consumption may inhibit brain repair functions. The basis for this concern arose when researchers documented a dampening effect of phytoestrogens on brain repair in rats.[22] Human studies appear to support this finding. A study with Japanese-Americans found a disturbing correlation between soy consumption and cognitive impairment.[23] I am not suggesting that soy = brain degeneration, but the issue certainly needs further study.

What doesn't need further study is the association between high soy consumption and growth and development. Here, the concern is that soy phytoestrogens may cause early puberty in girls and delayed physical maturation in boys. Mary G. Enig, Ph.D., president of the Maryland Nutritionists Association, states that the amount of phyto-estrogens in a day's worth of soy infant formula has the same estro-genic effect as five birth-control pills to an adult.[24] A study published in the British medical journal *Lancet* found that infants who were fed soy formula had levels of phytoestrogens that were thirteen thousand to twenty-two thousand times higher than natural estrogen concentrations in early life.[25]

There is also concern that protease inhibitors found in soy foods may inhibit normal growth and repair functions in children. At first, the soy industry claimed that these inhibitors were destroyed by cooking, but this has been disproved. Protease inhibitors have been shown to survive cooking and processing to a small but significant degree—certainly significant for a small child.[26]

The *thyroid factor* may also create problems for children and adults who consume high amounts of soy foods. The phytoestrogens genistein and daidzein have been found to interfere with thyroid function,[27] and although this would have no effect on a person eating a varied diet, those using soy as their primary source of protein may suffer, even to the point of thyroid disease.[28]

The Bottom Line on Soy

It's natural to jump on bandwagons. Nutrition is extremely complex, and we would all love a simple solution to the threats of heart disease and cancer. But I'd like to suggest that in regard to soy foods, as in all things, moderation is the key.

- If you eat a lot of meat, you can do yourself and the planet a huge favor by switching to vegetable proteins *at least* a few days a week. That's not just soy foods but any combination of beans, grains, low-fat dairy foods, nuts, and seeds.

- If you are pregnant or nursing, you should *not* make soy your sole source of protein. Three to five servings a week appear to be safe, but you should consult with your OB-GYN, midwife, or pediatrician.

- I would seriously reconsider using soy formula for babies. If you absolutely cannot breast-feed, consult a qualified health professional to work out a rotation strategy using soy milk, goat's milk, almond milk, and rice milk.

- If you have growing children, make sure they have a variety of proteins in their diet. Soy is fine, but if it is their sole protein, you may be limiting their adult height.

- Regarding soy and brain health, you'll have to stay tuned. This is a hot topic in nutrition research, and I will provide updates at www.TheMetabolicPlan.com as more information becomes available.

SUMMARY

Our eating habits—what we eat, when we eat, and how we eat—have been formed by the habits of our parents and of society as a whole, both of which have been heavily influenced by the enticing advertising of the huge processed-food industry. For baby boomers, you can throw in the insidious influence of the fast-food industry, our lifelong deadly habit.

To optimize the antiaging benefits of the Metabolic Plan, you need to take control of your eating habits and avail yourself of the extraordinary variety of organic natural foods that are available today. By incorporating longevity foods into your diet and optimizing digestion, you'll be delivering all the raw materials your body needs for peak anabolic repair.

Water:
Lifespring of the
Metabolic Plan

WATER, THE SOURCE OF LIFE

You've heard it so many times that it probably no longer registers. *Drink eight to ten glasses of water every day*. In virtually every magazine article you have ever read about general health or weight loss, you've probably read it: *Drink eight to ten glasses of water every day*. How well do we listen?

Well, what if I told you that you're dehydrating as you read this page, that we're all born grapes and we turn into raisins—that your body was once more than 70 percent water, and now, if you're like most Americans past age forty, you're lucky to have a hydration level above 60 percent. The bodies of most hospitalized elderly are less than 50 percent water.

Turboaging

As I've mentioned, Americans consume more coffee and soft drinks than water. If you do this, you might as well paste a sign on your forehead, AGING AS FAST AS I CAN. These beverages, along with tea and alcohol, are diuretics and dehydrate the body. To women consuming high levels of soft drinks and coffee, I ask, "Why bother putting moisturizer on your face, hoping to restore a youthful appearance, when you're pulling a hundred times as much water out of your skin through the urinary tract?" Of course, if it were just the skin that was dehydrating, it would be a small matter. Far more serious is the dehydration of the internal organs, connective tissue, and brain.

Dehydration and Disease

Even slight dehydration (caused by inadequate fluid intake and excessive water loss) can disrupt critical cell functions, and when you consider that most people experience this level of dehydration all day, nearly every day, you get a sense of the enormity of the problem. Water is essential for all anabolic repair functions, and conversely, dehydration accelerates catabolic damage.

Researchers at the Fred Hutchinson Research Center in Seattle found that women who drank two glasses of water a day had nearly twice the risk of colon cancer as women who drank four glasses per day. And what makes the data particularly convincing is that the few women in the study who drank eight or more glasses of water per day had less than half the risk of those who drank only four glasses. Even more impressive is the association of increased water intake and reduced risk for other types of cancer. In one study, the women who drank the most water were 80 percent less likely to develop bladder cancer than women who drank the least.[1]

Other conditions that often respond to increased water intake include headache, muscle aches, hangover, fatigue, constipation, heartburn, and even mitral valve prolapse. People with this common heart valve defect (possibly as many as one out of ten American adults) have been found to have low blood volume, which often results from dehydration. Advice from the Mitral Valve Prolapse Center in Birmingham, Alabama: drink more water, use a bit more salt, and avoid caffeine.

Drinking enough water will also reduce fluid retention and edema. It's sometimes hard for people to understand that drinking lots of water actually decreases water retention. However, if you provide your body with ample amounts of pure water, it will not have to retain water in the tissues.

Diuretic drugs offer only a temporary solution to water retention. Your body will compensate for diuretics as soon as you stop taking them. The real solution to a water-retention problem is to drink plenty of pure water. This makes it easy for your body to supply its metabolic needs and helps rapidly eliminate waste.

Water and Weight Management

Drinking water should also be an important part of a weight-loss program. The water you drink is essential for transporting and burning fat and for eliminating waste products that result from enhanced metabolic activity. In fact, water is vital to all your body's functions, including movement, digestion, and temperature regulation. Because most of us don't drink enough water to begin with, as you begin to exercise more, it is important that you pay attention to your body's increased need for water.

In addition, it is important to understand that the need for water does not always result in a clear signal to the brain. Sometimes, we simply experience a vague physiological need and we may interpret that signal as a call for food. Because most foods contain significant amounts of water, this practice generally fills our need for water, but we also end up eating when we aren't really hungry and consume more calories than we need. When we feel those vague cravings, our first response should be to drink a glass of water. If it was merely thirst, water will satisfy the need.

I'm OK. I Drink Whenever I'm Thirsty!

As it turns out, thirst is not a reliable indication of the need for water. Research shows that the body can become significantly dehydrated *before* we actually feel thirsty. To prevent this, you must develop a rote habit of drinking eight to ten glasses per day.

In the morning, you have a true metabolic need for water, but few people can feel it. The first liquid they consume is coffee, a beverage that sucks the water *out* of your cells.

Try this: When you get up, sip about four ounces of water—no more. You'll be surprised to see that in two to three minutes, your mouth will feel parched. You have unmasked your need for water. So have another four ounces, and in two to three minutes, you'll be thirsty again. You may have to repeat this six or more times before you are no longer thirsty. Add up all the four-ounce servings that you consumed, and you will discover your body's true metabolic need for water.

"ORGANIZED" WATER—OUR UNDERSTANDING DEEPENS

It used to be thought that water was merely the "environment" within which biochemical reactions took place. We now know that this is far from the truth, that water *participates* in all chemical reactions on multiple levels. It's becoming obvious that water plays a critical role in cell communication and that some of its actions and influences test our understanding of biology and physics. A recent study has shown that minute changes in cell hydration produce dramatic alterations in cellular metabolism and gene activity.[2] Because gene activity affects every cell of your body, including its ability to repair and reproduce, our intake of water has a direct and critically important bearing on the aging process.

Scientists have long known that water transports protein through the body but are now finding out that cell membranes use special proteins to transport water. Importantly, something *happens* to water once it enters the metabolism of living things. The molecules of water you drink from the faucet, bottle, or spring are arranged in random clusters. Once these molecules find their way into your cells, however, they become highly organized. Instead of the amorphous liquid that we all saw in Bio 101, water appears to exist within the cell in a complex, multilayered structure. Imagine that the water in your glass is like a box of Scrabble tiles. After you drink it, if you could look inside the cell with the right instruments, you'd see words and sentences. It is now "organized" water, ready to perform specific tasks just as words convey specific meaning in our speech.

Molecular biologist Gilbert Ling has shown that intercellular water is remarkably different from other forms of water.[3] Research at Rice University and the University of California has confirmed this using quasi-elastic neutron scattering,[4] and others have determined that thousands of biochemicals are channeled among enzymes through organized water.[5]

One of water's most important functions is to maintain and influence protein structure, thus the intimate connection with anabolic metabolism. In the past, researchers merely looked for the presence or absence of water, but a whole new world of biophysics has started to unfold. Drs. G. Alfred Gilman and Martin Rodbell won a Nobel Prize for their work with protein folding and G peptide, specifically for describing the role that proteins play in cell communication.

Remarkably, it has been shown that a matrix of clustered or organized water exists within these protein molecules.[6] In fact, Dr. Julia Goodfellow at Birbeck College in London has shown that it is the interaction of structured water with other molecules that *causes* the protein to fold and perform its strategic function.

How Cells Communicate

I was taking graduate courses in physiology in the mid-1970s and remember quite clearly that cell communication was limited to a discussion of receptor sites, hormones, and the intricate workings of the brain and nervous system. What no one seemed to want to tackle was the enormous question of how the *rest* of the body communicated. If 100 trillion cells contribute to human function, and hormone and nervous system pathways connect only a small fraction of those cells, there had to have been an enormous piece missing from a very important puzzle.

The transmission of information from DNA to RNA is a good case in point. I was perplexed by textbook drawings of DNA fragments "breaking off" and attaching to RNA, as if genetic communication were a mechanical process. "This is impossible," I protested, and my professor agreed. "It's just the way they choose to represent a process that is not understood," he replied.

We now know that the flow of information from DNA is *constant* and that the schematic textbook representations were utter nonsense. We know that in the core of that double helix is a column of organized water and that information is transmitted by that water at lightning speed via *resonant frequencies*. . . . That's right, *vibrations*.

The scientific support for this scenario is undeniable, involving principles of physics every bit as much as those of chemistry. It may sound weird to hear biochemists talking about semiconduction, electrical amplification, and resonant frequencies (typically the realm of the physicist), but that is the new frontier, and the implications of this research for aging and wellness are astounding.

Research demonstrates that cells possess individual and cooperative resonant patterns that change with a person's age and metabolic efficiency. These resonant patterns can be enhanced, producing beneficial effects on tissues and organs. After what we've discussed so far, you won't be surprised to learn that resonance is a part of anabolic and catabolic metabolism. Cell communication is enhanced in the anabolic state, and the disruption of cell and tissue function is clearly associated with catabolic decline.

In the early 1990s, research was published describing the role that organized water plays in the aging process. Japanese investigators using magnetic resonance imaging (MRI) found not only that aging results in dehydration but that the water that remains in the tissues undergoes significant structural changes.[7] Quite simply, much of the body's water gets bound into larger structures known as *macromolecules*. As levels of free or unbound water decrease, the dynamic activities of water—such as cell communication, protein folding, nutrient delivery, and detoxification—all decline.

Some have even suggested that the increased morbidity and mortality associated with obesity may stem in part from this decline in tissue levels of organized water. After all, hydration is related primarily to the muscle-to-fat ratio and the age of the body. An obese man may have a water content of approximately 45 percent, whereas a lean man of the same weight can have a water content of 70 percent or more. Likewise, the water content of an average forty-five-year-old man is 63 percent, but by age seventy, this decreases to approximately 47 percent.[8] Clearly, the ability to restore optimum levels of water to this system will have profound effects on the entire body. But there's even more.

The Fundamentals of Cellular Resonance

Resonance is a phenomenon that occurs throughout nature. At the atomic level, we know that electrons whirl about the nucleus in precise orbits. In order to move an electron from a lower to a higher orbit, a quantum of energy with very specific frequency characteristics is required. In fact, an electron will accept only energy of the appropriate frequency, and if the electron falls to a lower orbit, it will release energy of that very same frequency. This specific quantum of energy is known as the *resonant frequency*.

The phenomenon of resonance is the principle behind MRI scanning. Atoms and molecules have individual resonant frequencies, which will be excited only by energies of precise vibratory characteristics. With the correct electromagnetic stimulation, tissue systems respond with predictable resonant emission frequencies, which can be measured and converted to a computer image.

Medical researchers are now experimenting with *therapeutic*—as opposed to diagnostic—MRI devices. This represents a new paradigm in preventive health care: the normalization of subtle but now well-defined resonant frequencies in cellular systems. Inasmuch as we are talking about frequencies, you might think of this normalization as "fine-tuning."

MRI technology has revealed that catabolic activity will affect the primary tissue resonant frequency and create what's called an *emission phase shift phenomenon*. Current models of health care—or what I prefer to call "disease care"—initiate treatment only after symptoms develop, but symptoms are merely the *end result* of gross biochemical imbalances induced by many factors. In chronic degenerative disease, cellular imbalance usually produces no symptoms until the disease has reached an *advanced* stage. Before this stage is ever reached, however, disruptions in cell water multilayers will already have produced aberrant or incoherent information transfer that can be measured. Using a device known as a *magnetic resonance analyzer* (MRA), predisease conditions have been predicted, detected, and later confirmed. Even more exciting, of course, is the possibility of correcting those aberrant frequencies using noninvasive, safe, and inexpensive means.

WHAT, THEN, SHOULD WE DRINK?

We have discussed the incredible "organization" that is imparted to water after it enters your body. Unfortunately, as you age, this organization is not imparted nearly so well. Fortunately, there is something you can do about this aspect of aging. You can drink water that is already organized or clustered.

Clustered Water from Natural Sources

Remember that all living things organize water within their cells. Thus, the most reliable source of clustered water is fresh, raw vegetable and fruit juice. In addition to being excellent sources of vitamins and minerals, the water component of these juices has already been organized by the fruits and vegetables themselves.

Drinking these freshly made juices becomes more important as we age because aging itself involves a loss of clustering activity within the body. It's like a factory that has to assemble hundreds of pieces to make a product. Over time, parts on the assembly line wear out and break, making it increasingly difficult to create the product. Drinking clustered water is like delivering the product partly assembled.

Tap Water in America

Of course, it's not practical to think that we will always drink fresh vegetable and fruit juices. Thus, we need to consider other sources of water as well. The easiest way to get water, anytime and anywhere, is from the tap.

If we could all turn on the tap and drink water from high-mountain streams untouched by industrial and biological pollution, we wouldn't have to worry about the safety of the water we drink. But . . . alas!

How Bad Is Tap Water?

As cities grow and age, municipal water-treatment systems struggle to keep up. System resources are stretched to their limits, which can lead to contamination with organisms such as *Giardia* or *Cryptosporidium*. In the 1993 outbreak of cryptosporidiosis in Milwaukee, four hundred thousand people were affected, more than four hundred thousand were hospitalized, and as many as one hundred deaths were attributed to the disease.[9] While this intestinal parasite produces only transient (but often severe) diarrhea in healthy individuals, the complications of the disease can be fatal to children, the elderly, and those with gastrointestinal disease (such as colitis) or compromised immune systems.

Even if the water at the treatment plant is acceptable, the delivery system of pipelines may contribute to contamination before it arrives at your home or office. There are three broad categories of common contaminants, none of which is entirely removed by standard filtration and chlorine treatment:

1. Industrial and agricultural chemicals

2. Lead (still used in plumbing fixtures)

3. Biological organisms

Requirements to monitor chemicals, lead, or pesticides vary widely from state to state—in some areas, they are nearly nonexistent. According to a recent survey by the U.S. Environmental Protection Agency, the drinking water supplied to 30 million people in 819 cities contains lead levels above the recommended maximum. As I discussed in Chapter 6, this can be extremely damaging to children.

The Problem with Chlorine

Chlorine is used in the vast majority of water-treatment plants. A recent study by the U.S. Council on Environmental Quality has established a definite link between the chlorination of water and cancer risk. Chlorine can react with organic material in water to produce chemical compounds called trihalomethanes—known carcinogens that have also been found to increase risk for miscarriage.[10]

Treating Your Tap Water for Safe Drinking

Home water-filtration devices come in a variety of types. The National Sanitation Foundation, an independent, nonprofit organization founded in 1944, has developed standards, product testing, and certification services in the areas of public health, safety, and environmental protection. This foundation describes the common water-purification options as follows: solid carbon filtration, ceramic/particulate filtration, reverse osmosis, ultraviolet irradiation, and distillation.

The effectiveness of each system depends heavily on factors such as system design, manufacturing standards, quality control, and testing. Also of importance to system functionality are things like water flow in gallons per minute, the number of gallons the system can process between servicing and filter replacement, and the quality and temperature of the inlet water.

- *Solid carbon filtration* removes organic compounds, various liquids, gases, and dissolved or suspended matter through a physical process called *adsorption*, as contaminants adhere to the surface of or in the pores of the carbon medium.

- *Ceramic or particulate filters* will remove solids, perhaps even bacteria, down to a specific size (some down to .5 micron), depending on design.

- *Reverse osmosis* (RO) is a process by which water is forced through a semipermeable membrane. Most reverse-osmosis systems incorporate prefilters and postfilters along with the membrane itself. Unfortunately, RO units often require up to three quarts of water to produce one quart of purified water.

- *Ultraviolet irradiation* exposes the water to ultraviolet light (UV), which can kill microorganisms left unaffected by physical filtration systems. UV is generally used in combination with another filtering process and can be a rather expensive feature. Still, those living in areas where the water bacteria count is high—whether from a well or a municipal source—should seriously consider this option.

- *Distillation* is the process of condensing and collecting evaporated water. Some contaminants that convert readily into gases, such as volatile organic chemicals (VOCs), may be carried in the water vapor and re-collected. What's more, distilling enough water for consumption and cooking is a slow process, deterring more widespread use of this method.

    Distillation equipment can be expensive and slow and requires regular maintenance. However, unless you have significant VOCs present in your water source, distilled water is probably the purest form of drinking water. There have been many misconceptions regarding the consumption of distilled water. Some claim that distilled water will leach minerals from your body, but this is simply not true. Rainwater is essentially distilled, and entire cultures, including most Polynesians, rely heavily on collected rainwater and yet have some of the strongest bones in the world.

The overall cost of a drinking water treatment system can vary considerably depending on contaminant levels and includes the cost of the initial unit, its installation, and replacement elements. Replacement filters must be changed regularly, and this is often neglected. I have seen scores of old, contaminated filters sitting on countertops incubating untold numbers of bacteria and passing them into the water of health-conscious but forgetful people.

To select the appropriate water-treatment system, you might first wish to determine what's in the water you now drink. I recommend contacting your municipal water company for a copy of its Water Contaminant Analysis Report or contacting an independent laboratory to have your drinking water tested. Such labs are usually listed in the Yellow Pages under "Laboratories—Testing or Analytical."

Available systems can vary from small, portable units for hiking and camping to whole-house units. For the vast majority of families, three-part canister units that include a fiber filter, ceramic filter, and solid carbon core are effective and economical. Such a unit may be integrated into the plumbing system under the counter with its own faucet or on the countertop attached to the faucet. Look for a unit that tells you (via digital display or visual indicator) when it's time to change the filter cartridge.

There are also pour-through models that will produce limited volumes of water, from gallons a day to quart-sized carafe models. These are often convenient, but remember the limitations of applying only a single method of filtration.

Bottled Water: Is It Any Safer?

Is your bottled water safe? I recommend that you contact the bottler for a current independent assay. This assay should include not just bacteria levels (these are easy to control) but a comprehensive group of contaminants, including chlorine, known carcinogens, and heavy metals (lead, mercury, cadmium, arsenic). This report will include the safe range for each contaminant, and you want to see that the water you're drinking is either in the low end of this range or preferably ND (none detected). You can also visit the Web site for the National Sanitation Foundation at www.nsf.org, which rates popular bottled water brands for purity.

SUMMARY

Water exists in a variety of forms. In living things, water is transformed from randomly arranged H_2O molecules into a *highly organized system* that participates in or controls thousands of chemical and biophysical reactions. Water clusters vibrate at specific resonant frequencies, and these frequencies influence cell structure and function throughout life.

When clustered or organized water is consumed, high-frequency information is transmitted via proteins throughout the body. These proteins amplify the signal and send it in a cascading wave to other connected cells. This wave of information is carried throughout the body like a wake-up call to restore normal function.

Because of its important role in body function, adequate consumption of pure water is a critical part of any antiaging plan. The following Hydration Action Plan will help avoid the "raisin effect" brought on by the damaging habits of modern life.

Hydration Action Plan

1. Reduce or eliminate dehydrating beverages such as coffee, tea, and caffeinated soft drinks.

2. To the extent that you drink the unhealthy beverages mentioned in point 1, *don't* count them toward your goal of eight to ten cups of water for the day. In fact, if you drink thirty-two ounces of these beverages during the day, you should actually *add* sixty-four ounces of water to your goal to correct for the dehydrating effects of caffeine.

3. Eat lots of fresh fruits and vegetables. Melons are a great source of clustered water, as are fresh raw fruit and vegetable juices. Water from these sources could be called "living water," a significant benefit to aging people whose bodies are no longer efficient in organizing water.

4. Drink water all day long in small amounts.

   - If you're in one place most of the day, remembering to drink water will be easy. Simply take a twenty-four-ounce tumbler and fill it up in the morning. Be sure that it's empty by mid-morning. Refill it and make sure that's gone by midafternoon. Fill it again and make sure the last twenty-four ounces are consumed before 5:00 P.M.

   - If you're on the road, keep a water bottle handy. Sporting goods stores sell a variety of water carriers, from simple shoulder bags to backpack containers with over-the-shoulder straws.

   - Drink a glass of water slowly as you prepare your meal.

   - Put a sign on the refrigerator that reads CHOOSE WATER!

   - Remind yourself that the more water you drink, the better you will feel.

   - To make sure you turn to natural sources of water when you are thirsty, do not keep soft drinks in your home.

   - For variety, flavor your water with a squeeze of lemon or lime or with a small amount of fruit juice.

- Don't try to "simplify" the above steps into a routine of gulping half a quart three times a day. Not only will such a practice produce dramatic changes in your urination habits, but it will also fail to provide the full benefit you get from sipping water throughout the day.

5. Remember that the absence of a sense of thirst is *not* a reliable indicator of the need for water. Drink your eight to ten cups every day, whether thirsty or not.

Metabolic Issues for Women and Men

FOR WOMEN

I am not a doctor and I am not a woman, and I am not going to attempt to discuss all the complex issues that women face as they grow older. As a biochemist, however, I have access to information that I believe is critically important and that may prove valuable for a woman to discuss with her physician.

Regarding Hormones

Most people think men make testosterone and women make estrogen. In reality, men and women make *both* hormones, just in different quantities. Another myth is that the sex drive is a "testosterone thing." In fact, studies show that many hormones, including estrogen and progesterone, are involved in the sexual response. What's so attractive about the Metabolic Plan is that it does not rely on a single hormone factor. Even though I have focused a great deal on DHEA, you'll remember that DHEA is converted to testosterone and estrogen and raises growth hormone, pregenolone, and progesterone levels as well. As such, it appears to play a conductor role in the hormone symphony of life.

You'll remember from Chapter 7 that exercise is also a critical factor in healthy aging, and this is especially true for women. Studies have shown that functional ability (the ability to take care of yourself) is first and foremost a function of muscle mass and fitness. This, in turn, depends on levels of DHEA.[1] Women tend to have a more difficult time maintaining these longevity factors because they lose *two* powerful anabolic hormones as they grow older, DHEA and testosterone. In fact, between age twenty and age forty, the average American woman will see her testosterone levels drop by nearly 50 percent.

Notice that this happens a decade or more before anyone notices that her estrogen levels are changing, yet doctors have been slow to recognize the critical importance of DHEA and testosterone. A report in the *American Journal of Medicine* states:

> Women who are androgen [DHEA and testosterone] depleted develop physical and behavioral symptoms referred to as female androgen deficiency syndrome. . . . Women who . . . are deprived of endogenous ovarian androgens have consistently been shown to have impairment of sexual functioning, loss of energy, depression, and headaches. . . . Androgen replacement therapy is a neglected area of medical practice and further research is needed to identify all women who will benefit from it since studies in menopausal women have shown [oral] administration to be well tolerated and safe. Such therapy is underused and very much under researched.[2]

"Impairment of sexual functioning, loss of energy, depression, and headaches." Sound like anyone you know? For centuries, women were told that after age forty, these feelings were just part of the program. In other words, "Learn to live with it." Then, drugs were developed to combat depression, but they had significant side effects. One drug after another came and went until the advent of a class of drugs known as selective serotonin reuptake inhibitors (SSRIs), the best known being Prozac, Paxil, and Zoloft.

What's wrong with these drugs? While they can be very helpful in alleviating depression, the most common side effect (and by common, I mean almost 50 percent of users) is sexual dysfunction, including disturbances in sexual desire, arousal, and orgasm.[3] Other common side effects of SSRIs are gastrointestinal disturbances, headache, fatigue, insomnia, weight gain, and impaired memory.[4] Aren't those the very things women are trying to avoid?

Solution: I described in Chapter 5 how DHEA improves memory, abolishes depression, and at the same time *enhances* sexual function. Recently, researchers gave DHEA to a group of postmenopausal women, and in just seven days, the women experienced a remarkable restoration of endorphin metabolism.[5] Endorphins are the feel-good biochemicals that are normally part of the enthusiasm of youth. In other words, you don't have to replace one set of symptoms for another; you can actually turn back your biological clock and feel (and act) young again. We are not talking about masculinizing women but restoring the DHEA and testosterone levels that they enjoyed at about age thirty. This has been accomplished with moderate daily doses of DHEA.[6]

In addition to muscle mass, libido, strength, confidence, and functional ability, new research highlights yet another reason for maintaining testosterone levels. Testosterone appears to delay brain degeneration. We've known that estrogen helps maintain anabolic (repair and rebuild) functions of the brain, but it now appears that testosterone may also help by reducing the secretion of amyloid β-peptide (Aβ-peptide). The accumulation of Aβ-peptide can cause plaque deposits to form in the brain and is believed to play a major role in the development of Alzheimer's disease.[7]

From Brains to Bones—The Osteoporosis Time Bomb ✓

In their thirties and forties, few women are concerned about the strength of their bones. But a few short decades later, there is hardly a more dramatic impact on the quality of life for older women than osteoporosis and bone fractures. In fact, a recent survey of women aged seventy-five years and above revealed that 80 percent would rather die than experience the loss of independence, social isolation, depression, and other quality-of-life factors resulting from a bad hip fracture.[8]

The bad news: More than 28 million Americans are affected by osteoporosis, a disorder in which the bones become thin and brittle. The disease will cripple and kill more than 1.6 million people this year. More women die from the complications of osteoporosis than from cancer of the breast, cervix, and uterus combined.

The good news: Osteoporosis can be prevented, and the progressive loss of bone can be arrested.

The shocking news: Americans are still in the dark about measures to combat osteoporosis. Perhaps a new look at your bones would be appropriate. Where did you learn about bones? In biology or anatomy class. And what were you looking at? Either a picture of a skeleton in a book or, at best, a real skeleton hanging on a stand in the corner. The fundamental difference between these images and your skeleton, of course, is that they are dead and your bones are very much alive.

You see, there's only one way that nature could maintain an extraordinary, living, and dynamic structure like your skeleton over a lifetime. After all, bone gets old and has to be replaced just like every other part of your body. So you have cells known as *osteoclasts*, which excavate old bone (catabolic), and *osteoblasts*, which fill in new bone (anabolic). This works extremely well until the anabolic signal generated by DHEA, testosterone, estrogen, progesterone, and growth hormone weakens, resulting in excessive osteoclast breakdown and insufficient osteoblast repair. Thus, osteoporosis is fundamentally a metabolic disease.

Oh, I know, you thought it was a calcium deficiency.

The Calcium Connection

Today, you can wake up to a glass of calcium-fortified orange juice, pour high-calcium milk on your calcium-fortified breakfast cereal, and prepare toast (made with calcium-fortified flour) with calcium-fortified margarine or calcium-rich butter. Doctors often tell their patients to eat TUMS, and the limestone, dolomite, bonemeal, and oyster shell business has never been better. Is this the solution to the osteoporosis problem?

Research and common sense say no. We know there are societies that consume less calcium than Americans and yet have a much lower incidence of osteoporosis.[9] At the same time, countries with greater intake of calcium show no significant benefit. An excellent review article in the *Canadian Medical Association Journal* states, "Epidemiologic studies have failed to support the hypothesis that larger amounts of calcium are associated with increased bone density or a decreased incidence of fractures."[10]

The calcium craze has two dangerous consequences. First, believing that calcium supplements will eliminate osteoporosis risk, women may ignore the underlying metabolic issue and the need for exercise and broad-spectrum nutritional support. Second, excessive calcium supplementation can have significant health risks, including impaired absorption of magnesium, iron, zinc, and other minerals.

Is Calcium Unimportant?

Obviously, because calcium makes up the major portion of bone tissue, it *is* an important factor in optimizing bone growth and repair. It must also be remembered that better than half of all adult American women have calcium intakes less than 500 milligrams per day.[11] What is needed is a balanced perspective that considers not only the *amount* of calcium but also the *source* of calcium and other important raw materials needed to build and maintain strong bones.

How Much Calcium Do You Need?

Presently, the RDI (reference daily intake) for calcium is 1,000 milligrams per day. Some experts believe this should be increased to 1,200 to 1,500 milligrams per day. Because the average intake of American women appears to be in the range of 500 to 600 milligrams, I believe supplementation of an additional 800 to 1,000 milligrams is prudent. Ideally, this should be delivered in divided doses for optimal absorption.

What Are the Best Sources of Calcium?

I think you will agree that the amount of calcium on the label is not as important as the amount that gets into your bones. Thus, I recommend you avoid calcium phosphate products, which the body does not absorb well. Use some calcium carbonate, which is better absorbed, but focus on the highly bioavailable compounds such as calcium citrate, calcium aspartate, and calcium hydroxyapatite.[12] These are found in better-quality nutritional supplements designed to support bone health.

Beyond Calcium: The Role of Companion Nutrients

There are a number of other nutrients critical for bone health. In one study, intake of zinc and magnesium was shown to have a stronger influence on bone density than the intake of calcium.[13] Boron, manganese, silicon, folic acid, and vitamins B_6, D, C, and K are additional cofactors.[14]

Magnesium deserves special mention because it is in short supply in the American diet.[15] Analysis of national diet surveys shows that the intake of calcium by adult females has increased significantly since the 1980s, whereas the intake of magnesium has remained relatively constant. This has resulted in an imbalance of the intake ratio of these two nutrients.[16] There is also evidence that high calcium intake can reduce absorption of magnesium, especially in diets in which fiber is low.[17]

Good sources of magnesium include dark green vegetables, nuts, beans, whole grains, and seafood. Magnesium supplements are available in health food stores (usually in 400-milligram tablets), and high-quality bone-support formulas will always include this important mineral.

Drugs or Metabolism?

I am not an antipharmaceutical fanatic. It may be that at a certain stage of osteoporosis, the new bisphosphonate drugs can play an important role in decreasing risk for fracture. But that's pretty far down the road, and what is happening presently is that drugmakers are trying to persuade women to use these drugs at the first sign of decreased bone density. Because that includes over 45 million potential customers, you can understand the motive. If the drugs were effective and safe, I might even relax about it. But the effectiveness of these drugs is questionable, the adverse effects can be serious, and you have to take them for the rest of your life.

I explained earlier that maintaining the strength and flexibility of your bones requires a continual rebuilding process (called *remodeling*) in which osteoclasts excavate old bone and osteoblasts fill it in. In conventional aging—in which metabolism is ignored—increasing catabolic activity results in excessive osteoclast activity, thus weakening the bone.

The drug approach is predictable: kill the osteoclasts. Thus, bisphosphonates, which are basically target-specific poisons. This works for a while, but there have been no studies on the safety of long-term (decade-long) ingestion of these synthetic toxins. Recent reports suggest that bisphosphonates can cause liver damage,[18] and you also have to ask what the net result of impairing normal bone remodeling will be.

And what about side effects? Upper gastrointestinal (stomach and esophagus) damage appears to be the worst side effect, in which irritation of these tissues can become ulcerative.[19] Physicians are instructed to emphasize the importance of taking these drugs with a *full glass of water,* and by all means, *don't lie down* after you take it because the drug will damage any sensitive tissue that it touches. Is this something you want to do for the rest of your life?

Compare that to the metabolic approach, in which you restore anabolic metabolism and your body clicks into rebuild-and-repair mode. Once again, DHEA is the star because it performs double duty: stopping bone loss and stimulating new bone growth. What's more, DHEA can be converted to testosterone, estrogen, and indirectly to progesterone, all of which have anabolic, bone-building activity.

Many studies with postmenopausal women have illustrated the bone-strengthening effect of restoring DHEA.[20] The DHEAge study often referenced in this book found remarkable benefits in just six months.[21] A landmark Harvard study showed that DHEA supplementation restored normal bone growth and hormone balance in women with anorexia.[22]

Question: If I'm postmenopausal, will taking DHEA restore a normal menstrual cycle?
Answer: No. You went through menopause because the eggs in your ovaries were depleted by time and the quality-control mechanisms of your body. It is conceivable that a very large *overdose* of DHEA (hundreds of milligrams) could be converted to enough estrogen to restimulate uterine bleeding, but this has not been seen in any study using a physiological dose—that is, the amount of DHEA natural to the body—of between 5 and 50 milligrams per day.

If you are *approaching* menopause—the period known as *perimenopause*, in which hormone fluctuations are causing mood swings, hot flashes, insomnia, and irregular periods—DHEA or a combination of DHEA and progesterone may reset your clock back into normal cycling. The advantage, of course, is freedom from perimenopausal symptoms. You can, in other words, pause menopause. Some women, however, may want to "get it over with" and would not want to employ this strategy. Clearly, this is something to discuss with your health care professional.

Question: Should I take estrogen?
Answer: This is something you should discuss with your physician. There are a number of important issues to put on your discussion list:

1. Estrogen is a term used to describe a group of hormones, including estradiol, estrone, and estriol. Estradiol and estrone have anabolic benefits, but they also have side effects, including increased risk for breast and uterine cancer. Estriol, on the other hand, may actually reduce a woman's cancer risk. The optimal strategy appears to use a natural combination of these three compounds, with most of the hormone coming from estriol. Your physician can order effective preparations from any compounding pharmacy (a pharmacy that not only dispenses drugs but actually creates formulations to the physician's specifications). One well-known formulation is called *triple estrogen*.

2. Importantly, such preparations are natural. The giant pharmaceutical companies, on the other hand, have spent billions of dollars convincing physicians and the public to use unnatural hormones. Why? Because unnatural hormones can be patented. No woman produces only estradiol, so why create such a drug? And the alternative, Premarin, is not even a human hormone. It is extracted from the urine of pregnant mares (thus the name). A gynecologist friend of mine says that if she ever starts a veterinary practice, she'll consider prescribing Premarin. But in the meantime, she refuses to recommend horse hormones to human beings.

3. A woman's ovaries produce estrogens and progesterone. Replacing only the estrogen makes no sense. So remember to discuss the very real benefits of progesterone creams and patches.

4. Whichever hormone replacement strategy you work out with your physician, it should include DHEA for the comprehensive anabolic effect. DHEA contributes to all of the beneficial effects of hormone therapy—restored bone density; better sex; improvements in skin, hair, and nails; improved memory; better mood; and decreased risk for cardiovascular disease.

Summary

With the megamillions spent by pharmaceutical companies pushing treatments for the special problems faced by women as they age, it's not surprising that so many women equate their later decades with an expensive and frustrating state of perpetual decline and legal drug dependency. But there are better options. In response to the changing hormones, for instance, there is the leveling effect of DHEA. In response to the ticking time bomb of osteoporosis, a more comprehensive approach is required.

If a woman is deficient in calcium and other essential minerals, her bones will become weak. If she takes supplemental minerals, the weakening of her bones may slow down, but because the underlying problem is actually *metabolic,* just taking handfuls of calcium will not stop bone loss and certainly will not restore bone density. To do that, you have to alter the metabolic environment. Research shows conclusively that the weakening of a woman's skeleton with age is directly related to her loss of DHEA as well as testosterone, estrogen, and progesterone.[23] In other words, mineral deficiency is a biochemical need that can be met by proper diet and mineral supplements. But osteoporosis is a catabolic disease, and you must deal with it in metabolic terms.

Action Plan

1. Get a bone scan *before* menopause (at about age forty-five; earlier if you have a family history of osteoporosis) to determine future risk and appropriate preventive measures.

2. Restore anabolic metabolism with DHEA, 7-Keto, and possibly progesterone and natural estrogens.

3. Perform regular weight-bearing exercise such as weight training or Nautilus machines. The pressure of muscle against bone sends an anabolic signal to the bone to get stronger.[24]

4. Eat a highly varied natural foods diet including low-fat dairy products in order to obtain the full range of bone-support minerals.

5. Supplement the diet with a comprehensive bone and joint formula containing calcium, magnesium, manganese, boron, silica, vitamin D, vitamin C, glucosamine, and chondroitin sulfate.

6. Decrease intake of "bone-busting" beverages (caffeine and soft drinks), which are acid-forming and deplete calcium and magnesium.

7. Eat less meat and more vegetarian proteins. A diet high in meat protein accelerates bone loss.

8. Adopt a hunter-gatherer style of eating (frequent small meals versus two or three large meals). In animal research, this has been shown to dramatically improve bone density, most likely because of increased mineral absorption and decreased mineral loss, even when the same number of calories were consumed.[25]

FOR MEN

On the surface, it looks as if men have it relatively easy. They don't have menopause to dramatically alter hormone levels. And because men start out with higher bone mass, they are at lower risk for osteoporosis. The really intriguing thing, of course, is that women on average live longer than men—roughly six to eight years in America and Western Europe. This cannot be explained solely by sociological factors, even though men *are* more aggressive and therefore more prone to damage from stress, accidents, and warfare. There must be biological factors, too, because the female longevity advantage is seen worldwide, in developing nations and high-tech societies, and in most animals as well. What's more, we know that not only do men die from violent causes (murder, auto accidents, suicide) more often than women, but they also die more often from cancer, heart disease, stroke, and even pneumonia.

Why Do Women Have a Longevity Advantage?

Is there some clue that we can derive from this phenomenon that might help men live longer? I believe the answer is to be found in anatomy, biochemistry, and genetics. You see, women live longer than men not because they age more slowly but because, at every stage of life from infancy onward, women die at lower rates. What are the most likely factors?

Accumulation of Iron

Women do not accumulate iron until after menopause. That's because menstrual blood loss reduces iron every month. As I explained in Chapters 3 and 6, excess iron is a tremendous factor in cardiovascular disease and cancer. Excess iron catalyzes or accelerates production of free radicals, which affects virtually all known disease states.

Advice for men:

- Have a serum ferritin test as part of your yearly physical exam. If it is higher than 180 micrograms per liter, donate blood on a regular basis and decrease your intake of iron-rich red meat.

- Maintain optimum blood and tissue levels of antioxidants through a highly varied natural foods diet and comprehensive nutritional supplements (see Chapter 3).

Cholesterol Levels

Woman on average have lower total cholesterol levels, higher levels of protective high-density lipoprotein (HDL) cholesterol, and lower levels of artery-clogging low-density lipoprotein (LDL) cholesterol.

Advice for men:

- Keep a watchful eye on your cholesterol level and keep it below 180 milligrams per deciliter. Remember that it is far easier to keep it low than to lower cholesterol once it is in the high range (greater than 200 milligrams per deciliter).

- Maintain optimum blood and tissue levels of antioxidants (see the preceding subsection).

The X Chromosome

Women have an extra copy of the X chromosome. As the maternal part of you (your mother's egg) tumbled down her fallopian tube, it was neither male nor female. It carried an X chromosome. If the sperm that found its way to that egg also carried an X chromosome, you became a female. If the winning sperm carried a Y chromosome, you became a male. Every cell of a woman's body therefore has an extra copy of the X chromosome, which is presumably turned off. Scientists are beginning to think, however, that women may be able to use this extra copy when a genetic error occurs—sort of like having a backup disk if your computer crashes. This would make women less prone to accumulated genetic error. Remember that you are replacing roughly 300 billion cells every day, which necessitates making 300 billion copies of your DNA. As anabolic repair declines with advancing age, the error rate in this massive biochemical process increases, ultimately leading to impaired tissue function and accelerated catabolic damage.

Advice for men: There's nothing to be done about it now, except to:

- Minimize genetic error by maintaining optimal levels of intracellular antioxidants such as glutathione, SOD, and catalase (see Chapter 3 and 6).

- Maintain high levels of DNA repair enzymes by restoring and maintaining anabolic metabolism (Chapter 2).

The Prostate Gland

Women do not have a prostate gland. I've reported the bad news about abnormal prostate growth leading to cancer. Estimates are that it is found in 60 percent of sixty-year-old men, 70 percent of seventy-year-olds, and so forth. Presumably, every male centenarian has prostate cancer.

Advice for men: There's so much to talk about on this subject, we really ought to set aside some room for it.

The Prostate and DHEA: What's All the Buzz?

Because the prostate issue is inextricably tied to androgenic hormones—testosterone (T) and dihydrotestosterone (DHT)—this requires significant discussion. First, it is important to understand that testosterone does not cause prostate cancer, though removing sources of testosterone (testosterone blockade) slows the disease. This conclusion comes from common sense (if testosterone caused prostate cancer, all eighteen-year-old men would have the disease) and from research that finds no association between prostate cancer and blood levels of testosterone, dihydrotestosterone, or DHEA.[26]

Still, ever since the introduction of DHEA into the marketplace, debate has raged as to whether it is a beneficial hormone for those who have prostate cancer or whether it is potentially harmful. A number of rodent studies have indicated that DHEA has potent antitumor effects. It has also been proposed that DHEA, being a weak androgen, could potentially attach to receptors in prostate tissue and prevent the influence of more potent androgens. On the other hand, DHEA can convert into testosterone, and testosterone can convert to dihydrotestosterone. Because these hormones are believed to stimulate prostate tissue, many fear that DHEA could be counterproductive in men with prostate gland enlargement or prostate tumors.

The DHEA controversy has spanned the globe, through virtually all sectors of the medical and scientific community. Dr. Étienne-Émile Baulieu, one of the world's preeminent hormone biochemists and a leader in DHEA research, summarized his position in a cogent and compelling editorial published in the *Journal of Clinical Endocrinology and Metabolism:*

> Cancers, atherosclerosis, and decrease of immunological responses and brain functions are frequently observed in aging, along with global changes of metabolism (decrease of lean tissues, increase of fat mass, osteoporosis, etc.). . . . Logic pleads in favor of oral administration of DHEA at a dose that provides so called young DHEA levels in the blood and no T/DHT and estradiol concentrations superior to those of normal people of 30 to 40 years of age.[27]

Dr. Sam Yen and his colleagues at the University of California at San Diego made a similar statement:

> DHEA in *appropriate replacement doses* appears to have remedial effects with respect to its ability to induce an anabolic growth factor, increase muscle strength and lean body mass, activate immune function, and enhance quality of life in aging men and women [italics mine].[28]

The question, then, is what exactly is an appropriate replacement dose? In order to obtain maximum benefit and minimal risk, there are three important principles:

First Principle: Stay at a Physiological Dose

I have suggested a dose range of 10 to 25 milligrams of DHEA per day. This is roughly one-quarter to one-half of the amount of DHEA produced by a man at age thirty. Data supports the safety of this small dose, in that larger doses of 50 milligrams per day have resulted in no significant increase in T or DHT in male volunteers.[29]

The important point is that we are not elevating anabolic activity to a level above that seen in youthful adults. As such, there is no data, experimental or clinical, to suggest that there will be an increased risk for abnormal growth of any type, including tumors. Previous studies that suggested a causative influence of serum IGF-1 on prostate cancer have been disproved.[30] On the contrary, a recent animal study reported in the *European Journal of Urology* concluded that:

> Dehydroepiandrosterone (DHEA) and 9-cis-retinoic acid are the most active [cancer-preventive] agents identified to date. DHEA inhibits prostate cancer induction both when chronic administration is begun prior to carcinogen exposure, and when administration is delayed until preneoplastic prostate lesions are present.[31]

The goal, once again, is to create a metabolic signal to the brain indicating that the body is growing younger. This does not require—nor would we want—a dramatic alteration of hormone levels. A moderate hormone signal—combined with proper diet and exercise—restores anabolic metabolism, which, in turn, creates specific antiaging benefits, including enhanced immunity. Because 10 to 25 milligrams of DHEA may not be sufficient to generate this critical longevity signal in all individuals, I've proposed adding an important new analog of DHEA known as 7-Keto DHEA.

Second Principle: Use 7-Keto

As described in Chapter 2, 7-Keto (3-acetyl-7-keto DHEA) is not converted to testosterone and therefore serves as an anabolic signal "amplifier" with a remarkable safety profile. Because 7-Keto is a natural metabolite of DHEA and is produced from DHEA, it is easy to see the advantage of this combination. It has been shown that 7-Keto produces a wide range of benefits, including enhancement of immunity, body composition, mood, memory, and cognition.[32]

Rigorous investigation has also established that 7-Keto DHEA is extremely safe even in high doses. Clinical evaluation of a 200-milligram daily dose with male and female volunteers found no alteration of liver or kidney functions, no adverse effects on blood chemistry, and most important, no increase *at all* in serum testosterone, dihydrotestosterone, or estrogens.[33] Recommended dose: 25 to 100 milligrams per day.

Third Principle: Inhibit Conversion of Testosterone to Estradiol

After the decline in DHEA, the most significant age-related hormonal change occurring in males is a decline in free or biologically active testosterone. At the same time, estrogen levels increase, producing a remarkable shift in the testosterone-to-estrogen balance.

Estrogen levels increase as part of the catabolic cycle. The liver is responsible for detoxifying excess estrogen. As we have already discussed, aging is associated with a dramatic *decline* in liver function, accelerated by immoderate alcohol intake and the use of multiple prescription drugs. What's more, muscle mass declines, and body fat accumulates—and body fat converts testosterone to estrogen via an enzyme known as aromatase. Even lean men tend to produce more aromatase as they age, but the conversion of testosterone to estrogen may be ten to twenty times higher in the obese.

These factors all contribute to a situation in which the estrogen levels of the average fifty-four-year-old man are higher than those of the average fifty-nine-year-old woman.[34] There is growing evidence that estrogen is a primary factor in abnormal prostate growth, just as it fosters abnormal cell proliferation in a woman's breasts.[35]

The third principle, therefore, is to block the conversion of testosterone to estrogen. This is done by maintaining a high muscle-to-fat ratio and inhibiting the aromatase enzyme. Fortunately, natural aromatase inhibitors are found throughout a highly varied natural foods diet. It is now believed that a diet high in fruits, vegetables, beans, and seeds (such as the traditional Asian diet) helps to explain the reduced risk Asian cultures have for hormone-sensitive cancers.

Natural Aromatase Inhibitors	Source
Soy isoflavones	Soybeans, tofu, soy protein
Flavonoids	Vegetables, fruits, whole grains
Polyphenols	Green tea
Carotenoids	Vegetables, orange and yellow fruits
Lignans	Flaxseeds
Phytochemicals	White button mushrooms
Zinc	Nutritional supplements (10 to 30 milligrams per day)

Talking with Your Doctor

Obviously, if you have prostate disease (benign prostatic hypertrophy [BPH] or prostate cancer), you need to consult a physician regarding treatment options and the extraordinary developments in this area of men's health. Every month, more information is available to help us unravel the knot of prostate health. There are presently two new issues for any man over forty to discuss with his physician. You can follow future research at www.TheMetabolicPlan.com.

• **The Prostaglandin Connection** We know that when testosterone enters the prostate, some is converted to dihydrotestosterone (which stimulates growth), and some stimulates prostaglandin (PG) synthesis. The released PGs inhibit further bonding of testosterone to prostate cells, thus limiting abnormal cell proliferation.

But with aging, PG synthesis is known to become less efficient, resulting in a reduction of this braking action of PGs on abnormal prostate growth. Decreased PG synthesis is thought to result from inadequate intake of essential fats.

Action step: Decrease intake of nonessential fats from meat and dairy products. Increase intake of essential fats from vegetables, cold-water fish, olive oil, flaxseed oil, and perhaps an essential fatty acid nutritional supplement.

• **The Cyclooxygenase Connection** Cyclooxygenase, otherwise known as COX-2, is an inflammatory enzyme that has recently been found to be elevated in men with prostate cancer.[36] This is intriguing because COX-2 has been associated with a raft of disease states, and a number of COX-2–inhibiting drugs are now available. Unfortunately, the adverse effects from the drugs may include damage to the gastrointestinal tract and even increased risk for heart disease. On the other hand, nature already put plenty of COX-2 inhibitors in (*all together now*) a highly varied natural foods diet.

Action step: A number of flavonoids and carotenoids found in fruits and vegetables inhibit COX-2, which may help to explain why vegetarians have a lower risk for prostate cancer. In addition, green tea, resveratrol from red wine and grape concentrates, quercetin from onions, and a number of herbs can also be quite effective, including Chinese skullcap, holy basil, turmeric, ginger, rosemary, and oregano.[37] One especially effective natural COX-2 inhibitor is a flavonoid known as silymarin, derived from the milk thistle herb.[38] Silymarin actually does double duty here, as it also enhances liver function. And finally, omega-3 fats found in cold-water fish also dampen the inflammatory action of COX-2.

Summary
Although men don't face the trials of menopause and are much better protected against osteoporosis than women, they face some significant disadvantages in the longevity battle. As discussed, these include a tendency to accumulate iron, increases in serum cholesterol, and abnormal prostate growth. All three of these potential problems respond very well to nutritional therapy, regular exercise, and a prudent lifestyle. By following the advice and action items described above, men can go a long way toward overcoming their built-in anatomical and biochemical disadvantages. Now, let's take an important look at ways to monitor your progress.

ELEVEN

Keeping Score, Staying Motivated, and Taking Action

In any game, you need a way to keep score. In the old paradigm of aging, this was done with candles on a cake. But now you know that the chronology of life is not nearly as important as the biology of life—and that's determined by your metabolism, not by the year you were born.

Thus, scientists are now speaking in terms of one's *biological age,* which is a measure of how one looks, feels, and performs. While there is no universal agreement as to how biological age is determined, a number of important biomarkers have been identified.

Biomarkers of aging are those factors that show predictable and significant changes over the course of one's life. Data regarding these factors is not merely academic. Today, it is understood that altering biomarkers can produce changes in the aging process itself. When you support anabolic repair and/or reduce catabolic damage, you and your doctor can document the resulting benefit with reliable tests.

A COMPASS FOR THE JOURNEY

There are plenty of tests to measure the aging process. An ophthalmologist can measure failing eyesight. Internists use a battery of tests to document the decline in liver and kidney function. And cardiologists can provide a stunning picture of a weakened heart and occluded arteries. In fact, twenty-one cents out of every health care dollar is spent on tests to measure the breakdown process of aging. Conventional medicine, in other words, merely waits for sufficient bad news and then launches into fix-it mode. Health-conscious baby boomers are recognizing that this is insane. They want a proactive approach that *prevents the problems from occurring.*

Auto maintenance is a perfect analogy. No one waits for his or her engine to seize up before changing the oil. We balance our tires, lube every three thousand miles, change wiper blades, and carefully follow a tune-up schedule. People have been looking for a preventive-maintenance strategy for the human body, but until now, there has been no way to evaluate interventions like stress management, nutrition, exercise, and mind-body tools. You do not, in other words, feel yourself not getting cancer. You can't feel your bones getting stronger or brain cells regenerating. With the biomarker tests that I will describe, however, you will have a way to measure rejuvenation—to validate and quantify the Metabolic Plan.

OVERALL STRATEGY

The goal is to become aware of how you are changing as you grow older. A lot of this has to do with information derived from tests, but it's also important to chronicle the changes that occur in your attitudes, goals, and dreams. I strongly recommend that you keep a narrative journal to go along with a physical record. Your journal can be audiotaped, video, or written (or a combination), but make sure that it's something you do on a regular basis, at least once a week. You'll be surprised how it helps put things into clear focus.

To go along with this journal, create a three-ring binder labeled MY BODY, so that you don't end up with a drawer filled with loose papers. Here are the major divisions that will help you chart your progress.

THE ANABOLIC/CATABOLIC INDEX

In September of 1998, I was reviewing my weekly computerized biomedical update—a service that collects all of the scientific literature published anywhere in the world containing any of my keywords. A study came up in Japanese, and I was about to scroll through it to the next study when I recognized the chemical term *17-ketosteroid sulfate.* I knew that DHEA was metabolized to a 17-ketosteroid, so I was intrigued and went to find a Japanese lab technician to translate. I learned that the research was conducted by a highly respected endocrinologist and his colleagues at the University of Hokkaido, focusing on anabolic metabolism in humans.

Professor Oasmu Nishikaze was intrigued by the ability of the body to rebuild, repair, and restore itself. More important, he wanted to learn why this ability was different from person to person and why it changed during periods of stress, illness, and injury. So for two decades, he and his team tried to find a biomarker that would accurately reflect anabolic activity.

Their method was very innovative. They collected urine samples at a number of hospitals from patients as they were admitted and continued to gather daily samples until the patients were released. After years of painstaking work, they identified a group of metabolites that were uniformly low when people were first hospitalized. These same compounds rose in parallel to recovery and were at the highest point when the patients were released. Amazingly, this held true whether the patients were suffering from illness, injury, or even psychological stress.[1]

The compounds were a group of anabolic metabolites known as *17-ketosteroid sulfates,* biochemicals that appear in the urine whenever the body shifts into high-gear repair-and-heal mode—thus Nishikaze's announcement that he had identified the unitive or comprehensive biomarker for anabolic metabolism.[2]

From my research on metabolism and aging, I realized that 17-ketosteroid sulfate (17-KS-S) levels would tend to indicate one's rate of aging—not only one's position on the line from anabolic youth to catabolic old age but the speed at which one was approaching the brick wall.

Development

In 1999, my research group began development of a practical metabolic profile based on Nishikaze's four urinary biomarkers. First, the test method had to be automated and the sensitivity improved to the level required for a full-scale clinical trial. Both tasks were accomplished using advanced technology that could measure 17-KS-S levels down to one billionth of a gram. We named this assay the Anabolic/Catabolic Index, or ACI. Next, we had to run enough tests to confirm that ACI levels declined with advancing age. With that data (known as a *proof-of-principle study*), we went to an independent research organization for supervision of a clinical trial that would test the ability of a nutritional formula to enhance anabolic metabolism.

The design was placebo-controlled and double-blind, meaning that no one, neither the study participants nor the people administering the test, knew who was getting a placebo and who was getting the anabolic-support formula. The active ingredients of this formula included a small 10-milligram dose of DHEA, with 25 milligrams of 7-Keto, 1,000 milligrams of an amino acid known as *L-arginine,* and a group of botanical extracts designed to support liver function.

After thirty days, the codes were broken and I received the data. This is always nervous time for a scientist—a great deal of hard work can go down the drain, and although negative outcomes are still valuable, they are rarely publishable. So I turned first to the placebo groups. A significant effect there would invalidate my data; they had taken look-alike capsules with no nutritional value, and they should experience no significant effect. I was relieved to find that the anabolic activity in the placebo groups had declined slightly.

Comparing the before-and-after scores for the active group revealed a remarkable improvement. The group on the nutritional formula had increased their 17-KS-S levels in just thirty days. Equally impressive were the results from a corroborating lab that measured a different anabolic biomarker known as IGF-1.

Our methodology paper was published in the *Journal of Chromatography,* and a follow-up paper is pending publication in *Spectroscopy, the International Journal.*[3] To my knowledge, this is the first clinical trial proving that anabolic metabolism can be restored by nutritional means. Of course, study participants didn't immediately look younger. Metabolism works *over time* as cells and ultimately entire tissues are replaced in the natural process of renewal. You'll remember that this amounts to about 300 billion cells a day.

We predicted that this metabolic improvement would translate, over the course of weeks and months, to improved energy, higher muscle mass, greater stamina, better skin tone—all the things that we associate with young metabolic efficiency. But it was even better than that. People reported sleeping deeper, waking up feeling more alert, having better sex, more frequent sex, better moods, and even better digestion. They reported, in other words—I *know* this sounds trite—getting a new lease on life.

Case Study—The Boomer Dilemma

Marissa and John were a baby boomer couple experiencing a very common dilemma. They were smart, educated, professional, and motivated people. When they came to my office, I knew at once that what they *didn't* need was information. "We know what to do," sighed Marissa. "It's just that all of a sudden, everything has become so *difficult*. Exercise used to be something I looked forward to, and now it's a chore. John has gained twenty pounds in the last few years, and he's drinking eight cups of coffee a day. He used to be a health nut!"

I explained that what had changed was their metabolism and that until something was done about that, they could not expect to look or feel much better. I turned to John and asked, "What if I told you that you had to quit coffee? Would you do it?" "Well, no," said John. "I've tried to do that a dozen times already." "Exactly," I replied, "but what if you suddenly found that you had more energy and mental clarity and didn't *need* the caffeine?" That, of course, was a different story.

To Marissa, I posed a similar question: "What if I told you that you had to increase the intensity of your exercise routine?" "Well," she replied, "I'd think that was good advice but impossible to follow. I'm already experiencing muscle and joint pain and have to resort to ibuprofen three or four times a week." "That's because you're in the catabolic downward spiral," I explained, "but you know quite well that you don't have muscle pain because of an ibuprofen deficiency." She laughed and listened to my explanation of what would take place if she restored her anabolic repair-and-rebuild metabolism. I was confident in my predictions because this was a woman who *wanted* to exercise. It just didn't feel good, and let's face it, no matter how motivated someone might be, at some point, pain or fatigue will force him or her to give up. Both Marissa and John were on the edge of that precipice.

I showed them the results of the clinical trial, and they got it immediately. "This is the first time," said Marissa, "that someone has offered me a scientific way to monitor my progress. With everyone else, it's 'Here, take this pill, herb, exercise equipment, book . . . and *trust* me.' "

Marissa's first ACI test came back at 159, which was normal for a fifty-four-year-old woman. "Well," she said, "I'm normal." "That's right," I replied, "and there's no time to lose." The point, of course, is that a normal fifty-four-year-old is hurtling toward the brick wall. The goal is to find the brakes and support anabolic repair. After sixty days on the Metabolic Plan, she scored 201 (the level of an average forty-year-old), and six months later, her score was 380, what I consider the optimal range.

But those are just numbers. You want to know what happened in her life. As predicted, she started to experience greater energy and found that increasing the duration and intensity of her workout was easy. No more joint and muscle pain. Her skin tone improved to the point that everyone she met wanted to know what cosmetic line she was using. "Actually," she'd reply, "I'm working on it from the inside."

Marissa started noticing better muscle tone at the two-month mark, and about the same time, she began seducing John at night. "It's like we're back in college," said John, and it was a good thing they embarked on the Metabolic Plan together because he was able to match her energy and excitement. John lost the twenty pounds and, more important, gained muscle at the same time. The only downside, he told me later, was that they both had to go and buy new clothes. Not only smaller sizes but different styles to fit their young, anabolic attitudes.

I want to emphasize that John and Marissa didn't experience these dramatic results by sitting on the couch, eating doughnuts, and watching television. In addition to the anabolic-support formula, they exercised regularly, ate a highly varied natural foods diet, and supplemented with additional antioxidants. The point is, they were doing all of this before (minus the anabolic support) but were aging "normally," sliding down the catabolic spiral. What turned them around was a shift in their metabolism.

Getting a Handle on Stress

The Anabolic/Catabolic Index is reliable and sensitive—sometimes perhaps a bit too sensitive. I get a few calls every month from people—usually men—who tell me that the test couldn't possibly be accurate. "Well," I respond politely, "the research base for the test was written up in two medical journals, the test method has been published in a leading laboratory science journal, the test is performed with rigid quality controls and has been awarded a U.S. patent. Why do *you* think it's inaccurate?"

"Because I got a low score" is the common reply. "I eat right, exercise regularly, take handfuls of vitamins. How could my score be 85?" "Hmm," I reply. "What's your stress level like?"

Silence.

Then, the slower response: "Well, I'm getting a divorce, and I'm taking this company public, my dog died, and actually, I do have an ulcer. So you think that could be the problem?"

"Bingo," I say. "Think of stress as a catabolic turbocharger. You can do everything right, and stress can undo it all. Do something about the stress and then retest. I'm sure you'll see a significant difference."

Importantly, the ACI test is very sensitive to something that has been overlooked for decades, and that's stress. "Stress overlooked?" you ask. "There are *scores* of books on stress. Everybody's talking about it." And that's my point. All too often, people just talk about it. The average doctor visit today lasts twelve minutes. There's time for only a brief discussion of obvious symptoms, but the issue of stress is rarely touched. "I can't open that Pandora's box," admitted an internist friend, so patients leave with the impression that they are "normal," when in fact many have a time bomb called stress ticking away in their body. Because stress is such a catabolic influence, the ACI test represents a quick and effective way to evaluate the degree to which stress may be accelerating the aging process. It can be an important wake-up call.

How to Obtain an ACI Test

You can send for a test kit from the laboratory listed in Appendix A. Each kit contains a urine-collection container with a lock cap, instructions, and a self-addressed, prepaid overnight mailer. The sample is returned to the lab, and results are sent back within ten days. Results include your ACI score, the "normal" for your age group, and the optimal range that research suggests will indicate a more youthful capacity for anabolic repair.

OTHER IMPORTANT TESTS

The Anabolic/Catabolic Index is a very useful screening tool. It provides a snapshot view of your anabolic drive—the ability of your body to repair and rebuild itself—but it cannot tell your biological age. That requires additional tests to evaluate other important biomarkers:

General Health

These standard blood tests are part of a routine physical:

- *Chem 24:* A comprehensive blood chemistry, including glucose, electrolytes, blood proteins, cholesterol, triglycerides, and indicators of liver and kidney function.

- *CBC (complete blood count):* This is a comprehensive analysis of red and white blood cells, including their number, size, and characteristics. Three important CBC measurements (red blood cell number, hemoglobin, and hematocrit) are discussed in Chapter 3, in the "Testing for Anemia" subsection.

- *Urinalysis:* This is a general screen of the urine looking at characteristics that might indicate health problems such as diabetes, kidney disease, or infection.

Body Composition and Performance

These tests can be performed at a human performance lab, physical therapist's office, or sports medicine clinic:

- Percentage body fat.

- Fat-free mass.

- Hydration.

- Basal metabolic rate.

- Body mass index.

- Maximum oxygen extraction (VO_2 max). Rather than measuring the amount of air your lungs can hold, VO_2 max tells you how much oxygen you are extracting from a given volume of air. This has to do not only with the health of your lungs but with the amount of hemoglobin in your blood and the ability of your heart to pump that blood to the working muscles.

Related Metabolic Biomarkers

These tests can be performed in a physician's office:

- Serum hormone panel (For men and women after age forty), which should include:
    Serum DHEAS (the blood level of DHEA sulfate, the stored form of DHEA).
    Testosterone, estrogen, progesterone, and SHBG (sex steroids and their bioavailability).
    IGF-1 (insulinlike growth factor-1), an anabolic hormone

produced primarily in the liver in response to signals from the adrenals (via DHEA) and the pituitary (via growth hormone). Your doctor may also want to measure IGFBP, the protein that binds (and inactivates) IGF-1 for storage.

- PSA (for men after age forty: prostate-specific antigen, indicates abnormal growth of the prostate and risk for prostate cancer).

- Bone metabolism (for women after age forty):
  PTH (parathyroid hormone, a blood test)
  Pyridinium and deoxypyridinium (biomarkers of bone loss, a urine test)

Oxidative Stress and Glycation

These tests indicate damage from free radicals and simple sugars:

- Oxidative stress (a urine test to measure indicators of free-radical damage)

- Glycated (glycosylated) hemoglobin A1c (a blood test to measure hemoglobin that is bound to—and inactivated by—glucose and other simple sugars)

Immune Panel

This panel, which can be done in a physician's office, measures some sensitive markers of aging, because immune competence invariably falls with age, leading to increased incidence of all major diseases. A good immune panel will provide the ratio of helper to suppressor cells, measure autoantibodies (antibodies to your own tissues), and give you the number and activity of key defenders such as NK (natural killer) cells.

Nutrition Factors

These tests can be performed in a physician's office:

- WBC glutathione (the glutathlone level of the white blood cell— a better indicator of glutathione levels than a serum level, although serum glutathione is better than nothing)

- Serum ferritin (see Chapter 3)

- RBC magnesium (the magnesium level of the red blood cell)

- Serum vitamin E

- Homocysteine (an important risk factor for heart disease and an indirect measure of adequacy for vitamins B_{12}, B_6, and folic acid)

H-Scan

The H-scan (named after the inventor, Robert Hochschild) is a computerized system that measures twelve performance biomarkers of aging, including auditory reaction time, highest audible pitch, vibrotactile sensitivity, visual reaction time, muscle movement speed, vital lung capacity, forced expiratory volume, decision reaction time, short-term memory, alternate button tapping, and visual accommodation. It provides an excellent view of a number of important aspects of biological age and is available at many antiaging clinics.

Tests You Can Do at Home (for Free!)

Skin Elasticity

As we age, free radicals damage the collagen and elastin under the skin, which causes a loss of elasticity. In addition, the subdermal level of the skin dehydrates. These two factors produce wrinkling. An indirect measure of your ability to neutralize dangerous free radicals is the snap-back test.

Lay your hand palm down on a firm surface such as a tabletop. Pinch the skin on the back of your hand for five seconds. Let go and measure how long it takes the skin to resume its normal smooth appearance.

For a teenager (unless he or she smokes), the skin will snap back immediately. For someone forty-five years of age, there will be no snap at all, but in three to five seconds, the skin will regain its smooth appearance. By age sixty, that will normally take ten to fifteen seconds, and by age seventy, the pinch will be visible for thirty-five seconds to a minute.

This is a visual test for cross-linked (age-damaged) skin. But you have to understand that it also indicates damage that you can't see: the collagen in our arteries, for example, also loses flexibility as we age. When the heart pumps, these arteries are supposed to expand. When they lose this elastic quality, blood vessels become damaged, and this is a contributing cause of heart disease. The good news? Your body is re-building this connective tissue all the time. With adequate antioxidant protection, you can prevent excess cross-linking and improve the integrity of the collagen and elastin throughout your body.

Reaction Time

Have a friend hold a wooden eighteen-inch ruler vertically from the one-inch line. Position your thumb and forefinger about three inches apart equidistant from the eighteen-inch line. Have your friend let go of the ruler without warning, and you catch it between your finger and thumb as fast as you can. The number at the point where you catch the ruler is your score. Take the average of three tries. A twenty-year-old will average about twelve inches, and that generally decreases progressively to about five inches by age sixty-five.

Again, don't worry if your score is fairly high (biologically old). You can improve reaction times with games like Ping-Pong, in which the action/reaction demands are high. Tennis is almost as good if you're playing a partner of equal or better skill. Even repeating the ruler test a few times a day will quickly improve your reaction time. Remember, your brain and body function on a "use it or lose it" basis. The Think-FAST software listed in Appendix A also includes an excellent (and more precise) way to measure reaction time.

Static Balance

The static balance test is very valuable because it measures a number of neurological parameters of aging. Have you ever gone on a roller-coaster ride (or even a high swing) with your kids and felt uncomfortable afterward? Your kids are tugging at your arm to go again, and you feel nauseated and dizzy. That's because, as we age, the mechanism that maintains balance becomes less efficient. Communication from the inner ear to the brain and from the brain to the body is impaired.

Now, that's interesting—but here's the really intriguing part. You can improve your sensory-motor balance ability, and this appears to have a positive effect on other unrelated brain functions such as memory. This underscores our understanding of the mind-body connection and how important it is to challenge our limitations. If you accept the obsolete and erroneous notion that aging is immutable, you'll miss exciting opportunities like this to become biologically younger.

To test static balance, stand without shoes on a level, uncarpeted surface. With your feet together, close your eyes and raise one foot about six inches off the ground (if you are right-handed, raise the right foot). See how many seconds you can stand on one foot with your eyes closed before you have to open your eyes or move your supporting foot. Again, test three times and take the average.

Most twenty-year-olds will have no trouble standing for thirty seconds or more. But every decade shows a considerable drop in scores until, at age sixty-five, most people can stand for only three to five seconds. By age eighty, many people can't stand with their eyes closed even on two feet. The cause of this deterioration is more than just the inner ear: neurologists now believe that this test reflects a fundamental deterioration of brain-body communication.

The good news, as I said, is that *this can be improved.* As it turns out, the balancing postures that have been an important part of yoga practice for five thousand years are powerfully effective in improving this important neurological skill. Because balance is now recognized as an important part of any conditioning program, many health clubs now use balance boards. You can also purchase a balance board from a physical therapy supply company or construct your own with a sturdy plank and a two-by-four. For five to ten minutes a day, try to balance on the board. As you improve, move your feet farther apart. When that becomes easy, stand on one foot or round off the edges of the two-by-four. All the while, you'll be improving not only your balance but your memory and learning skills.

Vital Lung Capacity

There are many high-tech ways of measuring the capacity of your lungs, but simply holding your breath is accurate and inexpensive. Take three deep breaths. Hold the fourth breath for as long as you can. Do not force this. Don't get bug-eyed or pass out. Just hold your breath. Healthy twenty-year-olds will have no trouble holding their breath for two minutes. That will decrease by about 15 percent per decade, so that a sixty-year old will be doing well if he can hold his breath for forty-five seconds. What increases vital lung capacity? As you might have guessed, physical activity that forces you to breathe deeply. Exercise stimulates and strengthens the muscles and reflexes that pump air into and out of the lungs. Yoga deep-breathing techniques (in which you learn to breathe using the diaphragm) can also help.

Hand-Grip Strength

Hand-grip strength is measurable with an instrument known as a *hand dynamometer*, available from medical supply companies. Because there are fourteen muscles in your hand, the coordinated strength of these muscles is a good indicator of overall bioenergetics, which includes not only strength but communication between the nervous system and the muscles—known as neuromuscular fitness. A hand dynamometer is useful for measuring this important facet of anabolic metabolism over the years.[4]

Memory/Cognition

As we age, short-term memory declines, as does our ability to work with information stored in this area of the brain. One useful way to evaluate these functions is known as the reverse sequential number test. Have a friend write down three seven-digit numbers. Be sure that the person to be tested cannot see this list. The tester says the first seven-digit number twice. The person taking the test must now repeat the number backward. Do the same with the second and third numbers and average the results for an accurate test.

A thirty-year-old will have no trouble at all. By age fifty, most people will miss one digit out of seven. At age sixty, chances are high that someone will miss two digits. The average seventy-year-old will only be able to repeat four digits. The last three numbers will have disappeared from his or her short-term memory. And the average eighty-year-old will be hard-pressed to accurately reverse-order more than three numbers out of seven.

Improvements in this test may be seen not only in terms of accuracy but also in terms of the speed and ease with which the reverse order is given. Be sensitive to all three measures, and understand that improvements indicate a younger-functioning brain. Again, the ThinkFAST software listed in Appendix A includes excellent (and fun) tests for long-term memory, short-term memory, and decision-making time.

MOTIVATION

Measurable progress toward any goal is a great motivator. When children experience the satisfaction of mastering new skills, they are motivated to learn more. When employees are promoted or rewarded, they are motivated to keep developing and using their skills to the best of their ability. When athletes achieve better scores, they are motivated to stick with difficult training regimens.

In the past, however, we had no convenient way to measure the benefits of good food choices and the use of nutritional supplements. We were guided largely by logic: it just made good *sense* to eat right and supplement with vitamins and minerals. When the scientific literature started to accumulate regarding the benefits of supplementation, we were further motivated to do what we had sensed was right. But even then, we didn't *know* with any certainty that our efforts were paying off for *us* as individuals, as opposed to the average person represented by studies. If we lived to be one hundred, we would have a pretty good idea that our efforts had not been in vain; but while we were moving toward old age, we couldn't be sure.

Now, however, we have the ability to measure our progress month by month and year by year. With this comprehensive battery of tests, we can get a clear picture of the inner health of our bodies down to the cellular level and *know* that what we are doing is working—that we are moving backward on the biological age time line. And that's powerful motivation.

ACTION

It's been said that motivation without action is the height of folly. So at this point, we need a clear way to implement the Metabolic Plan. Following is a decade-by-decade summary guide to help you achieve the best results.

Caution: These recommendations are intended for generally healthy individuals without major medical problems. If you have any symptoms you are concerned about, or significant medical problems, you should consult with a physician to receive personal guidance regarding each of these suggestions.

Action Steps for Those Aged Twenty-five to Thirty-five

Top Five Causes of Death

Motor vehicle accidents
Homicide
Suicide
Nonvehicle accidents
Cancer

Overview

At this age, you still have the anabolic advantage. The idea is to keep it as long as possible. This is where you assemble your baseline data that you'll be looking to maintain or improve for the next century.

Major Focus

- Clearly, the major focus is to develop good habits. This includes not only exercise and diet but stress-management activities that will serve you well for many decades. Consider learning yoga or Tai Chi.

- Minimize exposure to chemicals and radiation. Remember that every sunburn will greatly increase your chance of skin cancer later on.

- Care for your teeth. If you have no fillings, great! If you have some mercury amalgam fillings, consider having them replaced with a more durable, nontoxic material (see Chapter 6).

Major Concerns

Bones and joints: This is your *best chance* to pack minerals into your bones. The bone mineral density you achieve now will have to last you for what may be another century of active living. Review Chapter 8 ("Optimal Nutrition") and beware of the "bone-busters," caffeine and soft drinks.

Physical activity: This is the turning point for millions of people who are just leaving an active lifestyle and becoming immersed in career and family responsibilities. Don't fall into a sedentary trap. Stay active and strong.

Sexually transmitted diseases: AIDS is now the sixth leading cause of death among men aged twenty-five to forty-four. The incidence of hepatitis, herpes, syphillis, gonorrhea, and chlamydia are all on the rise. If you need guidance regarding reducing your risk for STDs, contact your local health department or the National Center for HIV, STD, and TB Prevention (hot line: [800] 227–8922, Web site: www.cdc.gov/nchstp/dstd/dstdp.html). Review Chapters 3 and 6 for additional information.

Sleep hygiene: Now is the time to develop good sleeping habits, although many in your age group are still in party mode. Health experts agree that seven to eight hours of sleep is best and that less than six and a half hours is insufficient to completely restore the body and brain. Review sleep suggestions in Chapter 4.

Childbearing
Statistically speaking, if you're a woman, this is a good time to have a baby and breast-feed. Women who have a child between ages twenty and thirty and nurse the baby for at least six months have a significantly decreased lifelong risk for cancer of the breast, cervix, ovary, and uterus compared to women who have no children or who have their first child after age thirty.[5]

Tests

Yearly

- Complete physical exam, with blood pressure, heart rate, reflexes, and so forth.

- Complete blood count (CBC) and chem 24.

- HIV.

- Homocysteine. Get a baseline of this metabolite in your blood, which has been shown to be a risk factor in cardiovascular disease and brain degeneration. *Note for women:* High homocysteine has recently been linked to *poor pregnancy outcome,* a term that includes miscarriage, birth defects, and stillbirths.[6]

- Urinalysis.

- Anabolic/Catabolic Index (ACI) for baseline data.

- *Men:* Clinical testicular exam.

- *Women:* Clinical breast exam and pelvic exam.

- Dental checkup and cleaning (twice a year).

- Body composition: percentage body fat, fat-free mass, hydration, and basal metabolic rate.

- Time to have a comprehensive toxic metal evaluation, including hair, urine, and blood levels of lead, mercury, and cadmium. If levels are low and you have no significant environmental or occupational exposure, no need to retest for another ten years. It is especially important for women to have this screen before conceiving a child.

Monthly Self-Check

- *Women:* Breast self-exam

- *Men:* Testicular self-exam

Exercise

- Aim for 200 points a week but make sure to earn at least 150 (see Chapter 7 for point system).

- Resistance training with hand weights or machines two to three times a week.

- Range-of-motion stretching or yoga two to three times a week.

Nutritional Supplements

- High-potency multiple-dose multivitamin with minerals

- Comprehensive antioxidant (see Chapter 3)

- Bioenergetic formula (see Chapter 7)

- *For women:* Comprehensive bone-building formula (see Chapter 10)

- Stage 1 immune-support formula (see Chapter 6)

- Aloe concentrate: one ounce a day

Action Steps for Those Aged Thirty-five to Forty-five

Top Five Causes of Death

Motor vehicle accidents
Cancer
Heart disease
Nonvehicle accidents
Suicide

Overview

For most people, the balance point at which anabolic and catabolic forces are roughly equal is age thirty, after which, metabolism becomes progressively more catabolic. If you've remained physically fit, you have extended the balance point a full five years, but you may still need help. You have a tremendous opportunity to determine your own metabolic destiny and chart a new course in human potential. Be bold.

Major Focus

Maintain good habits. Particularly important is your dedication to regular exercise and a natural foods diet. This is a busy decade as you strengthen family and career paths. Become immune to the workaholic virus by keeping your eye on the prize: a balanced life!

Major Concerns

Bones and joints: Women: It may still be possible to strengthen bones, but this time, the operative words are *metabolism* and *weight-bearing exercise.* Make sure you have both well in hand.

Physical activity: Stay active and strong. If you can maintain the same muscle mass throughout this decade, you will have won an important metabolic victory. If you're starting from an unfit or overweight state, this is your golden opportunity to turn your life around.

Tests

Yearly

- Complete physical exam, with blood pressure, heart rate, reflexes, and so forth.

- Complete blood count (CBC) and chem 24.

- HIV if you have changed sex partners.

- Homocysteine.

- Urinalysis.

- Anabolic/Catabolic Index (ACI).

- *Men:* Clinical testicular exam.

- *Women:* Clinical breast exam and pelvic exam.

- Dental checkup and cleaning (twice a year).

- Body composition: percentage body fat, fat-free mass, hydration, and basal metabolic rate.

Monthly Self-Check

- *Women:* Breast self-exam

- *Men:* Testicular self-exam

- *Both:* Skin self-exam

Exercise

- Aim for 200 points a week but make sure to earn at least 150 (see Chapter 7 for point system).

- Resistance training with hand weights or machines two to three times a week.

- Range-of-motion stretching or yoga two to three times a week.

Nutritional Supplements

- High-potency multiple-dose multivitamin with minerals

- Comprehensive antioxidant (see Chapter 3)

- Bioenergetic formula (see Chapter 7)

- *For women:* Comprehensive bone-building formula (see Chapter 10)

- Stage 1 immune-support formula (see Chapter 6)

- Aloe concentrate: two ounces a day

- DHEA: 5–20 milligrams per day before bed

- 7-Keto DHEA: 25 milligrams soon after waking up

- Alpha lipoic acid: 100 milligrams per day

- N-acetyl-cysteine (NAC): 300 milligrams per day

Action Steps for Those Aged Forty-five to Fifty-five

Top Five Causes of Death

Heart disease
Cancer
Stroke
Motor vehicle accidents
Nonvehicle accidents

Overview

This is the decade of the greatest metabolic change. I know that may surprise you, but if you have attended reunions regularly, you'll agree. At your tenth high school reunion, people looked more . . . mature. But at your twenty-fifth or thirtieth reunion, everyone was between forty and fifty, and the change was dramatic—so dramatic that you probably had to look at people's name tags.

For a woman, the greatest increase in fracture risk is in her fourth decade of life. Conventional "wisdom" says that it is now impossible to increase bone density, but you know better. You know that if you maintain the anabolic drive that got you here and maintain a healthy diet and a habit of regular weight-bearing exercise, you can move into your sixties with strong bones and high muscle mass.

If you're looking in the mirror and wondering if it's possible to regain your "lost" youth, there's no better time to start growing younger. You're at an important crossroads and can go either way. Many of your friends have given up, but you don't have to.

Major Focus

You're going to have to make a conscious decision to take the anabolic path to a more youthful body and mind. With the tools provided in this book, it won't be arduous or painful. All that's required is knowledge and perseverance.

Major Concerns

Cardiovascular health: Notice that heart disease is now the number one cause of death for your age group. As more and more people get on the Metabolic Plan, this will change, but for now, take heed. Your heart has already pumped about 50 million gallons of blood, and to make it last as long as possible, you have to keep your blood vessels clean and flexible. If your cholesterol is over 200 milligrams per deciliter, it's time to get it under 200 (preferably between 160 and 180). In a large clinical trial measuring cardiovascular risk factors in men with high cholesterol, participants enjoyed a 10 percent decrease in risk for coronary heart disease for every 5 percent reduction in cholesterol. What's more, those who made significant alterations in diet by decreasing meat and dairy fat and increasing fresh fruits and vegetables had a risk factor reduction of 24 percent![7]

Bones and joints: It's time to give nature a hand by providing greater amounts of glucosamine and chondroitin (see Chapter 7). But you can also make these important structural proteins yourself by engaging in range-of-motion (ROM) exercise along with weight-bearing exercise such as walking, jogging, cycling, or weight lifting.

Physical activity: A significant challenge in this area is conventional thinking, especially as it relates to a woman's "role." If you've been on the Metabolic Plan, you already know that you have more energy and a higher sex drive than most thirty-five-year-olds. You understand, perhaps more than at any other time in your life, the maxim "Use it or lose it." So go ahead, get that bikini, take that dream vacation, and "act your age" . . . your *biological* age.

Teeth and gums: Alveolar bone loss starts showing up in the fourth decade of life. Make sure you are taking good care of your teeth and gums. Daily flossing and twice-a-day brushing are essential. Ask your dentist about recent research on sonic and ultrasonic toothbrushes.

Tests

Yearly

- Complete physical exam, with blood pressure, heart rate, reflexes, and so forth

- Complete blood count (CBC) and chem 24

- HIV if you have changed sex partners

- Homocysteine

- Urinalysis

- Hemoccult (test for blood in the stool)

- Anabolic/Catabolic Index (ACI)

- Dental checkup and cleaning (twice a year)

- Body composition: percentage body fat, fat-free mass, hydration, and basal metabolic rate

- *Men:*
  Clinical testicular exam
  PSA
  Digital rectal exam

- *Women:*
  Clinical breast exam and pelvic exam
  Bone scan (dual-photon absorptiometry)

Once Every Two Years

- Stress cardiogram (in which you jog on a treadmill or ride an ex-ercycle while a cardiologist watches your EKG). Your goal is to reach 80 percent of your maximal heart rate with no irregularities in heart function.

Monthly Self-Check

- *Women:* Breast self-exam

- *Men:* Testicular self-exam

- *Both:* Skin self-exam

Exercise

- Aim for 150 points a week but make sure to earn at least 100 (see Chapter 7 for point system).

- Start taking 1,000 milligrams of branched-chain amino acids (BCAAs), available in capsules, after strenuous exercise.

- Resistance training with hand weights or machines two to three times a week.

- Range-of-motion stretching or yoga two to three times a week.

Nutritional Supplements

- High-potency multiple-dose multivitamin with minerals

- Additional vitamin E to total 400 international units per day

- Additional vitamin C to total 500 milligrams per day

- Comprehensive antioxidant (see Chapter 3)

- Bioenergetic formula (see Chapter 7)

- Stage 1 immune-support formula (see Chapter 6)

- Aloe concentrate: two ounces a day

- DHEA: 10–20 milligrams per day before bed

- 7-Keto DHEA: 25 milligrams soon after waking up

- Alpha lipoic acid: 100 milligrams per day

- N-acetyl-cysteine (NAC): 300 milligrams per day

- Acetyl-L-carnitine: 250 milligrams per day

- During periods of physical or emotional stress, L-glutamine: 500 milligrams per day

- Comprehensive bone- and joint-support formula containing glucosamine and chondroitin sulfate.

Action Steps for Those Aged Fifty-five to Sixty-five

Top Five Causes of Death

Heart disease
Cancer
Stroke
Chronic obstructive pulmonary disease (COPD)
Pneumonia and influenza

Overview

You've got your retirement organization membership card in your wallet. So what? You only retire if you want to. Many of you are looking at grandchildren (late bloomers are dealing with teenagers), and the world seems different. Most have lost one or both parents. You always thought you'd feel crotchety at sixty, but the Metabolic Plan works. In reality, it is entirely possible for a sixty-year-old man or woman to have the strength and stamina of a thirty-year-old. Are you willing to work for it?

Major Focus

You'll realize, looking at your friends who are not on the Metabolic Plan, that aging is no picnic. Make sure that this is a motivating factor and not a discouraging one. It's now time to create a support system if you haven't already so that the possibilities remain in sight.

Major Concerns

Cardiovascular health: Heart disease is still the number one cause of death for your age group and will remain so. The importance of regular exercise shifts from wanting to look good on the beach to wanting to stay in good cardiovascular shape. Of course, you can *also* look great on the beach . . .

Bones and joints: Range-of-motion (ROM) exercise becomes critically important. This is the decade when arthritis becomes common, and you can both prevent and treat this painful disease with ROM and the COX-2 inhibitors listed in Chapter 6. Think of your back when you lift or carry heavy objects: remember to lift with your legs.

Physical activity: Notice that chronic obstructive pulmonary disease is the fourth leading cause of death and that influenza (often fatal due to respiratory complications) is the fifth. All the more reason to maintain high respiratory efficiency through regular aerobic exercise and deep-breathing techniques.

Memory and cognition: You may notice that you're losing your car keys or forgetting things more frequently. Now's the time to protect and restore brain function. Blueberries work great fresh, frozen, in a smoothie, or in a nutritional concentrate. Ginkgo biloba effectively improves cerebral circulation and glucose metabolism. Also, less television and more crossword puzzles, chess, or playing piano will help a great deal. Use it or lose it.

Nutrition/hydration: Fresh fruit and vegetable juices become more important. Make sure you're getting your money's worth from that juicer or blender. In addition to your eight to ten glasses of water each day, make sure you're getting five glasses of fresh-squeezed or freshly juiced fruit and vegetables per week. Another valuable and more convenient option is to use a powdered "green drink" (see Chapter 8) mixed with a tall glass of water every day.

Tests

Yearly

- Complete physical exam, with blood pressure, heart rate, reflexes, and so forth.

- Complete blood count (CBC) and chem 24.

- HIV if you have changed sex partners.

- Homocysteine.

- Urinalysis.

- Hemoccult (test for blood in the stool).

- Respiratory efficiency (forced exhalation volume [FEV] and maximum oxygen extraction [VO_2 max]).

- Anabolic/Catabolic Index (ACI).

- Dental checkup and cleaning (twice a year).

- Body composition: percentage body fat, fat-free mass, hydration, and basal metabolic rate.

- Sigmoidoscopy (every four to five years if first exam is normal).

- Consider hepatitis vaccine.

- Men:
    Clinical testicular exam
    PSA
    Digital rectal exam

- Women:
    Clinical breast exam (may include mammogram) and pelvic exam
    Bone scan (dual-photon absorptiometry)

Once Every Two Years

- Stress cardiogram (in which you jog on a treadmill or ride an exercycle while a cardiologist watches your EKG). Your goal is to reach 80 percent of your maximal heart rate with no irregularities in heart function.

Monthly Self-Check

- *Women:* Breast self-exam

- *Men:* Testicular self-exam

- *Both:* Skin self-exam

Exercise

- Aim for 150 points a week but make sure to earn at least 100 (see Chapter 7 for point system).

- Continue taking 1,000 milligrams of branched-chain amino acids (BCAAs) after strenuous exercise.

- Resistance training with hand weights or machines two to three times a week.

- Range-of-motion stretching or yoga two to three times a week.

Nutritional Supplements

- High-potency multiple-dose multivitamin with minerals

- Additional vitamin E to total 400 international units per day

- Additional vitamin C to total 500 milligrams per day

- Comprehensive antioxidant (see Chapter 3)

- Bioenergetic formula (see Chapter 7)

- Comprehensive bone- and joint-support formula containing chondroitin and glucosamine sulfate

- Stage 1 immune-support formula (see Chapter 6)

- Aloe concentrate: two ounces a day

- DHEA: 15–25 milligrams per day before bed

- 7-Keto DHEA: 25–50 milligrams soon after waking up

- Alpha lipoic acid: 150 milligrams per day

- N-acetyl-cysteine (NAC): 300 milligrams per day

- Acetyl-L-carnitine: 250 milligrams per day

- During periods of physical or emotional stress, L-glutamine: 500 milligrams per day

- *Men:* Prostate formula providing selenium, zinc, and standardized concentrates of saw palmetto, silymarin, pygeum, and nettles

- Melatonin: 0.25–0.50 milligram before bed

Action Steps for Those Aged Sixty-five to Seventy-five

Top Five Causes of Death

Heart disease
Cancer
Stroke
Chronic obstructive pulmonary disease (COPD)
Pneumonia and influenza

Overview

If you've been on the Metabolic Plan, you might be feeling like a "stranger in a strange land"—thus the importance of the support group mentioned earlier. It's hard to relate to many in your age group because they are aging on a completely different schedule. By now, you've probably figured out that it works best to hang out with the forty-year-olds. In fact, if you've been on "the plan," comprehensive testing will reveal that you're not much different in functional ability or blood chemistry from that age group. If you're just starting, welcome aboard. You can expect to experience dramatic changes in your energy level, followed by more gradual but no less important changes in skin tone, muscle tone, immunity, memory, and mood. The watchword is patience. You thought time was running out, but research suggests that you can, through diligent effort, "buy" more time. How many decades would you like?

Major Focus

Again, one of the biggest challenges in this decade is conventional thinking. Our society expects you to retire and move to Florida or Arizona. Go ahead, if you want to, but *stay active!*

Major Concerns

Cardiovascular health: If you scan the obituaries, you'll see that the vast majority are still dying of heart disease. With all that we know about antioxidants, iron overload, stress, exercise, and metabolism, it's hard to believe. Renew your commitment to ageless living. That magnificent heart within your chest is quite capable of pumping nonstop for at least another four decades.

Bones and joints: Range-of-motion (ROM) exercise remains critically important. You may find water aerobics to be easier on your joints than a regular aerobics class. The warmth of the water and the support it provides create a very enjoyable experience.

Memory and cognition: In addition to the blueberries and ginkgo, you might want to purchase brain-building software (see Appendix A) that challenges, trains, and tests your mental ability.

Kidney and liver function: Keep a watchful eye on your kidney and liver function tests (chem 24). This is the decade in which you typically start to see impaired detox function. If you've been on the Metabolic Plan, this may not occur at all, but if it does, or if you are just starting on the plan, you'll want to discuss therapeutic options with a prevention-oriented physician. Preventive steps will include:

- Staying adequately hydrated. You should be consuming very little caffeine, no soft drinks, and only moderate amounts of alcohol (one glass of wine per day).

- You may want to increase fresh-squeezed or fresh-juiced vegetable and fruit juice to ten glasses per week.

- Add liver-support herbs (silymarin, wolfberry) to your supplement schedule.

- Give special attention to glutathione-support nutrients such as N-acetyl-cysteine (NAC).

Nutrition/hydration: It's time to move closer to a vegetarian diet if you're not already there. Cold-water fish remains an excellent protein choice, but red meat and poultry should be limited to a few servings a month. A high-protein meal-replacement shake in the morning may be a good idea, but make sure that the protein is coming from a *mix* of protein sources, starting with ultrafiltrated (easy-to-digest) whey and including soy protein.

Tests

Yearly

- Complete physical exam, with blood pressure, heart rate, reflexes, and so forth.

- Complete blood count (CBC) and chem 24.

- Homocysteine.

- White blood cell assay for glutathione.

- Urinalysis.

- HIV if you have changed sex partners.

- Hemoccult (test for blood in the stool).

- Respiratory efficiency (forced exhalation volume [FEV] and maximum oxygen extraction [VO_2 max]).

- Anabolic/Catabolic Index (ACI).

- Dental checkup and cleaning (twice a year).

- Body composition: percentage body fat, fat-free mass, hydration, and basal metabolic rate.

- Sigmoidoscopy (every four to five years if first exam is normal).

- B-vitamin serum levels, including B_{12}, folic acid, B_1, B_2, B_3, B_5 (pantothenic acid), and B_6.

- Discuss flu vaccine with your doctor.

- Discuss hepatitis vaccine.

- *Men:*
    Clinical testicular exam
    PSA
    Digital rectal exam

- *Women:*
    Clinical breast exam (may include mammogram) and pelvic exam
    Bone scan (dual-photon absorptiometry)

Once Every Two Years

- Stress cardiogram (in which you jog on a treadmill or ride an exercycle while a cardiologist watches your EKG). Your goal is to reach 80 percent of your maximal heart rate with no irregularities in heart function.

Monthly Self-Check

- *Women:* Breast self-exam

- *Men:* Testicular self-exam

- *Both:* Skin self-exam

Exercise

- Aim for 150 points a week but make sure to earn at least 100 (see Chapter 7 for point system).

- Start taking 1,000 milligrams of branched-chain amino acids (BCAAs) after all exercise.

- Resistance training with hand weights or machines two to three times a week.

- Range-of-motion stretching or yoga two to three times a week.

Nutritional Supplements

- High-potency multiple-dose multivitamin with minerals

- Additional vitamin E to total 400 international units per day

- Additional vitamin C to total 500 milligrams per day

- Sublingual B_{12} formula (health food store) and B-complex capsules

- Comprehensive antioxidant (see Chapter 3)

- Bioenergetic formula (see Chapter 7)

- Comprehensive bone and joint-support formula containing glucosamine and chondroitin sulfate

- Stage 1 immune-support formula (see Chapter 6)

- Aloe concentrate: three ounces a day

- DHEA: 15–25 milligrams per day before bed

- 7-Keto DHEA: 25–50 milligrams upon arising

- Alpha lipoic acid: 100 milligrams twice per day

- N-acetyl-cysteine (NAC): 250 milligrams twice per day

- Acetyl-L-carnitine: 500 milligrams per day

- During periods of physical or emotional stress, L-glutamine: 1,000 milligrams per day

- Melatonin: 0.50–1.0 milligram before bed

- Liver-support formula (standardized concentrates of silymarin and wolfberry)

- *Men:* Prostate formula providing selenium, zinc, and standardized concentrates of saw palmetto, silymarin, pygeum, and nettles

Action Steps for Those Older Than Seventy-five

Top Five Causes of Death

Heart disease
Cancer
Stroke
Chronic obstructive pulmonary disease (COPD)
Pneumonia and influenza

Overview

If you've been on the Metabolic Plan, you're now experiencing a "second wind." It's a wonderful feeling to know that the "wall" of life expectancy (76.7 years) was just a curtain. Of course, you have not only special knowledge but a remarkably different *experience* of aging. If you're just starting, the motto "Better late than never" was never more appropriate. Research has conclusively demonstrated that you can significantly increase muscle mass, bone strength, immunity, memory, mood, and overall functional ability (including balance and coordination). You have a great deal more control over aging than you ever imagined. The choice is yours.

Major Focus

Your challenge is to chart your own course when people all around you are pulling down their sails and heading to port.

Major Concerns

Cardiovascular health: As long as you don't stop moving, your cardiovascular system will be just fine. Your heart has pumped more than 70 million gallons of blood by age seventy-five, and while that may seem like a Herculean task, this magnificent organ has been rebuilding and rejuvenating itself the whole time.

Bones and joints: Range-of-motion (ROM) exercise remains critically important. Water exercise is highly recommended.

Physical activity: The operative word is *activity.* If you're moving, you're exercising, but don't get lazy. Set new goals and enjoy new triumphs. How many mountains have you climbed in your life?

Memory and cognition: Keep at it. Learning to play the piano, accordion, or guitar is a great idea.

Teeth and gums: These can be a significant problem if you have not been paying careful attention to oral health. Make sure that you are doing everything possible to keep your teeth intact and strong. One of the most significant nutritional problems for seniors is that many simply cannot chew well.

Nutrition/hydration: The same suggestions as for the previous decade, with renewed emphasis on limiting meat. A high-protein meal-replacement shake in the morning is convenient and essential for optimal anabolic repair-and-rebuild functions. If you have trouble chewing, now is a good time to invest in a high-quality blender (such as Vita Mix) and start pureeing vegetables into soup and fruit into smoothies. The "green drink" mentioned previously is essential. Try to get two servings a day in a tall glass of water.

An added nutritional problem in this age group is eating alone. It's difficult and not much fun to cook and eat alone. Try to share at least one meal a day with friends or family.

Tests

Yearly

- Complete physical exam, with blood pressure, heart rate, reflexes, and so forth.

- Complete blood count (CBC) and chem 24.

- Homocysteine.

- White blood cell assay for glutathione.

- Urinalysis.

- HIV if you have changed sex partners.

- Respiratory efficiency (forced exhalation volume [FEV] and maximum oxygen extraction [VO_2 max]).

- Hemoccult (test for blood in the stool).

- Anabolic/Catabolic index (ACI).

- Dental checkup and cleaning (twice a year).

- Body composition: percentage body fat, fat-free mass, hydration, and basal metabolic rate.

- Sigmoidoscopy (every four to five years if first exam is normal).

- B-vitamin serum levels, including B_{12}, folic acid, B_1, B_2, B_3, B_5 (pantothenic acid), and B_6.

- Discuss flu vaccine with your doctor.

- Discuss hepatitis vaccine.

- *Men:*
  Clinical testicular exam
  PSA
  Digital rectal exam

- *Women:*
  Clinical breast exam (may include mammogram) and pelvic exam
  Bone scan (dual-photon absorptiometry)

Once Every Two Years

- Stress cardiogram. You're going to have a hard time finding a cardiologist who's willing to do a stress EKG on an eighty-year-old, but perhaps when the doctor sees that you've got a 20 percent body fat level, he or she will relent. No need to get up to 80 percent of maximal heart rate, but it would be great to compare your results with previous tests. Onward and upward.

Monthly Self-Check

- *Women:* Breast self-exam

- *Men:* Testicular self-exam

- *Both:* Skin self-exam

Exercise

- Aim for 150 points a week but make sure to earn at least 100 (see Chapter 7 for point system).

- Start taking 1,000 milligrams of branched-chain amino acids (BCAAs) twice a day as well as before and after all exercise.

- Resistance training with hand weights or machines two to three times a week.

- Range-of-motion stretching or yoga two to three times a week.

Nutritional Supplements

- High-potency multiple-dose multivitamin with minerals.

- Additional vitamin E to total 400 international units per day.

- Additional vitamin C to total 500 milligrams per day.

- Monthly B-vitamin injections are highly recommended, including folic acid, B_{12}, B_1, B_2, and B_6.

- Comprehensive antioxidant (see Chapter 3).

- Bioenergetic formula (see Chapter 7).

- Comprehensive bone- and joint-support formula containing glucosamine and chondroitin sulfate.

- Stage 1 immune-support formula (see Chapter 6).

- Aloe concentrate: three ounces a day.

- DHEA: 15–25 milligrams per day before bed.

- 7-Keto DHEA: 25–50 milligrams soon after waking up.

- Alpha lipoic acid: 100 milligrams twice per day.

- N-acetyl-cysteine (NAC): 500 milligrams twice per day.

- Acetyl-L-carnitine: 500 milligrams per day.

- During periods of physical or emotional stress, L-glutamine: 1,000 milligrams per day.

- Melatonin: 1–2 milligrams before bed.

- Liver-support formula (standardized concentrates of silymarin and wolfberry).

- *Men:* Prostate formula providing selenium, zinc, and standardized concentrates of saw palmetto, silymarin, pygeum, and nettles.

TWELVE

Conclusion:
A Question of Balance,
the Nature of Time

How old would you be if you didn't know how old you are?

By now, you are keenly aware that there are no magic bullets (darn), and perhaps the Metabolic Plan feels a bit daunting. I've tried to cut it into digestible bites, but it bears repeating that the core principles are actually quite simple. Think, eat, and exercise like a hunter-gatherer while taking advantage of the blessings of modern biochemistry. I'm sure that Russell E. Marker had no idea what a wonderful door he opened in 1935 when he discovered how to obtain the human hormone DHEA from a plant.

The question is, what will you do with this remarkable opportunity? In my presentations, I always end by asking my audience to reflect on a couple of important questions: "Why do I want to live longer?" and "What will I do with the extra years?"

You don't have to answer right now. But I'd suggest that as you get "into" antiaging, you keep in touch with your core desires and motivations. The process of self-reflection is different for everyone and can involve anything from long walks on the beach to sitting quietly in church. Two things, however, are certain. Self-reflection takes time and personal space. Wherever you are, it's taken you a while to get there, so if you are thinking about changing directions, you will have to invest some time.

STAGE 1: REFLECTION

Here are a few ideas to give your thoughts focus. Over the next few weeks, make some simple notes on the following questions:

- Who am I?

- Where am I going?

- How am I going to get there?

Who Am I?

This question is not about your job or relationships to others. Who is the real you? What are your talents and interests? What excites you? What activities make you feel good about yourself? Don't worry about spelling or order. This is for you and you alone.

Where Am I Going?

Are you making the best use of your talents and interests? Are the things that you do each day fulfilling on a deep level? Take a look at which parts of your life resonate with your inner self and which parts don't. This exercise is not intended to suggest that you quit your job and move to Tahiti. It's just the beginning of looking at ways to align the person you are with your goals and taking small steps to get there.

How Am I Going to Get There?

How can you align your activities with what makes you feel fulfilled? Instead of "Try it. You'll like it," my motto is "You like it? Try it!" Develop a list of possible activities, such as volunteering, coaching a kids' sports team, listening to music for thirty minutes, or listening to an audiobook. List activities that are totally within your control.

Small steps in the right direction are better than lofty goals with no movement. If you wish you were a concert pianist, start with one lesson. Over the next few weeks, try just a few things on the list. Consider them experiments in change. By the third week of this process, you will be ready for the last step—the development of a personal mission.

Take an hour or so to reflect on the "Who am I?" question and what felt right about the experiments of the last few weeks. Look forward five years and develop a mission statement for the person you would like to be at that time. Try to keep it simple and on one piece of paper. Once you know where you are going, you will be amazed at how almost magically—or through apparent coincidence—you will find activities and relationships that support your direction.

It might be useful to create a pie chart of your life right now and how you might prefer it. On the left side of a blank sheet of paper, draw a circle. Within the circle, create six or eight pie-shaped slices, each of which will represent one of the important areas of life. Your slices might include work/career, education, family, exercise, spirituality, recreation, investments, and relationships. The size of each "slice" represents the importance that aspect of your life has, as judged by the weekly hours spent in that area or any other measure you choose. By evaluating each area honestly, you can gain insight into where your life is out of balance. Remember, this is your pie and your life, so be honest.

Now, on the right, draw another pie as you would like your life to be. You may be the exception, but I have never known anyone to draw both pies and slices the same. Look at both sides and reflect upon the implications of what you see. Is your life in balance? Are you living life to the fullest? "So," you ask, "what can I do about it? I have to work I have to pay bills What about the kids' college? I have no time to exercise."

As with all the pieces of the Metabolic Plan, the secret to success is in small, achievable steps that are within your control. Take action to focus more on the small slices and less on the big slices to the extent that they exclude or limit the others. For example, you likely need to work, and work can be gratifying and fulfilling, but if work consumes your whole life, you will ultimately lose out on what you are working for. At life's end, you will probably not say, "I wish I could have one more day at work."

Don't underestimate the power of recreation Many people think of it as just "goofing off." Instead, look at the word as *re-creation*. Smiling, laughing, playing, and enjoying yourself are essential parts of your renewal . . . living life to its fullest. See a movie, take a walk, write to your sister, read a book.

Each of your slices is important, but it is your commitment to the balance that will have your wheel rolling smoothly and straight. Make a brief personal plan for each area that needs to grow or shrink in its focus and importance.

This final step of the Metabolic Plan can be the most life-changing and rejuvenating. Taking even small steps will create a sense of move-ment and a restoration of balance. This balance, when combined with the other steps we've outlined, can create a sense of optimism and youthful vitality that help you feel that years have virtually melted away.

Where to Go for Help

Remember that you're not in this alone. There are resources, many of which are listed in Appendix A, to which you can turn for assistance in this exciting endeavor. Www.TheMetabolicPlan.com will provide an ongoing resource and forum.

You may also benefit from the guidance of a sympathetic and knowl-edgeable health professional. So many people complain that their doc-tor doesn't "believe" in antiaging—but in reality, it is the hype and hoopla to which the doctor is probably reacting. All physicians practice some form of antiaging. Your job is to find one who is as excited about this information as you are, who understands the importance of nutri-tion and metabolism, and who is willing to assist you in whatever ways you require. Fortunately, the number of these pioneers is increasing every day. Appendix A lists organizations of health care professionals who specialize in preventive care.

STAGE 2: THE VALUE OF A REASONED RETREAT

When I speak of retreat, I'm not talking about weekend retreats to the woods, although I'm all in favor of those, too. Such retreats help put things in perspective and give us opportunities to know ourselves and our loved ones better. Nor am I talking about sticking your head in the sand to artificially blind yourself to life's stresses. Blindness does not equal serenity.

What I'm talking about is using our hearts and minds to evaluate whether there are things in our lives that are not serving us, things that are hindering our advancement instead of helping us get where we really want to go. It can be helpful to scan our relationships, work, and habits to evaluate whether they are helping or hurting us. Do they bring a sense of joy and peace to our lives?

I suggest you unplug yourself from the pop-culture idea that you have to know everything that is happening in the world all the time.

Take a look at how television and the Internet have commandeered our time and attention and ask yourself if this is helping you become a happier or better person.

You might say that what I'm suggesting is the equivalent of burying your head in the sand, but I don't think it is. My question to you is this: How does it improve your life to know that a ferryboat capsized in a far-off land today, killing 356 people? What will you do differently today because of that knowledge? How are you made stronger, or how are you now able to contribute to the world, because of the footage you saw on the evening news? You are informed, yes, but so what? Random bits of information by themselves, robbed of a context in which you are actually able to do something about them, are useless. In reality, the endless barrage of tragic news from every corner of the earth wears us down, adds to our stress, and creates a feeling of helplessness. I believe we tend to do *less* in our communities because we have been anesthetized by daily exposure to the incredible worldwide volume of pain and suffering that is beyond our reach.

In his excellent book on the modern entertainment culture *Amusing Ourselves to Death,* Neil Postman argues that the way in which information is delivered in the modern world introduces "on a large scale irrelevance, impotence, and incoherence." The value of information, he suggests, is no longer "tied to any function it might serve in social and political decision-making and action, but may attach merely to its novelty, interest, and curiosity."[1] And through television, it comes at us in such unending waves that we are swamped.

Most of the information we receive is *irrelevant* because it holds no value for what we do in our lives. It contributes to a sense of *impotence* because, in most cases, there is nothing we can do with the information. And it manifests as *incoherence* because of the way in which it is delivered— sandwiched in rapid succession between two completely unconnected stories, which are themselves sandwiched by commercial messages filled with beautiful people living the good life via their purchases. This leaves us no time for the sort of assimilation and contemplation that might allow us to be truly affected by the story—and certainly no practical way in which we might learn something useful or take action.

Television affects our bodies as well as our minds by interfering with our natural cycles of sleep—cycles that are critically important in the body's anabolic repair. The modern television "habit" thus has an enormous effect on stress and aging.

I'm sorry, but to deprive yourself of sleep in order to watch a television show that you won't remember in the morning is nothing short of lunacy. Bill McKibben, author of *The Age of Missing Information,* offers a useful suggestion: "Those of us who live in the north know that every few years a big snowstorm immobilizes us and turns off the power—and turns the world spectacularly peaceful. We forget that we have the power, and the right, to simulate the effects of a snowstorm as often as we want to."[2]

McKibben suggests that the reason we often feel guilty about watching television is that "it's time out of life. Which is okay if you're really winded—TV as white-noise therapy has its occasional value. But the time-outs soon last longer than the game, which at some level you realize is passing you by."[3]

Have you ever wondered what people did with their time before they spent four to five hours of every day spaced out in front of the tube? Have you ever thought about how much you could learn during those hours; what skills you could acquire; what you might do to improve your physical, emotional, or spiritual condition; what bonds of trust, love, and respect you might build with your children if you used the television for occasional entertainment rather than as a baby-sitter or constant companion?

Habits die hard, and many people fear the silence of a home that doesn't have the constant distraction of television. We have crowded so much into our lives that many of us have forgotten how to quietly contemplate our own emotional interiors. It's much safer, in a way, to occupy ourselves with the endless stream of information (so-called news), immature sitcoms (so-called comedy), and unrealistic cop/doctor/lawyer shows (so-called drama).

I have a friend who fell into this trap and kept to his habit faithfully every day. Television is just so *easy;* it doesn't demand anything of you. He turned on the morning news as soon as he got up and the evening news as soon as he got home from work. Then, the set stayed on until bedtime.

When a close friend of his became critically ill, however, he set upon a dedicated program of prayer and fasting, including fasting from popular culture. In addition to using the extra time in his day for prayer, he also started to read again. At first, he read murder mysteries, looking for that entertainment fix, but as he began to feel comfortable with the new, quiet pace of his evenings and weekends, he began to read books that touched him deeply, that brought tears to his eyes and led him into contemplation of his own condition, that challenged his habits of thinking and living.

Guess what he discovered? He didn't miss the tube a bit. He learned that while he could scarcely recall *any* details from the news and entertainment shows he had watched in a fog over the previous years, the lives of those he was *reading* about stayed with him. He felt richer, long after finishing a good book, for having had the opportunity to indelibly paint their lives and worlds on the canvas of his own imagination.

When his fast was over, the television remained off, for the most part. He found that when he did sit down to watch shows he used to enjoy, most now seemed empty and juvenile. He quickly became irritated by the sound of his set and turned it off. He now watches very selectively—two to three hours a week—and continues to enjoy the abundance of free time that appeared seemingly out of nowhere.

Try it. Not for a night or two but for long enough to become accustomed to the silence. Long enough to figure out what to do with the time. Long enough to learn how to live with yourself without ever-present distractions. You might be astounded at what you learn.

And finally, I want to acknowledge that making changes in your life is never an easy task. The key, however, is not to get caught up in the distance you have to go to get to where you want to be. Nor should you despair over the amount of control you have over your circumstances. Progress is made in the small, intentional steps, and chances are, you have more power than you think. By focusing on the little steps that you can take every day, the progress you make will motivate you to continue your journey, and eventually, you can get to wherever you want to go. The important thing is simply to begin!

APPENDIX A

Resources

PRIMARY RESOURCE: WWW.THEMETABOLICPLAN.COM

TheMetabolicPlan.com is the leading Internet site for up-to-the-minute information, research breakthroughs, and exciting discussion concerning wellness and longevity. If TheMetabolicPlan.com cannot answer your question, the site will direct you via hot link to additional resources.

MEDICAL ORGANIZATIONS OF NUTRITIONALLY ORIENTED/ANTIAGING PHYSICIANS

American Academy of Anti-Aging Medicine (A4M)
World Health Network
Web site: www.worldhealth.net
An organization with a membership of ten thousand physicians and scientists from sixty countries, the American Academy of Anti-Aging Medicine is a registered 501(c)3 nonprofit organization that is dedicated to the advancement of therapeutics related to the science of longevity medicine.

American Board of Holistic Medicine (ABHM)
Web site: www.amerboardholisticmed.org
The practice of holistic medicine integrates conventional and complementary therapies to promote optimal health and to prevent and treat disease. It focuses on physician-patient cooperation, balances the mitigation of causes with the relief of symptoms, and empowers patients to create a condition of wellness that goes far beyond merely the absence of illness to an experience of being fully alive. A list of board-certified members can be found at the organization's Web site.

American College for Advancement in Medicine (ACAM)
23121 Verdugo Dr., Suite 204
Laguna Hills, CA 92653
Fax: (949) 455-9679
Web site: www.acam.org
Founded in 1973, the American College for Advancement in Medicine is a
not-for-profit medical society dedicated to educating physicians and other
health care professionals on the latest findings and emerging procedures in
preventive/nutritional medicine. ACAM's goals are to improve skills, knowledge, and diagnostic procedures as they relate to complementary and alternative medicine; to support research; and to develop awareness of alternative
methods of medical treatment.

Life Extension Foundation (LEF)
1100 W. Commercial Blvd.
Fort Lauderdale, FL 33309
Phone: (800) 544-4440, (954) 766-8433
Web site: www.lef.org
Incorporated in 1980, the Life Extension Foundation is a nonprofit organization whose long-range goal is the extension of the healthy human life
span. In seeking to control aging, our objective is to develop methods
to enable us to live in health, youth, and vigor for unlimited periods of
time.

LABORATORIES OFFERING LEAD AND MERCURY TESTING AND/OR COMPREHENSIVE TESTING FOR PARASITES

The following laboratories should be used (in conjunction with your physician).

Great Smokies Laboratory
63 Zillicoa St.
Asheville, NC 28801
Phone: (800) 522-4762

Meridian Valley Clinical Laboratory
515 West Harrison St., Suite 9
Kent, WA 98032
Phone: (253) 859-8700

Metametrix Clinical Laboratory
4855 Peachtree Blvd.
Norcross, GA 30092

Phone: (800) 221-4640
Fax: (770) 441-2237

Pinnacle Laboratories
6965 Union Park Center, Suite 100
Salt Lake City, UT 84047
Phone: (888) 556-5567

HOW TO OBTAIN AN ACI (ANABOLIC/CATABOLIC INDEX) TEST

Unigen Pharmaceuticals, Inc.
100 Technology Dr.
Broomfield, CO 80021
Phone: (303) 438-8666
Web site: www.unigenpharma.com

RESOURCES (TAPES AND VIDEOS) FOR STRESS MANAGEMENT AND DEEP RELAXATION

Association for Applied Psychophysiology and Biofeedback
10200 W. 44th Ave., Suite 304
Wheat Ridge, CO 80033-2840
Phone: (303) 422-8436
Fax: (303) 422-8894
E-mail: AAPB@resourcenter.com
Web site: www.aapb.org

Institute of HeartMath
14700 W. Park Ave.
Boulder Creek, CA 95006
Phone: (831) 338-8500
Fax: (831) 338-8504
E-mail: info@heartmath.org
Web site: www.heartmath.org

Preventive Medicine Research Institute
900 Bridgeway, no. 1
Sausalito, CA 94965
Phone: (415) 332-2525
Fax: (415) 332-5730
Web site: www.pmri.org
President: Dean Ornish, M.D.

Tools for Wellness
9755 Independence Ave.
Chatsworth, CA 91311-4318
Phone: (800) 456-9887
Fax: (818) 407-0850
Web site: www.toolsforwellness.com

RECOMMENDED READING ON MINDFULNESS AND LIFE BALANCE

The Art of Happiness: A Handbook for Living,
    by the Dalai Lama and Howard Cutler
Loving What Is, by Byron Katie
Peace in Every Step: The Path of Mindfulness in Everyday Life,
    by Thich Nhat Hahn
The Power of Now, by Eckhart Tolle

CERTIFYING ORGANIZATIONS FOR FITNESS TRAINERS

Aerobics and Fitness Association of America
15250 Ventura Blvd., Suite 310
Sherman Oaks, CA 91403
Phone: (800) 446-2322

American College of Sports Medicine
P.O. Box 1440
Indianapolis, IN 46206
Phone: (317) 637-9200

IDEA International Association of Fitness Professionals
6190 Cornerstone Court E, Suite 204
San Diego, CA 92121-3773
Phone: (800) 999-4332

SOURCES FOR HERBAL COFFEE

Abundant Earth
Orders Department
762 W. Park Ave.
Port Townsend, WA 98368
Phone: (888) 513-2784
Web site: www.abundantearth.com

Abundant Earth has a growing selection of organic and natural delicious coffee alternatives, with no caffeine.

Oasis Wellness Network
Oasis AM—Caffeine Free Coffee
100 Technology Dr., Suite 130
Broomfield, CO 80021
Phone: (877) 627-4787
Web site: www.oasisnetwork.com
Specially formulated with Oasis Bio-Energy supplements, this rich, robust, good-for-you coffee replacement is made from the finest herbs, grains, fruits, and nuts, which are roasted, ground, and brewed just like coffee.

Teeccino Caffe, Inc.
P.O. Box 42259
Santa Barbara, CA 93105
Phone: (800) 498-3434
E-mail: Teeccino@aol.com
Web site: www.teeccino.com
Teeccino is the "no-caf" alternative to regular and decaf. Teeccino is distributed to natural foods stores in the United States, Britain, and Canada but also sells directly to consumers via catalog and the Internet.

INFORMATION ABOUT THE VITA-MIX BLENDER:

Vita-Mix Foodservice
Household Division
8615 Usher Rd.
Cleveland, OH 44138
Phone: (800) 848-2649 (United States and Canada)
Fax: (440) 235-3726 (United States and Canada)
E-mail: household@vitamix.com, international@vitamix.com

WHERE TO PURCHASE: BRAIN FITNESS/THINKFAST SOFTWARE

Brain.com
c/o Hot Brain, Inc.
3535 E. Coast Highway
P.O. Box 319

Corona del Mar, CA 92625
Web site: www.brain.com

INFORMATION ON THE PREVENTION OF SEXUALLY TRANSMITTED DISEASES (STDs)

Centers for Disease Control and Prevention
National Center for HIV, STD, and TB Prevention
Division of Sexually Transmitted Diseases
Web site: www.cdc.gov/nchstp/dstd/dstdp.html

FOOD AND WATER SAFETY

EPA Safe Drinking Water Hotline
Phone: (800) 426-4791

National Sanitation Foundation
Web site: www.nsf.org

Water Quality Association
Phone: (800) 749-0234
Web site: www.wqa.org

Research Summary

Short-Term Metabolic Effect of Nutritional Intervention in Human Volunteers as Measured by Two Biomarkers of Anabolic Drive
S. Cherniske, Q. Jia, M. F. Hong, and X. P. Zhao.

OBJECTIVE: To determine the effect of a nutritional intervention program on anabolic (repair and rebuild) metabolism in healthy adults.

HYPOTHESIS: A two-tiered nutritional intervention program produces greater improvements in anabolic drive than a placebo.

Study type: Thirty-five-day intervention trial.

Subjects: Seventy-five.

Inclusion Criteria
- Males/females aged forty to seventy
- Good general health
- A willingness to stop using current vitamins and to use only the test formulation throughout the course of the study

Exclusion Criteria
- Known sensitivity to DHEA or DHEA derivatives
- Severe, chronic asthma
- Diabetes
- Immunological disorders such as AIDS or SLE (systemic lupus erythematosus)
- Participation in any oral drug study within the last four weeks

- Pregnant or lactating women
- Any condition for which the investigator determined that the subject could be placed under undue risk

Supervision: An institutional review board (IRB) approved the protocol, obtained informed consent, and provided subject instructions and study schedule in accordance with Title 21 of the Code of Federal Regulations, parts 50 and 56.

Investigator: California Skin Research Institute (CSRI).

Subject randomization to group A or B: Assignments were made via computer-based random number generator.

Group A (active; *n* = 60): Group A received nutritional formulas twice a day.

A.M. nutritional formula containing:

DHEA (dehydroepiandrosterone)	5.0 mg
7-Keto (3-acetyl-7-oxo-dehydroepiandrosterone)	12.5 mg
Lycium barbarum (wolfberry)	200.0 mg
Chlorella	150.0 mg
Polygonum multiflorum (fo-ti) (cured root extract, 12:1)	100.0 mg
Aloe vera (spray-dried gel powder, 200:1)	30.0 mg

P.M. nutritional formula containing:

L-arginine HCl	1,000.0 mg
DHEA (dehydroepiandrosterone)	5.0 mg
7-Keto (3-acetyl-7-oxo-dehydroepiandrosterone)	12.5 mg
Lycium barbarum (wolfberry)	200.0 mg
Chlorella	150.0 mg
Polygonum multiflorum (fo-ti) (cured root extract, 12:1)	100.0 mg
Aloe vera (spray-dried gel powder, 200:1)	30.0 mg

Group B (placebo; *n* = 15): Group B received look-alike placebo capsules containing microcrystalline cellulose.

Laboratories: Anabolic/Catabolic Index was performed at Unigen Pharmaceuticals, Inc., Broomfield, Colorado. IGF-1 assay was conducted at Diagnos-Techs Laboratory, Osceola, Wisconsin.

Test protocol: In both laboratories, the test protocol was blind, with all samples being number-coded. Neither sequence nor sample identity was known to either testing facility.

Duration: The study started on June 23, 1999, and was completed on August 30, 1999.

Data points:
1. ACI tests conducted at baseline and on days 7, 14, 21, 28, and 35.
2. IGF-1 assay conducted at baseline and upon completion.
3. Outcome-based data point was a before-and-after subject questionnaire designed by statisticians from the University of Colorado.

Results data points:
1. In the course of thirty days, ACI scores for the placebo group B declined slightly, while scores in the active group A showed a mean increase of 198 percent. (chart A)
2. In the course of thirty days, IGF-1 scores for the placebo group B declined very slightly, while IGF-1 levels in the active group A showed a mean increase of 106 percent. (chart B)

Chart A

Study Results: ACI Test
After 30 Days on a Nutritional Anabolic Support Formula

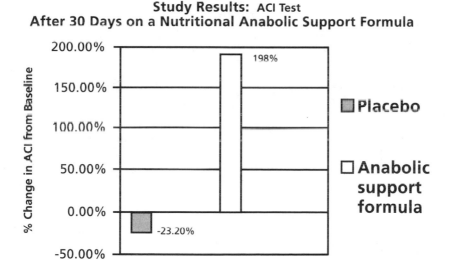

Appendix B

Chart B

Study Results: IGF-1 Test
After 30 Days on a Nutritional Anabolic Support Formula

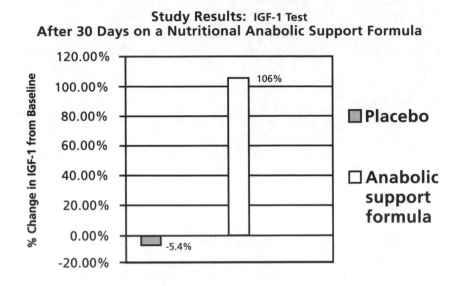

Notes

INTRODUCTION

1. G. Ravaglia et al., "Determinants of Functional Status in Healthy Italian Nonagenarians and Centenarians: A Comprehensive Functional Assessment by the Instruments of Geriatric Practice," *Journal of the American Geriatrics Society* 45, no. 10 (October 1997): 1196–1202.

CHAPTER 1: FOUNDATIONS

1. Leonard Hayflick, a gerontologist at the University of California, San Francisco, states: "Nature designed humans to peak physically at about age 20, to assure reproduction and survival. After that, humans 'coast' for another four or five decades and it is the length of that coast that determines longevity."

Actually, DHEA levels—a useful measure of "youth"—peak in women between sixteen and nineteen years of age, while men reach this peak between ages twenty and twenty-four. (N. Orentreich et al., "Age Changes and Sex Differences in Serum DHEA Concentrations throughout Adulthood," *Journal of Clinical Endocrinology and Metabolism* 59 [1984]: 551–55).

2. G. Ravaglia et al., "Determinants of Functional Status in Healthy Italian Nonagenarians and Centenarians: A Comprehensive Functional Assessment by the Instruments of Geriatric Practice," *Journal of the American Geriatrics Society* 45, no. 10 (October 1997): 1196–1202.

3. I. Kim et al., "Vitamin and Mineral Supplement Use and Mortality in a U.S. Cohort," *American Journal of Public Health* 83, no. 4 (April 1993): 546–50.

R. D. Lipman et al., "Disease Incidence and Longevity Are Unaltered by Dietary Antioxidant Supplementation Initiated during Middle Age," *Mechanisms of Ageing and Development* 103, no. 3 (July 15, 1998): 269–84.

4. Ravaglia et al., "Determinants of Functional Status in Healthy Italian Nonagenarians and Centenarians."

G. Ravaglia et al., "The Relationship of Dehydroepiandrosterone Sulfate (DHEAS) to

Endocrine-Metabolic Parameters and Functional Status in the Oldest-Old: Results from an Italian Study on Healthy Free-Living over-Ninety-Year-Olds," *Journal of Clinical Endocrinology and Metabolism* 81, no. 3 (March 1996): 1173–78.

5. S. B. Solerte et al., "Dehydroepiandrosterone Sulfate Enhances Natural Killer Cell Cytotoxicity in Humans via Locally Generated Immunoreactive Insulin-like Growth Factor I," *Journal of Clinical Endocrinology and Metabolism* 84, no. 9 (September 1999): 3260–67.

6. R. H. Straub et al., "Serum Dehydroepiandrosterone (DHEA) and DHEA Sulfate Are Negatively Correlated with Serum Interleukin-6 (Il-6), and DHEA Inhibits Il-6 Secretion from Mononuclear Cells in Man in Vitro: Possible Link between Endocrinosenescence and Immunosenescence," *Journal of Clinical Endocrinology and Metabolism* 83, no. 6 (June 1998): 2012–17.

7. K. Landin-Wilhelmsen, L. Wilhelmsen, and B. A. Bengtsson, "Postmenopausal Osteoporosis Is More Related to Hormonal Aberrations Than to Lifestyle Factors," *Clinical Endocrinology* (Oxford) 51, no. 4 (October 1999): 387–94.

P. Gamero, E. Sornay-Rendu, and P. D. Delmas, "Low Serum IGF-1 and Occurrence of Osteoporotic Fractures in Postmenopausal Women," *Lancet* 355, no. 9207 (March 11, 2000): 898–99.

É.-É. Baulieu et al., "Dehydroepiandrosterone (DHEA), DHEA Sulfate, and Aging: Contribution of the DHEAge Study to a Sociobiomedical Issue," *Proceedings of the National Academy of Sciences of the United States of America* 97, no. 8 (April 11, 2000): 4279–84.

8. A. Aleman et al., "Insulin-like Growth Factor-I and Cognitive Function in Healthy Older Men," *Journal of Clinical Endocrinology and Metabolism* 84, no. 2 (February 1999): 471–75.

A. L. Markowska, M. Mooney, and W. E. Sonntag, "Insulin-like Growth Factor-1 Ameliorates Age-Related Behavioral Deficits," *Neuroscience* 87, no. 3 (December 1998): 559–69.

CHAPTER 2: RESTORING YOUR ANABOLIC POWER

1. "Benefits of Fruits, Vegetables Still Go Unrealized," *Los Angeles Times,* August 16, 1990, H54.

G. W. Comstock et al., "Serum Retinol, Beta-Carotene, Vitamin E and Selenium as Related to Subsequent Cancer of Specific Sites," *American Journal of Epidemiology* 135 (1992): 115–21.

A. Bendich, "Vitamin E Status of U.S. Children," *Journal of the American College of Nutrition* 11 (1992): 441–44.

L. E. Cleveland, "Dietary Intake of Whole Grains," *Journal of the American College of Nutrition* 19, no. 3, supplement (2000): 331–38S.

2. R. Lappalainen, M. Knuuttila, and R. Salminen, "The Concentrations of Zinc and Manganese in Human Enamel and Dentine Related to Age and Their Concentrations in the Soil," *Archives of Oral Biology* 26 (1981): 1.

H. A. Schroeder, "Losses of Vitamins and Trace Minerals Resulting from Processing and Preservation of Foods," *American Journal of Clinical Nutrition* 24 (1971): 562.

R. J. Shamberger and C. E. Willis, "Selenium Distribution and Human Cancer Mortality," *Critical Review Clinical Chemistry* 2 (1971): 211.

3. R. A. Anderson et al., "Chromium Intake, Absorption and Excretion of Subjects Consuming Self-Selected Diets," *American Journal of Clinical Nutrition* 41 (1985): 1177–83.

4. A. Drewnowski and C. Gomez-Carneros, "Bitter Taste, Phytonutrients, and the Consumer: A Review," *American Journal of Clinical Nutrition* 72, no. 6 (December 2000): 1424–35.

5. H. J. Naurath et al., "Effects of Vitamin B_{12}, Folate, and Vitamin B_6 Supplements in Elderly People with Normal Serum Vitamin Concentrations," *Lancet* 346, no. 8967 (July 8, 1995): 85–89.

K. M. Koehler et al., "Folate Nutrition and Older Adults: Challenges and Opportunities," *Journal of the American Dietetic Association* 97, no. 2 (February 1997): 167–73.

B. B. Alford and M. L. Boyle, *Nutrition during the Life Cycle* (Englewood Cliffs, N.J.: Prentice Hall, 1982).

6. R. S. Kuzdenbaeva, V. E. Kurakina, and M. K. Iztleuov, "Effect of Anabolic Substances on the State of the Individual Components of the Glutathione–Ascorbic Acid System," *Farmakologiya i Toksikologiya* 43, no. 5 (September–October 1980): 607–9.

M. Jeevanandam et al., "Altered Plasma Cytokines and Total Glutathione Levels in Parenterally Fed Critically Ill Trauma Patients with Adjuvant Recombinant Human Growth Hormone (rhGH) Therapy," *Critical Care Medicine* 28, no. 2 (February 2000): 324–29.

7. R. Chopra and T. Anastassiades, "Specificity and Synergism of Polypeptide Growth Factors in Stimulating the Synthesis of Proteoglycans and a Novel High Molecular Weight Anionic Glycoprotein by Articular Chondrocyte Cultures," *Journal of Rheumatology* 25, no. 8 (August 1998): 1578–84.

8. I. Setnikar et al., "Pharmacokinetics of Glucosamine in Man," *Arzneimittel Forschung* 43, no. 10 (1993): 1109–13.

9. R. Ruane and P. Griffiths, "Glucosamine Therapy Compared to Ibuprofen for Joint Pain," *British Journal of Community Nursing* 7, no. 3 (March 2002): 148–52.

10. The five research organizations were:

- The Department of Molecular and Cell Biology, University of California, Berkeley
- The Children's Hospital Oakland Research Institute
- The Department of Biochemistry and Biophysics, Linus Pauling Institute, Oregon State University, Corvallis
- The Department of Pharmacology and Pathobiology, Royal Veterinary and Agricultural University, Copenhagen, Denmark
- Lawrence Berkeley National Laboratory, Berkeley, California

11. T. M. Hagen et al., "Feeding Acetyl-L-Carnitine and Lipoic Acid to Old Rats Significantly Improves Metabolic Function While Decreasing Oxidative Stress, Mitochondrial-Supported Bioenergetics Decline and Oxidative Stress Increases during Aging," *Proceedings of the National Academy of Sciences of the United States of America* 99, no. 4 (February 19, 2002): 1870–75.

12. www.berkeley.edu/news/berkeleyan/2002/02/27_ames.html.

13. J. E. Nestler et al., "Dehydroepiandrosterone Reduces Serum Low Density Lipoprotein Levels and Body Fat but Does Not Alter Insulin Sensitivity in Normal Men," *Journal of Clinical Endocrinology and Metabolism* 66, no. 1 (January 1988): 57–61.

14. G. Aimarettiet al., "DHEA-S Levels in Hypopituitaric Patients with Severe GH Deficiency Are Strongly Reduced across Lifespan: Comparison with IGF I Levels before and during rhGH Replacement," *Journal of Endocrinological Investigation* 23, no. 1 (January 2000): 5–11.

15. G. A. Orner et al., "Dehydroepiandrosterone Is a Complete Hepatocarcinogen and Potent Tumor Promoter in the Absence of Peroxisome Proliferation in Rainbow Trout," *Carcinogenesis* 16, no. 12 (December 1995): 2893–98.

16. C. Metzger, P. Bannasch, and D. Mayer, "Enhancement and Phenotypic Modulation of N-Nitrosomorpholine-Induced Hepatocarcinogenesis by Dehydroepiandrosterone," *Cancer Letters* 121, no. 2 (December 23, 1997): 125–31.

17. S. S. Yen and G. A. Laughlin, "Aging and the Adrenal Cortex," *Experimental Gerontology* 33, nos. 7–8 (November–December 1998): 897–910.

18. P. Diamond et al., "Metabolic Effects of 12 Month Percutaneous Dehydroepiandrosterone Replacement Therapy in Postmenopausal Women," *Journal of Endocrinology* 150 (1996): S43–50.

19. O. Khorram, L. Vu, and S. S. Yen, "Activation of Immune Function by Dehydroepiandrosterone (DHEA) in Age-Advanced Men," *Journal of Gerontology* 52A, no. 1 (1997): M1–M7.

20. O. M. Wolkowitz et al., "Dehydroepiandrosterone (DHEA) Treatment of Depression," *Biological Psychiatry* 41 (1997): 311–18.

21. É.-É. Baulieu, "Dehydroepiandrosterone (DHEA): A Fountain of Youth?" *Journal of Clinical Endocrinology and Metabolism* 81, no. 9 (1996): 3147–51.

22. A. Heinz et al., "Severity of Depression in Abstinent Alcoholics Is Associated with Monoamine Metabolites and Dehydroepiandrosterone-Sulfate Concentrations," *Psychiatry Research* 89, no. 2 (December 20, 1999): 97–106.

23. O. M. Wolkowitz et al., "Double-Blind Treatment of Major Depression with Dehydroepiandrosterone," *American Journal of Psychiatry* 156, no. 4 (April 1999): 646–49.

24. M. Stomati et al., "Endocrine, Neuroendocrine and Behavioral Effects of Oral Dehydroepiandrosterone Sulfate Supplementation in Postmenopausal Women," *Gynecological Endocrinology* 13, no. 1 (February 1999): 15–25.

25. W. J. Reiter et al., "Dehydroepiandrosterone in the Treatment of Erectile Dysfunction: A Prospective, Double-Blind, Randomized, Placebo-Controlled Study," *Urology* 53, no. 3 (March 1999): 590–94; discussion 594–95.

26. N. E. Eaton et al., "Endogenous Sex Hormones and Prostate Cancer: A Quantitative Review of Prospective Studies," *British Journal of Cancer* 80, no. 7 (1999): 930–34.

27. K. Okamoto, "Distribution of Dehydroepiandrosterone Sulfate and Relationships between Its Level and Serum Lipid Levels in a Rural Japanese Population," *Journal of Epidemiology* 8, no. 5 (December 1998): 285–91.

28. C. M. Gordon et al., "Changes in Bone Turnover Markers and Menstrual Function after Short-Term Oral DHEA in Young Women with Anorexia Nervosa," *Journal of Bone and Mineral Research* 14, no. 1 (January 1999): 136–45.

29. P. De Becker et al., "Dehydroepiandrosterone (DHEA) Response to I.V. ACTH in Patients with Chronic Fatigue Syndrome," *Hormone and Metabolic Research* 31, no. 1 (January 1999): 18–21.

30. W. M. Jefferies, "The Etiology of Rheumatoid Arthritis," *Medical Hypotheses* 51, no. 2 (August 1998): 111–14.

M. Cutolo et al., "Hypothalamic-Pituitary-Adrenocortical Axis Function in Premenopausal Women with Rheumatoid Arthritis Not Treated with Glucocorticoids," *Journal of Rheumatology* 26, no. 2 (February 1999): 282–88.

31. I. H. Zwain and S. S. Yen, "Dehydroepiandrosterone: Biosynthesis and Metabolism in the Brain," *Endocrinology* 140, no. 2 (February 1999): 880–87.

R. Rupprecht and F. Holsboer, "Neuropsychopharmacological Properties of Neuro-active Steroids," *Steroids* 64, nos. 1–2 (January–February 1999): 83–91.

32. S. Bastianetto et al., "Dehydroepiandrosterone (DHEA) Protects Hippocampal Cells from Oxidative Stress-Induced Damage," *Brain Research. Molecular Brain Research* 66, nos. 1–2 (March 20, 1999): 35–41.

J. Herbert, "Neurosteroids, Brain Damage, and Mental Illness," *Experimental Gerontology* 33, nos. 7–8 (November–December 1998): 713–27.

33. L. Milewich et al., "Induction of Murine Hepatic Glutathione S-Transferase by Dietary Dehydroepiandrosterone," *Journal of Steroid Biochemistry and Molecular Biology* 46, no. 3 (September 1993): 321–29.

34. K. M. Chiu et al., "Correlation of Serum L-Carnitine and Dehydro-epiandrosterone Sulphate Levels with Age and Sex in Healthy Adults," *Age and Ageing* 28, no. 2 (March 1999): 211–16.

35. M. Stomati et al., "Six-Month Oral Dehydroepiandrosterone Supplementation in Early and Late Postmenopause," *Gynecological Endocrinology* 14, no. 5 (October 2000): 342–63.

36. R. H. Straub et al., "Serum Dehydroepiandrosterone (DHEA) and DHEA Sulfate Are Negatively Correlated with Serum Interleukin-6 (Il-6), and DHEA Inhibits Il-6 Secretion from Mononuclear Cells in Man in Vitro: Possible Link between Endocrinosenescence and Immunosenescence," *Journal of Clinical Endocrinology and Metabolism* 83, no. 6 (June 1998): 2012–17.

37. M. Bloch et al., "Dehydroepiandrosterone Treatment of Midlife Dysthymia," *Biological Psychiatry* 45, no. 12 (June 1999): 1533–41.

38. É.-É. Baulieu et al., "Dehydroepiandrosterone (DHEA), DHEA Sulfate, and Aging: Contribution of the DHEAge Study to a Sociobiomedical Issue," *Proceedings of the National Academy of Sciences of the United States of America* 97, no. 8 (April 11, 2000): 4279–84.

39. S. S. Yen, A. J. Morales, and O. Khorram, "Replacement of DHEA in Aging Men and Women: Potential Remedial Effects," *Annals of the New York Academy of Sciences* 774 (December 29, 1995): 128–42.

40. 7-Keto is a trademark of the Humanetics Corporation.

41. P. R. Casson, A. Morales, and J. E. Buster, "The Use and Effects of DHEA in Humans," in *DHEA: A Comprehensive Review*, ed. J.H.H. Thijssen and H. Nieuwenhuyse (New York: Parthenon, 1999), 127–52.

42. S. Manglik et al., "Serum Insulin but Not Leptin Is Associated with Spontaneous and Growth Hormone (GH)-Releasing Hormone-Stimulated GH Secretion in Normal Volunteers with and without Weight Loss," *Metabolism* 47, no. 9 (September 1998): 1127–33.

L. Denti et al., "Effects of Aging on Dehydroepiandrosterone Sulfate in Relation to Fasting Insulin Levels and Body Composition Assessed by Bioimpedance Analysis," *Metabolism* 46 (1997): 826–32.

43. X. Xu, R. L. Ingram, and W. E. Sonntag, "Ethanol Suppresses Growth Hormone-Mediated Cellular Responses in Liver Slices," *Alcoholism—Clinical and Experimental Research* 19, no. 5 (October 1995): 1246–51.

44. B. Eto et al., "Glutamate-Arginine Salts and Hormonal Responses to Exercise," *Archives of Physiology and Biochemistry* 103, no. 2 (May 1995): 160–64.

45. E. Van Cauter, R. Leproult, and L. Plat, "Age-Related Changes in Slow Wave Sleep and REM Sleep and Relationship with Growth Hormone and Cortisol Levels in

Healthy Men," *JAMA—Journal of the American Medical Association* 284, no. 7 (August 16, 2000): 861–68.

46. S. Loth et al., "Improved Nasal Breathing in Snorers Increases Nocturnal Growth Hormone Secretion and Serum Concentrations of Insulin-like Growth Factor 1 Subsequently," *Rhinology* 36, no. 4 (December 1998): 179–83.

CHAPTER 3: PUTTING THE BRAKES ON CATABOLIC METABOLISM

1. www.methodisthealth.com/Skin/stats.htm.

2. U. Ravnskov, "Cholesterol Lowering Trials in Coronary Heart Disease: Frequency of Citation and Outcome," *British Medical Journal* 305 (1992): 15–19.

3. M. J. Stampfer et al., "Vitamin E and the Risk of Coronary Disease in Women," *New England Journal of Medicine* 328 (1993): 1444–49.

E. B. Rimm et al., "Vitamin E Consumption and the Risk of Coronary Heart Disease in Men," *New England Journal of Medicine* 328 (1993): 1450–56.

4. S. Stolberg, "Studies Show Vitamin E May Reduce Heart Disease Risk," *Los Angeles Times,* May 20, 1993, A21.

K. Gey, G. Brubacher, and J. Stahelin, "Plasma Levels of Antioxidant Vitamins in Relation to Ischemic Heart Disease and Cancer," *American Journal of Clinical Nutrition* 45 (1987): 1368.

M. S. Menkes et al., "Serum Beta-Carotene, Vitamins A and E, Selenium, and the Risk of Lung Cancer," *New England Journal of Medicine* 315, no. 20 (1986): 1250.

G. McKeowne-Eysses et al., "A Randomized Trial of Vitamin C and Vitamin E Supplementation in the Prevention of Recurrence of Colorectal Polyps," *Preventive Medicine* 16 (1987): 275.

5. T. M. Hagen et al., "Mitochondrial Decay in the Aging Rat Heart: Evidence for Improvement by Dietary Supplementation with Acetyl-L-Carnitine and/or Lipoic Acid," *Annals of the New York Academy of Sciences* 959 (April 2002): 491–507.

6. J. Lykkesfeldt et al., "Age-Associated Decline in Ascorbic Acid Concentration, Recycling and Biosynthesis in Rat Hepatocytes—Reversal with (R)-a-Lipoic Acid Supplementation," *FASEB Journal* 12 (1998): 1183–89.

T. M. Hagen et al. "(R)-a-Lipoic Acid-Supplemented Old Rats Have Improved Mitochondrial Function, Decreased Oxidative Damage, and Increased Metabolic Rate," *FASEB Journal* 13 (1998): 411–18.

C. K. Sen, "Redox Signaling and the Emerging Therapeutic Potential of Thiol Antioxidants," *Biochemical Pharmacology* 55, no. 11 (June 1998): 1747–58.

7. M. de A. Smith et al., "Investigation of the Effect of Hydrogen Peroxide on the Chromosomes of Young and Elderly Individuals," *Mechanisms of Ageing and Development* 56, no. 2 (November 1990): 107–15.

8. P. R. Heaton et al., "Role of Dietary Antioxidants to Protect against DNA Damage in Adult Dogs," *Journal of Nutrition* 132, no. 6 (June 2002): 1720–24S.

9. G. A. Homandberg, F. Hui, and C. Wen, "Fibronectin Fragment Mediated Cartilage Chondrolysis. II. Reparative Effects of Anti-oxidants," *Biochimica et Biophysica Acta* 1317, no. 2 (November 15, 1996): 143–48.

O. Sangha and G. Stucki, "Vitamin E in Therapy of Rheumatic Diseases," *Zeitschrift fur Rheumatologie* 57, no. 4 (August 1998): 207–14.

T. E. McAlindon et al., "Do Antioxidant Micronutrients Protect against the Development and Progression of Knee Osteoarthritis?" *Arthritis and Rheumatism* 39, no. 4 (April 1996): 648–56.

M. Sowers and L. Lachance, "Vitamins and Arthritis: The Roles of Vitamins A, C, D, and E," *Rheumatic Disease Clinics of North America* 25, no. 2 (May 1999): 315–32.

10. J. A. Joseph et al., "Reversals of Age-Related Declines in Neuronal Signal Transduction, Cognitive and Motor Behavioral Deficits with Blueberry, Spinach or Strawberry Dietary Supplementation," *Journal of Neuroscience* 19, no. 18 (September 15, 1999): 8114–21.

11. P. Mecocci et al., "Lymphocyte Oxidative DNA Damage and Plasma Antioxidants in Alzheimer Disease," *Archives of Neurology* 59, no. 5 (May 2002): 794–98.

12. S. Rajan et al., "Screening for Cobalamin Deficiency in Geriatric Outpatients: Prevalence and Influence of Synthetic Cobalamin Intake," *Journal of the American Geriatrics Society* 50, no. 4 (April 2002): 624–30.

13. O. Stanger, "Physiology of Folic Acid in Health and Disease," *Current Drug Metabolism* 3, no. 2 (April 2002): 211–23.

L. Le Marchand et al., "B-Vitamin Intake, Metabolic Genes, and Colorectal Cancer Risk (United States)," *Cancer Causes and Control* 13, no. 3 (April 2002): 239–48.

A. J. Alberg et al., "The Risk of Cervical Cancer in Relation to Serum Concentrations of Folate, Vitamin B$_{12}$, and Homocysteine," *Cancer Epidemiology Biomarkers and Prevention* 9, no. 7 (July 2000): 761–64.

M. P. Mattson, I. I. Kruman, and W. Duan, "Folic Acid and Homocysteine in Age-Related Disease," *Ageing Research Reviews* 1, no. 1 (February 2002): 95–111.

A. McCaddon et al., "Functional Vitamin B(12) Deficiency and Alzheimer Disease," *Neurology* 58, no. 9 (May 14, 2002): 1395–99.

I. I. Kruman et al., "Folic Acid Deficiency and Homocysteine Impair DNA Repair in Hippocampal Neurons and Sensitize Them to Amyloid Toxicity in Experimental Models of Alzheimer's Disease," *Journal of Neuroscience* 22, no. 5 (March 1, 2002): 1752–62.

14. J. W. Eichenbaum, "Vitamins for Cataracts and Macular Degeneration," *Journal of Ophthalmic Nursing and Technology* 15, no. 2 (1996): 65–67.

B. Villeponteau, R. Cockrel, and J. Feng, "Nutraceutical Intervention May Delay Aging and the Age-Related Diseases," *Experimental Gerontology* 35, nos. 9–10 (2000): 1405–17.

15. B. J. Diamond et al., "Ginkgo Biloba Extract: Mechanisms and Clinical Indications," *Archives of Physical Medicine and Rehabilitation* 81, no. 5 (May 2000): 668–78.

J. Cai et al., "Oxidative Damage and Protection of the RPE," *Progress in Retinal and Eye Research* 19, no. 2 (March 2000): 205–21.

16. J. C. Feghali, W. Liu, and T. R. Van De Water, "L-N-Acetyl-Cysteine Protection against Cisplatin-Induced Auditory Neuronal and Hair Cell Toxicity," *Laryngoscope* 111, no. 7 (July 2001): 1147–55.

C. Waters, "Molecular Mechanisms of Cell Death in the Ear," *Annals of the New York Academy of Sciences* 884 (November 28, 1999): 41–51.

M. D. Seidman et al., "Biologic Activity of Mitochondrial Metabolites on Aging and Age-Related Hearing Loss," *American Journal of Otology* 21, no. 2 (March 2000): 161–67.

17. R. I. Garcia, E. A. Krall, and P. S. Vokonas, "Periodontal Disease and Mortality from All Causes in the VA Dental Longitudinal Study," *Annals of Periodontology* 3, no. 1 (July 1998): 339–49.

18. T. Hanioka et al., "Effect of Topical Application of Coenzyme Q10 on Adult Periodontitis," *Molecular Aspects of Medicine* 15, supplement (1994): S241–48.

E. G. Wilkinson, R. M. Arnold, and K. Folkers, "Bioenergetics in Clinical Medicine. VI. Adjunctive Treatment of Periodontal Disease with Coenzyme Q10," *Research Communications in Chemical Pathology and Pharmacology* 14, no. 4 (August 1976): 715–19.

E. I. Weiss et al., "Inhibiting Interspecies Coaggregation of Plaque Bacteria with a Cranberry Juice Constituent," *Journal of the American Dental Association* 129, no. 12 (December 1998): 1719–23.

19. H. Y. Huang, K. J. Helzlsouer, and L. J. Appel, "The Effects of Vitamin C and Vitamin E on Oxidative DNA Damage: Results from a Randomized Controlled Trial," *Cancer Epidemiology Biomarkers and Prevention* 9, no. 7 (July 2000): 647–52.

B. L. Pool-Zobel et al., "Anthocyanins Are Potent Antioxidants in Model Systems but Do Not Reduce Endogenous Oxidative DNA Damage in Human Colon Cells," *European Journal of Nutrition* 38, no. 5 (October 1999): 227–34.

20. "Acrylamide in Food," *Weekly Epidemiological Record* 77, no. 20 (May 17, 2002): 166–67.

21. C. Gorman, "Do French Fries Cause Cancer?" *Time,* May 6, 2002, 73.

22. T. J. Smith et al., "How Can Carcinogenesis Be Inhibited?" *Annals of the New York Academy of Sciences* 768 (1995): 82–90.

23. N. Guthrie, Department of Biochemistry, University of Western Ontario. Reported at the Experimental Biology annual meeting, San Diego, 2000.

24. J. A. Joseph et al., "Reversals of Age-Related Declines in Neuronal Signal Transduction, Cognitive and Motor Behavioral Deficits."

25. M. Kretzschmar and D. Muller, "Aging, Training and Exercise: A Review of Effects on Plasma Glutathione and Lipid Peroxides," *Sports Medicine* 15, no. 3 (March 1993): 196–209.

26. D. G. Bostwick et al., "Antioxidant Enzyme Expression and Reactive Oxygen Species Damage in Prostatic Intraepithelial Neoplasia and Cancer," *Cancer* 89, no. 1 (July 1, 2000): 123–34.

27. G. Fassina et al., "Polyphenolic Antioxidant (-)-Epigallocatechin-3-Gallate from Green Tea as a Candidate anti-HIV agent," *AIDS* 16, no. 6 (April 12, 2002): 939–41.

28. K. A. Naidu and N. B. Thippeswamy, "Inhibition of Human Low Density Lipoprotein Oxidation by Active Principles from Spices," *Molecular and Cellular Biochemistry* 229, nos. 1–2 (January 2002): 19–23.

M. Martinez-Tome et al., "Antioxidant Properties of Mediterranean Spices Compared with Common Food Additives," *Journal of Food Protection* 64, no. 9 (September 2001): 1412–19.

29. P. B. Walter et al., "Iron Deficiency and Iron Excess Damage Mitochondria and Mitochondrial DNA in Rats," *Proceedings of the National Academy of Sciences* 99, no. 4 (2002): 2264–69.

30. G. H. Guyatt et al., "Diagnosis of Iron-Deficiency Anemia in the Elderly" (see comments), *American Journal of Medicine* 88, no. 3 (March 1990): 205–9.

G. H. Guyatt et al., "Laboratory Diagnosis of Iron-Deficiency Anemia: An Overview," *Journal of General Internal Medicine* 7, no. 2 (March–April 1992): 145–53.

31. W. C. Wu et al., "Blood Transfusion in Elderly Patients with Acute Myocardial Infarction," *New England Journal of Medicine* 345, no. 17 (October 25, 2001): 1230–36.

32. D. S. Abdalla, A. Campa, and H. P. Monteiro, "Low Density Lipoprotein Oxidation by Stimulated Neutrophils and Ferritin," *Atherosclerosis* 97, nos. 2–3 (December 1992): 149–59.

33. Jesus Pujol et al., "Biological Significance of Iron-Related Magnetic Resonance Imaging Changes in the Brain," *Archives of Neurology* 49 (1992): 711–17.

34. S. Y. Wang and H. Jiao, "Scavenging Capacity of Berry Crops on Superoxide Rad-

icals, Hydrogen Peroxide, Hydroxyl Radicals, and Singlet Oxygen," *Journal of Agricultural and Food Chemistry* 48, no. 11 (2000): 5677–84.

C. B. Pedersen et al., "Effects of Blueberry and Cranberry Juice Consumption on the Plasma Antioxidant Capacity of Healthy Female Volunteers," *European Journal of Clinical Nutrition* 54, no. 5 (2000): 405–8.

35. M. Turunen, P. Sindelar, and G. Dallner, "Induction of Endogenous Coenzyme Q Biosynthesis by Administration of Peroxisomal Inducers," *Biofactors* 9, nos. 2–4 (1999): 131–39.

F. Aberg et al., "Increases in Tissue Levels of Ubiquinone in Association with Peroxisome Proliferation," *Chemico-Biological Interactions* 99, nos. 1–3 (January 5, 1996): 205–18.

36. A. Cerami et al., "Glucose and Aging," *Scientific American* 256 (1987): 90–96.

37. M. A. Smith et al., "Advanced Maillard Reaction End Products Are Associated with Alzheimer Disease Pathology," *Proceedings of the National Academy of Sciences of the United States of America* 91, no. 12 (June 7, 1994): 5710–14.

38. D. B. Jiaan et al., "Age-Related Increase in an Advanced Glycation End Product in Penile Tissue," *World Journal of Urology* 13, no. 6 (1995): 369–75.

39. Y. J. Suzuki , M. Tsuchiya, and L. Packer, "Lipoate Prevents Glucose-Induced Protein Modifications," *Free Radical Research Communications* 17, no. 3 (1992): 211–17.

40. A. Bierhaus et al., "Advanced Glycation End Product–Induced Activation of NF-kappaB Is Suppressed by Alpha-Lipoic Acid in Cultured Endothelial Cells," *Diabetes* 46, no. 9 (September 1997): 1481–90.

41. P. A. Low, K. K. Nickander, and H. J. Tritschler, "The Roles of Oxidative Stress and Antioxidant Treatment in Experimental Diabetic Neuropathy," *Diabetes* 46, supplement 2 (September 1997): S38–42.

42. M. Nakayama et al., "Suppression of N(Epsilon)-(Carboxymethyl)Lysine Generation by the Antioxidant N-Acetylcysteine," *Peritoneal Dialysis International* 19, no. 3 (May–June 1999): 207–10.

43. H. M. Salzer, "Relative Hypoglycemia as a Cause of Neuropsychiatric Illness," *Journal of the National Medical Association* 58 (1966): 12.

44. S. Reiser and B. Szepesi, "SCOGS Report on the Health Aspects of Sucrose Consumption," *American Journal of Clinical Nutrition* 31, no. 1 (January 1978): 9–11.

45. V. J. Burley, "Sugar Consumption and Human Cancer in Sites Other Than the Digestive Tract," *European Journal of Cancer Prevention* 7, no. 4 (August 1998): 253–77.

46. W. L. Dills, "Protein Fructosylation: Fructose and the Maillard Reaction," *American Journal of Clinical Nutrition* 58, supplement (1993): 779–87S.

47. C. B. Hollenbeck, "Dietary Fructose Effects on Lipoprotein Metabolism and Risk for Coronary Artery Disease," *American Journal of Clinical Nutrition* 58, supplement (1993): 800–807S.

J. Hallfrisch et al., "The Effects of Fructose on Blood Lipid Levels," *American Journal of Clinical Nutrition* 37, no. 3 (1983): 740–48.

48. R. Ivaturi and C. Kies, "Mineral Balances in Humans as Affected by Fructose, High-Fructose Corn Syrup and Sucrose," *Plant Foods for Human Nutrition* 42, no. 2 (1992): 143–51.

49. T. Koschinsky et al., "Orally Absorbed Reactive Glycation Products (Glycotoxins): An Environmental Risk Factor in Diabetic Nephropathy," *Proceedings of the National Academy of Sciences of the United States of America* 94, no. 12 (June 10, 1997): 6474–79.

50. W. Zheng et al., "Well-Done Meat Intake and the Risk of Breast Cancer," *Journal of the National Cancer Institute* 90, no. 22 (November 18, 1998): 1724–29.

51. T. Nakagawa et al., "Protective Activity of Green Tea against Free Radical– and Glucose-Mediated Protein Damage," *Journal of Agricultural and Food Chemistry* 50, no. 8 (April 10, 2002): 2418–22.

52. C. H. van de Lest, B. M. van den Hoogen, and P. R. van Weeren, "Loading-Induced Changes in Synovial Fluid Affect Cartilage Metabolism," *Biorheology* 37, nos. 1–2 (2000): 45–55.

H. Langberg et al., "Type I Collagen Synthesis and Degradation in Peritendinous Tissue after Exercise Determined by Microdialysis in Humans," part 1, *Journal of Physiology—London* 521 (November 15, 1999): 299–306.

53. P. Chithra, G. B. Sajithlal, and G. Chandrakasan, "Influence of Aloe Vera on Collagen Characteristics in Healing Dermal Wounds in Rats," *Molecular and Cellular Biochemistry* 181, nos. 1–2 (April 1998): 71–76.

54. W. J. Kraemer et al., "Resistance Training Combined with Bench-Step Aerobics Enhances Women's Health Profile," *Medicine and Science in Sports and Exercise* 33, no. 2 (February 2001): 259–69.

55. J. S. Coombes and L. R. McNaughton, "Effects of Branched-Chain Amino Acid Supplementation on Serum Creatine Kinase and Lactate Dehydrogenase after Prolonged Exercise," *Journal of Sports Medicine and Physical Fitness* 40, no. 3 (September 2000): 240–46.

56. L. M. Castell et al., "The Role of Tryptophan in Fatigue in Different Conditions of Stress," *Advances in Experimental Medicine and Biology* 467 (1999): 697–704.

J. M. Davis, N. L. Alderson, and R. S. Welsh, "Serotonin and Central Nervous System Fatigue: Nutritional Considerations," part 2, *American Journal of Clinical Nutrition* 72, no. 2 (August 2000): 573–78S.

57. R. A. Bassit et al., "The Effect of BCAA Supplementation upon the Immune Response of Triathletes," *Medicine and Science in Sports and Exercise* 32, no. 7 (July 2000): 1214–19.

58. M. M. Kanter, L. A. Nolte, and J. O. Holloszy, "Effects of an Antioxidant Vitamin Mixture on Lipid Peroxidation at Rest and Postexercise," *Journal of Applied Physiology* 74, no. 2 (February 1993): 965–69.

59. C. K. Sen and L. Packer, "Thiol Homeostasis and Supplements in Physical Exercise," *American Journal of Clinical Nutrition* 72, no. 2, supplement (August 2000): 653–69S.

60. R. M. McAllister, M. D. Delp, and M. H. Laughlin, "Thyroid Status and Exercise Tolerance: Cardiovascular and Metabolic Considerations," *Sports Medicine* 20, no. 3 (September 1995): 189–98.

61. D. Defalque et al., "GH Insensitivity Induced by Endotoxin Injection Is Associated with Decreased Liver GH Receptors," part 1, *American Journal of Physiology* 276, no. 3 (March 1999): E565–72.

62. "Report of the U.S. Preventive Services Task Force: Screening for Alcohol and Other Drug Abuse," in *Guide to Clinical Preventive Services* (Washington, D.C.: U.S. Department of Health and Human Services, U.S. Government Printing Office, 1990).

63. N. A. Ivleva and Z. F. Sabirova, "Role of Risk Factors in the Development of Chronic Digestive System Diseases in Children," *Gigiena I Sanitariia,* no. 5 (September–October 2000): 5–7.

64. J. Harvey and D. G. Colin-Jones, "Mistletoe Hepatitis," *British Medical Journal* 282 (1981): 739.

F. Stirpe, "Mistletoe Toxicity," *Lancet* 2 (1983): 1442.

C. F. Weston, "Veno-Occlusive Disease of the Liver Secondary to Ingestion of Comfrey," *British Medical Journal* 295 (1987): 183.

F. B. MacGregor et al., "Hepatoxicity of Herbal Remedies," *British Medical Journal* 299 (1989): 1156–57.

M. Katz and F. Saibil, "Herbal Hepatitis: Subacute Hepatic Necrosis Secondary to Chaparral Leaf," *Journal of Clinical Gastroenterology* 12 (1990): 203–6.

D. Larrey et al., "Hepatitis after Germander (*Teucrium chamaedrys*) Administration: Another Instance of Herbal Medicine Hepatotoxicity," *Annals of Internal Medicine* 117 (1992): 129–32.

65. J. F. Fries, "Aging, Natural Death, and the Compression of Morbidity," *New England Journal of Medicine* 303, no. 3 (July 17, 1980): 130–35.

CHAPTER 4: STRESS AND THE AGING PROCESS

1. M. D. Majewska, "Neuronal Actions of Dehydroepiandrosterone: Possible Roles in Brain Development, Aging, Memory and Affect," *Annals of the New York Academy of Sciences* 774 (1995): 111–19.

M. D. Majewska, "Actions of Steroids on Neuron: Role in Personality, Mood, Stress, and Disease," *Integrative Psychiatry* 5 (1985): 258–73.

2. T. W. Uhde, L. C. Malloy, and S. O. Slate, "Fearful Behavior, Body Size, and Serum IGF-I Levels in Nervous and Normal Pointer Dogs," *Pharmacology Biochemistry and Behavior* 43, no. 1 (September 1992): 263–69.

3. C. L. Melchior and R. F. Ritzmann, "Dehydroepiandrosterone Is an Anxiolytic in Mice on the Plus Maze," *Pharmacology Biochemistry and Behavior* 47, no. 3 (March 1994): 437–41.

C. A. Frye and E. H. Lacey, "The Neurosteroids DHEA and DHEAS May Influence Cognitive Performance by Altering Affective State," *Physiology and Behavior* 66, no. 1 (March 1999): 85–92.

4. O. Zinder and D. E. Dar, "Neuroactive Steroids: Their Mechanism of Action and Their Function in the Stress Response," *Acta Physiologica Scandinavica* 167, no. 3 (November 1999): 181–88.

Y. Noda, H. Kamei, and T. Nabeshima, "Sigma-Receptor Ligands and Anti-stress Actions," *Nippon Yakurigaku Zasshi* 114, no. 1 (July 1999): 43–49.

Y. Akwa and É.-É. Baulieu, "Neurosteroids: Behavioral Aspects and Physiological Implications," *Journal de la Societe de Biologie* 193, no. 3 (1999): 293–98.

5. F. Holsboer et al., "Steroid Effects on Central Neurons and Implications for Psychiatric and Neurological Disorders," *Annals of the New York Academy of Sciences* 746 (November 30, 1994): 345–59; discussion 359–61.

6. L. E. Carlson, B. B. Sherwin, and H. M. Chertkow, "Relationships between Dehydroepiandrosterone Sulfate (DHEAS) and Cortisol (CRT) Plasma Levels and Everyday Memory in Alzheimer's Disease Patients Compared to Healthy Controls," *Hormones and Behavior* 35, no. 3 (June 1999): 254–63.

7. V. I. Reus et al., "Dehydroepiandrosterone (DHEA) and Memory in Depressed Patients," *Neuropsychopharmacology* 9 (1993): 66S.

8. G. Ceresini et al., "Evaluation of the Circadian Profiles of Serum Dehydroepiandrosterone (DHEA), Cortisol, and Cortisol/DHEA Molar Ratio after a Single Oral Administration of DHEA in Elderly Subjects," *Metabolism* 49, no. 4 (April 2000): 548–51.

A. Heinz et al., "Severity of Depression in Abstinent Alcoholics Is Associated with Monoamine Metabolites and Dehydroepiandrosterone-Sulfate Concentrations," *Psychiatry Research* 89, no. 2 (December 20, 1999): 97–106.

S. S. Yen and G. A. Laughlin, "Aging and the Adrenal Cortex," *Experimental Gerontology* 33, nos. 7–8, (November–December 1998): 897–910.

J. Herbert, "Neurosteroids, Brain Damage, and Mental Illness," *Experimental Gerontology* 33, nos. 7–8, (November–December 1998): 713–27.

9. O. T. Wolf and C. Kirschbaum, "Actions of Dehydroepiandrosterone and Its Sulfate in the Central Nervous System: Effects on Cognition and Emotion in Animals and Humans," *Brain Research Reviews* 30 (1999): 264–88.

10. H. Kuratsune et al., "Dehydroepiandrosterone Sulfate Deficiency in Chronic Fatigue Syndrome," *International Journal of Molecular Medicine* 1, no. 1 (January 1998): 143–46.

P. H. Dessein et al., "Hyposecretion of Adrenal Androgens and the Relation of Serum Adrenal Steroids, Serotonin and Insulin-like Growth Factor-1 to Clinical Features in Women with Fibromyalgia," *Pain* 83, no. 2 (November 1999): 313–19.

R. M. Bennett, "Disordered Growth Hormone Secretion in Fibromyalgia: A Review of Recent Findings and a Hypothesized Etiology," *Zeitschrift fur Rheumatologie* 57, supplement 2 (1998): 72–76.

11. W. Arlt et al., "Dehydroepiandrosterone Replacement in Women with Adrenal Insufficiency," *New England Journal of Medicine* 341, no. 14 (September 30, 1999): 1013–20.

12. O. M. Wolkowitz et al., "Double-Blind Treatment of Major Depression with Dehydroepiandrosterone," *American Journal of Psychiatry* 156, no. 4 (April 1999): 646–49.

O. M. Wolkowitz et al., "Dehydroepiandrosterone (DHEA) Treatment of Depression," *Biological Psychiatry* 41, no. 3 (February 1, 1997): 311–18.

13. O. M. Wolkowitz and V. I. Reus, "Treatment of Depression with Antiglucocorticoid Drugs," *Psychosomatic Medicine* 61, no. 5 (September–October 1999): 698–711.

14. C. N. Shealy, *DHEA: The Youth and Health Hormone* (New Canaan, Conn.: Keats Publishing, 1996), 43.

15. D. G. Cruess et al., "Cognitive-Behavioral Stress Management Buffers Decreases in Dehydroepiandrosterone Sulfate (DHEA-S) and Increases in the Cortisol/DHEA-S Ratio and Reduces Mood Disturbance and Perceived Stress among HIV-Seropositive Men," *Psychoneuroendocrinology* 24, no. 5 (July 1999): 537–49.

16. H. M. Helm et al., "Does Private Religious Activity Prolong Survival? A Six-Year Follow-up Study of 3,851 Older Adults," *Journals of Gerontology Series A—Biological Sciences and Medical Sciences* 55, no. 7 (July 2000): M400–405.

J. B. Meisenhelder and E. N. Chandler, "Prayer and Health Outcomes in Church Members," *Alternative Therapies in Health and Medicine* 6, no. 4 (July 2000): 56–60.

17. "Caffeine Reduction as an Adjunct to Anxiety Management," part 3, *British Journal of Clinical Psychology* 27 (September 1988): 265–66.

M. A. Lee et al., "Anxiogenic Effects of Caffeine on Panic and Depressed Patients," *American Journal of Psychiatry* 145, no. 5 (May 1988): 632–35.

18. H. Jaggy and E. Koch, "Chemistry and Biology of Alkylphenols from *Ginkgo biloba L.*," *Pharmazie* 52, no. 10 (October 1997): 735–38.

19. J. Haase, P. Halama, and R. Horr, "Effectiveness of Brief Infusions with Ginkgo Biloba Special Extract EGb 761 in Dementia of the Vascular and Alzheimer Type," *Zeitschrift fur Gerontologie und Geriatrie* 29, no. 4 (July 1996): 302–9.

20. M.V.R. Appa rao, K. Srinivasan, and R.T.L. Koteswara, "The Effect of *Centella asiatica* on the General Mental Ability of Mentally Retarded Children," *Indian Journal of Psychiatry* 19 (1977): 54–59.

K. Nalini et al., "Effect of *Centella asiatica* Fresh Leaf Aqueous Extract on Learning and Memory and Biogenic Amine Turnover in Albino Rats," *Phytotherapia* 63, no. 3 (1992): 232–37.

21. V. Florian, M. Mikulincer, and G. Hirschberger, "The Anxiety-Buffering Function of Close Relationships: Evidence That Relationship Commitment Acts as a Terror Management Mechanism," *Journal of Personality and Social Psychology* 82, no. 4 (April 2002): 527–42.

22. J. H. Medina et al., "Overview—Flavonoids: A New Family of Benzodiazepine Receptor Ligands," *Neurochemical Research* 22, no. 4 (April 1997): 419–25.

A. C. Paladini et al., "Flavonoids and the Central Nervous System: From Forgotten Factors to Potent Anxiolytic Compounds," *Journal of Pharmacy and Pharmacology* 51, no. 5 (May 1999): 519–26.

23. R. Manber et al., "The Effects of Regularizing Sleep-Wake Schedules on Daytime Sleepiness," *Sleep* 19, no. 5 (June 1996): 432–41.

CHAPTER 5: HOW GOOD DO YOU WANT TO LOOK AND FEEL?

1. R. Marks, "Seeing through the Stratum Corneum," *Keio Journal of Medicine* 49, no. 2 (June 2000): 80–83.

P. W. Wertz, "Lipids and Barrier Function of the Skin," *Acta Dermato-Venereologica* (Stockholm) 208, supplement (2000): 7–11.

2. É.-É. Baulieu et al., "Dehydroepiandrosterone (DHEA), DHEA Sulfate, and Aging: Contribution of the DHEAge Study to a Sociobiomedical Issue," *Proceedings of the National Academy of Sciences of the United States of America* 97, no. 8 (April 11, 2000): 4279–84.

3. K. S. Lee, K. Y. Oh, and B. C. Kim, "Effects of Dehydroepiandrosterone on Collagen and Collagenase Gene Expression by Skin Fibroblasts in Culture," *Journal of Dermatological Science* 23, no. 2 (June 1, 2000): 103–10.

4. C. L. Greenstock, "Related Articles. Radiation and Aging: Free Radical Damage, Biological Response and Possible Antioxidant Intervention," *Medical Hypotheses* 41, no. 5 (November 1993): 473–82.

5. Z. Qiu et al., "Modified *Aloe barbadensis* Polysaccharide with Immunoregulatory Activity," *Planta Medica* 66 (2000): 1–5.

6. A. Castillo-Richmond et al., "Effects of Stress Reduction on Carotid Atherosclerosis in Hypertensive African Americans," *Stroke* 31, no. 3 (March 2000): 568–73.

7. J. A. Joseph et al., "Long-Term Dietary Strawberry, Spinach, or Vitamin E Supplementation Retards the Onset of Age-Related Neuronal Signal-Transduction and Cognitive Behavioral Deficits," *Journal of Neuroscience* 18, no. 19 (October 1, 1998): 8047–55.

8. J. A. Joseph et al., "Reversals of Age-Related Declines in Neuronal Signal Transduction, Cognitive, and Motor Behavioral Deficits with Blueberry, Spinach, or Strawberry Dietary Supplementation," *Journal of Neuroscience* 19, no. 18 (September 15, 1999): 8114–21.

9. R. A. Yokel, D. D. Allen, and D. C. Ackley, "The Distribution of Aluminum into and out of the Brain," *Journal of Inorganic Biochemistry* 76, no. 2 (August 30, 1999): 127–32.

C. Struys-Ponsar, O. Guillard, and P. van den Bosch de Aguilar, "Effects of Aluminum Exposure on Glutamate Metabolism: A Possible Explanation for Its Toxicity," *Experimental Neurology* 163, no. 1 (May 2000): 157–64.

10. A. M. Robert et al., "Aging and Brain Circulation: Role of the Extracellular Matrix of Brain Microvessels," *Comptes Rendus des Seances de la Societe de Biologie et de ses Filiales* 191, no. 2 (1997): 253–60.

11. E. F. Binder, M. Storandt, and S. J. Birge, "The Relation between Psychometric Test Performance and Physical Performance in Older Adults," *Journals of Gerontology Series A—Biological Sciences and Medical Sciences* 54, no. 8 (August 1999): M428–32.

D. F. Hultsch et al., "Use It or Lose It: Engaged Lifestyle as a Buffer of Cognitive Decline in Aging?" *Psychology and Aging* 14, no. 2 (June 1999): 245–63.

12. Baulieu et al., "Dehydroepiandrosterone (DHEA), DHEA Sulfate, and Aging."

CHAPTER 6: ILLNESS, IMMUNITY, AND METABOLISM

1. D. Carmelli and T. Reed, "Stability and Change in Genetic and Environmental Influences on Hand-Grip Strength in Older Male Twins," *Journal of Applied Physiology* 89, no. 5 (November 2000): 1879–83.

K. Christensen et al., "Genetic and Environmental Influences on Functional Abilities in Danish Twins Aged 75 Years and Older," *Journals of Gerontology Series A—Biological Sciences and Medical Sciences* 55, no. 8 (August 2000): M446–52.

2. H. Gudmundsson et al., "Inheritance of Human Longevity in Iceland," *European Journal of Human Genetics* 8, no. 10 (October 2000): 743–49.

3. T. B. Harris et al., "Associations of Elevated Interleukin-6 and C-Reactive Protein Levels with Mortality in the Elderly," *American Journal of Medicine* 106, no. 5 (May 1999): 506–12.

4. K. James et al., "IL-6, DHEA and the Ageing Process," *Mechanisms of Ageing and Development* 93, nos. 1–3 (February 1997): 15–24.

5. M. McIntosh, H. Bao, and C. Lee, "Opposing Actions of Dehydroepiandrosterone and Corticosterone in Rats," *Proceedings of the Society for Experimental Biology and Medicine* 221, no. 3 (July 1999): 198–206.

K. L. Blauer et al., "Dehydroepiandrosterone Antagonizes the Suppressive Effects of Dexamethasone on Lymphocyte Proliferation," *Endocrinology* 129, no. 6 (December 1991): 3174–79.

M. May et al., "Protection from Glucocorticoid Induced Thymic Involution by Dehydroepiandrosterone," *Life Sciences* 46, no. 22 (1990): 1627–31.

D. Ben-Nathan et al., "Dehydroepiandrosterone Protects Mice Inoculated with West Nile Virus and Exposed to Cold Stress," *Journal of Medical Virology* 38, no. 3 (November 1992): 159–66.

6. S. E. Wiedmeier et al., "Thymic Modulation of IL-2 and IL-4 Synthesis by Peripheral T Cells," *Cellular Immunology* 135, no. 2 (July 1991): 501–18.

7. O. Khorram, L. Vu, and S. S. Yen, "Activation of Immune Function by Dehydroepiandrosterone (DHEA) in Age-Advanced Men," *Journals of Gerontology Series A—Biological Sciences and Medical Sciences* 52, no. 1 (January 1997): M1–7.

8. S. N. Han et al., "Vitamin E Supplementation Increases T Helper 1 Cytokine Production in Old Mice Infected with Influenza Virus," *Immunology* 100, no. 4 (August 2000): 487–93.

9. L. M. Castell, J. R. Poortmans, and E. A. Newsholme, "Does Glutamine Have a

Role in Reducing Infections in Athletes?" *European Journal of Applied Physiology* 73, no. 5 (1996): 488–90.

10. M. Heberer et al., "Role of Glutamine in the Immune Response in Critical Illness," *Nutrition* 12, nos. 11–12, supplement (November–December 1996): S71–72.

11. B. P. Bourgoin et al., "Lead Content in 70 Brands of Dietary Calcium Supplements," *American Journal of Public Health* 83, no. 8 (August 1993): 1155–60.

12. A. Laudat et al., "Changes in Systemic Gonadal and Adrenal Steroids in Asymptomatic Human Immunodeficiency Virus–Infected Men: Relationship with the CD4 Cell Counts," *European Journal of Endocrinology* 133, no. 4 (October 1995): 418–24.

13. E. Henderson, J. Y. Yang, and A. Schwartz, "Dehydroepiandrosterone (DHEA) and Synthetic DHEA Analogs Are Modest Inhibitors of HIV-1 IIIB Replication," *AIDS Research and Human Retroviruses* 8 (1992): 625–31.

14. P. A. Corley, "HIV and the Cortisol Connection: A Feasible Concept of the Process of AIDS," *Medical Hypotheses* 44, no. 6 (June 1995): 483–89.

15. D. J. Carr, "Increased Levels of IFN-Gamma in the Trigeminal Ganglion Correlate with Protection against HSV-1-Induced Encephalitis Following Subcutaneous Administration with Androstenediol," *Journal of Neuroimmunology* 89, nos. 1–2 (August 14, 1998): 160–67.

J. Daigle and D. J. Carr, "Androstenediol Antagonizes Herpes Simplex Virus Type 1–Induced Encephalitis through the Augmentation of Type I IFN Production," *Journal of Immunology* 160, no. 6 (March 15, 1998): 3060–66.

R. M. Loria, D. A. Padgett, and P. N. Huynh, "Regulation of the Immune Response by Dehydroepiandrosterone and Its Metabolites," *Journal of Endocrinology* 150, supplement (September 1996): S209–20.

16. R. J. Donaldson, ed., *Parasites and Western Man* (Baltimore: University Park Press, 1979).

17. T. J. Slom et al., "An Outbreak of Eosinophilic Meningitis Caused by *Angiostrongylus cantonensis* in Travelers Returning from the Caribbean," *New England Journal of Medicine* 346, no. 9 (February 28, 2002): 668–75.

18. K. O. Adams et al., "Intestinal Fluke Infection as a Result of Eating Sushi," *American Journal of Clinical Pathology* 86, no. 5 (1986): 688.

J. W. Hutchinson et al., "Diphyllobothriasis after Eating Raw Salmon," *Hawaii Medical Journal* 56, no. 7 (July 1997): 176–77.

J. T. Hiramoto and J. Tokeshi, "Anisakiasis in Hawaii. A Radiological Diagnosis," *Hawaii Medical Journal* 50, no. 6 (June 1991): 202–3.

19. E. E. Keighley, "Trichomonas in a Closed Community: Efficacy of Metronidazole," *British Medical Journal* 1 (1971): 207.

20. O. Jirovec and M. Petru, "*Trichomonas vaginalis* and Trichomonas," in *Advances in Clinical Pathology*, vol. 6, ed. B. Dawes (London: Academic Press, 1988).

21. J. M. Mansfield, ed., *Parasitic Diseases* (New York: Marcel Dekker, 1981).

22. A. C. Chester et al., "Giardiasis as a Chronic Disease," *Digestive Diseases and Sciences* 30, no. 3 (1985): 215.

23. N. S. Atkins et al., "Humoral Responses in Human Strongyloidiasis: Correlations with Infection Chronicity," *Transactions of the Royal Society of Tropical Medicine and Hygiene* 91, no. 5 (September–October 1997): 609–13.

24. R. L. Guerrant et al., "Evaluation and Diagnosis of Acute Infectious Diarrhea," *American Journal of Medicine* 78, no. 68 (1985): 91.

25. C. D. Mackenzie et al., "Inflammatory Response to Parasites," *Parasitology* 94, supplement (1987): 9.

26. K. F. Gey et al., "Inverse Correlation between Plasma Vitamin E and Mortality from Ischemic Heart Disease in Cross-Cultural Epidemiology," *American Journal of Clinical Nutrition* 53 (1991): 326–34S.

27. J. P. Moran et al., "Plasma Ascorbic Acid Concentrations Relate Inversely to Blood Pressure in Human Subjects," *American Journal of Clinical Nutrition* 57 (1993): 213–17.

28. D. Gavish and J. L. Breslow, "Lipoprotein(a) reduction by N-Acetylcysteine," *Lancet* 337, no. 8735 (January 26, 1991): 203–4.

29. E. Barret-Connor, K. T. Knaw, and S.S.C. Yen, "A Prospective Study of Dehydroepiandrosterone Sulfate, Mortality and Cardiovascular Disease," *New England Journal of Medicine* 315 (1986): 1519–24.

30. Y. Moriyama et al., "The Plasma Levels of Dehydroepiandrosterone Sulfate Are Decreased in Patients with Chronic Heart Failure in Proportion to the Severity," *Journal of Clinical Endocrinology and Metabolism* 85, no. 5 (May 2000): 1834–40.

31. A. N. Nafziger, D. M. Herrington, and T. L. Bush, "Dehydroepiandrosterone and Dehydroepiandrosterone Sulfate: Their Relation to Cardiovascular Disease," *Epidemiologic Reviews* 13 (1991): 267–93.

32. R. L. Jesse et al., "Dehydroepiandrosterone Inhibits Human Platelet Aggregation in Vitro and in Vivo," *Annals of the New York Academy of Sciences* 774 (December 29, 1995): 281–90.

33. N. A. Beer et al., "Dehydroepiandrosterone Reduces Plasma Plasminogen Activator Inhibitor Type 1 and Tissue Plasminogen Activator Antigen in Men," *American Journal of the Medical Sciences* 311, no. 5 (May 1996): 205–10.

34. H. S. Kim, S. Kacew, and B. M. Lee, "In Vitro Chemopreventive Effects of Plant Polysaccharides *(Aloe barbadensis miller, Lentinus edodes, Ganoderma lucidum* and *Coriolus versicolor)*," *Carcinogenesis* 20, no. 8 (August 1999): 1637–40.

35. C. Ho et al., "Antioxidative Effect of Polyphenols Extract Prepared from Various Chinese Teas," *Preventive Medicine* 21 (1992): 520–25.

36. C. S. Yang and Z. Y. Wang, "Tea and Cancer," *Journal of the National Cancer Institute* 85, no. 13 (1993): 1038–49.

37. H. F. Stich, "Teas and Tea Components as Inhibitors of Carcinogen Formation in Model Systems and Man," *Preventive Medicine* 21 (1992): 377–84.

38. U.S. National Cancer Institute, *Cancer Weekly* 12 (July 6, 1992).

39. N. E. Fleshner and O. Kucuk, "Antioxidant Dietary Supplements: Rationale and Current Status as Chemopreventive Agents for Prostate Cancer," *Urology* 57, no. 4, supplement 1 (April 2001): 90–94.

40. A. J. Costello, "A Randomized, Controlled Chemoprevention Trial of Selenium in Familial Prostate Cancer: Rationale, Recruitment, and Design Issues," *Urology* 57, no. 4, supplement 1 (April 2001): 182–84.

41. X. W. Mao, J. O. Archambeau, and D. S. Gridley, "Immunotherapy with Low-Dose Interleukin-2 and a Polysaccharopeptide Derived from *Coriolus versicolor,*" *Cancer Biotherapy and Radiopharmaceuticals* 6 (December 11, 1996): 393–403.

V. E. Ooi and F. Liu, "Immunomodulation and Anti-Cancer Activity of Polysaccharide-Protein Complexes," *Current Medicinal Chemistry* 7, no. 7 (July 2000): 715–29.

42. G. D. Stoner and H. Mukhtar, "Polyphenols as Cancer Chemopreventive Agents," *Journal of Cellular Biochemistry* 220, supplement (1995): 169–80.

43. Y. Zhang, "Molecular Mechanism of Rapid Cellular Accumulation of Anticarcinogenic Isothiocyanates," *Carcinogenesis* 22, no. 3 (March 2001): 425–31.

K. Singletary and C. MacDonald, "Inhibition of Benzo[a]pyrene- and 1,6-Dinitropyrene-DNA Adduct Formation in Human Mammary Epithelial Cells by Dibenzoylmethane and Sulforaphane," *Cancer Letters* 155, no. 1 (July 3, 2000): 47–54.

44. R. G. Clarke et al., "Effect of Eicosapentaenoic Acid on the Proliferation and Incidence of Apoptosis in the Colorectal Cell Line HT29," *Lipids* 34, no. 12 (December 1999): 1287–95.

C. P. Burns et al., "Phase I Clinical Study of Fish Oil Fatty Acid Capsules for Patients with Cancer Cachexia: Cancer and Leukemia Group B Study 9473," *Clinical Cancer Research* 5, no. 12 (December 1999): 3942–47.

A. E. Norrish et al., "Prostate Cancer Risk and Consumption of Fish Oils: A Dietary Biomarker-Based Case-Control Study," *British Journal of Cancer* 81, no. 7 (December 1999): 1238–42.

45. R. Bartoli et al., "Effect of Olive Oil on Early and Late Events of Colon Carcinogenesis in Rats: Modulation of Arachidonic Acid Metabolism and Local Prostaglandin E(2) Synthesis," *Gut* 46, no. 2 (February 2000): 191–99.

46. M. Cuendet and J. M. Pezzuto, "The Role of Cyclooxygenase and Lipoxygenase in Cancer Chemoprevention," *Drug Metabolism and Drug Interactions* 17, nos. 1–4 (2000): 109–57.

47. J. J. Caro et al., "Anemia as an Independent Prognostic Factor for Survival in Patients with Cancer: A Systemic, Quantitative Review," *Cancer* 91, no. 12 (June 15, 2001): 2211–21.

CHAPTER 7: ENERGY, EXERCISE, AND METABOLISM

1. D. N. Proctor, P. Balagopal, and K. S. Nair, "Age-Related Sarcopenia in Humans Is Associated with Reduced Synthetic Rates of Specific Muscle Proteins," *Journal of Nutrition* 128, no. 2, supplement (February 1998): 351–55S.

R. D. Starling, P. A. Ades, and E. T. Poehlman, "Physical Activity, Protein Intake, and Appendicular Skeletal Muscle Mass in Older Men," *American Journal of Clinical Nutrition* 70, no. 1 (July 1999): 91–96.

2. S. S. Yen, A. J. Morales, and O. Khorram, "Replacement of DHEA in Aging Men and Women: Potential Remedial Effects," *Annals of the New York Academy of Sciences* 774 (December 29, 1995): 128–42.

3. S. Marconi et al., "Alpha-Ketoglutarate-Pyridoxine Complex and Human Performance," *European Journal of Applied Physiology* 49 (1982): 307.

4. R. E. Olson and H. Rudney, "Biosynthesis of Ubiquinone," *Vitamins and Hormones* 40 (1983): 2–43.

5. R. A. Anderson et al., "Chromium Intake, Absorption and Excretion of Subjects Consuming Self-Selected Diets," *American Journal of Clinical Nutrition* 41 (1985): 1177–83.

6. B. W. Morris et al., "The Inter-relationship between Insulin and Chromium in Hyperinsulinaemic Euglycaemic Clamps in Healthy Volunteers," *Journal of Endocrinology* 139, no. 2 (November 1993): 339–45.

7. J. T. Hicks, "Treatment of Fatigue in General Practice: A Double Blind Study," *Clinical Medicine* 71 (1964): 85–90.

8. C. H. van de Lest, B. M. van den Hoogen, and P. R. van Weeren, "Loading-Induced Changes in Synovial Fluid Affect Cartilage Metabolism," *Biorheology* 37, nos. 1–2 (2000): 45–55.

9. H. Langberg et al., "Type I Collagen Synthesis and Degradation in Peritendinous Tissue after Exercise Determined by Microdialysis in Humans," part 1, *Journal of Physiology—London* 521 (November 15, 1999): 299–306.

M. J. Rennie, "Teasing Out the Truth about Collagen," *Journal of Physiology—London* 521 (November 15, 1999): 1.

10. J. O. Holloszy, W. M. Kohrt, and P. A. Hansen, "The Regulation of Carbohydrate and Fat Metabolism during and after Exercise," *Frontiers in Bioscience* 3 (September 15, 1998): D1011–27.

11. D. S. Kalman et al., "A Randomized, Double-Blind, Placebo-Controlled Study of 3-Acetyl-7-Oxo Dehydroepiandrosterone in Healthy Overweight Adults," *Current Therapeutic Research* 61, no. 7 (2000): 435–42.

CHAPTER 8: OPTIMAL NUTRITION: BUILDING BLOCKS
OF THE METABOLIC PLAN

1. H. F. Erbersdobler, "Food Quality and 'Health Nutrition': A Challenge for Agriculture and Food Processing," *Berliner und Munchener Tierarztliche Wochenschrift* 102, no. 4 (April 1, 1989): 112–17.

A. Drewnowski and C. Gomez-Carneros, "Bitter Taste, Phytonutrients, and the Consumer: A Review," *American Journal of Clinical Nutrition* 72, no. 6 (December 2000): 1424–35.

2. B. N. Ames, "Micronutrients Prevent Cancer and Delay Aging," *Toxicology Letters* 102–3 (1998): 5–18.

3. E. De Ritter, "Stability Characteristics of Vitamins in Processed Foods," *Food Technology* 30 (1976): 48–54.

4. W. Marusich et al., "Provitamin A Activity and Stability of Beta Carotene in Margarine," *Journal of the American Oil Chemists Society* 34 (1959): 217.

5. D. R. Jacobs et al., "Fiber from Whole Grains, but Not Refined Grains, Is Inversely Associated with All-Cause Mortality in Older Women: The Iowa Women's Health Study," *Journal of the American College of Nutrition* 19, no. 3, supplement (June 2000): 326–30S.

6. L. Brewster and M. F. Jacobson, *The Changing American Diet* (Washington, D.C.: Center for Science in the Public Interest, 1978).

7. P. E. Johnson, "Effect of Food Processing and Preparation on Mineral Utilization," *Advances in Experimental Medicine and Biology* 289 (1991): 483–98.

J. Hammink, "The Nutritional Value of Hot Meal Components Prepared in Different Ways," *Annales de la Nutrition et de l'Alimentation* 32, nos. 2–3 (1978): 459–65.

8. N. Mann, "Dietary Lean Red Meat and Human Evolution," *European Journal of Nutrition* 39, no. 2 (April 2000): 71–79.

9. L. Gay, "Meat from Diseased Animals Approved for Consumers," Scripps Howard News Service, July 14, 2000.

10. C. Fortes et al., "Diet and Overall Survival in a Cohort of Very Elderly People," *Epidemiology* 11, no. 4 (July 2000): 440–45.

11. Richard Behar and Michael Kramer, "Something Smells Fowl," *Time*, October 17, 1994, 42. Jane Brody, "Personal Health," *New York Times*, October 5, 1994.

12. C. Smith and J. D. DeWaal, "Playing Chicken: The Human Cost of Inadequate Regulation of the Poultry Industry," Center for Science in the Public Interest, March 1996, 2.

M. E. Berrang, R. J. Buhr, and J. A. Cason, "Campylobacter Recovery from External and Internal Organs of Commercial Broiler Carcasses Prior to Scalding," *Poultry Science* 79, no. 2 (February 2000): 286–90.

13. L. J. Appel et al., "A Clinical Trial of the Effects of Dietary Patterns on Blood Pressure," DASH Collaborative Research Group, *New England Journal of Medicine* 336, no. 16 (April 17, 1997): 1117–24.

D. W. Harsha et al., "Dietary Approaches to Stop Hypertension: A Summary of Study Results," DASH Collaborative Research Group, *Journal of the American Dietetic Association* 99, no. 8, supplement (August 1999): S35–39.

F. M. Sacks et al., "A Dietary Approach to Prevent Hypertension: A Review of the Dietary Approaches to Stop Hypertension (DASH) Study," *Clinical Cardiology* 22, no. 7, supplement (July 1999): III6–10.

14. D. A. Mackie and R. M. Pangborn, "Mastication and Its Influence on Human Salivary Flow and Alpha-Amylase Secretion," *Physiology and Behavior* 47, no. 3 (March 1990): 593–95.

15. *Tufts University Diet & Nutrition Letter* 9, no. 4 (1991): 1–2.

16. K. E. Kwast and S. C. Hand, "Oxygen and pH Regulation of Protein Synthesis in Mitochondria," part 1, *Biochemical Journal* 313 (January 1, 1996): 207–13.

17. S. J. Evans et al., "Acid-Base Homeostasis Parallels Anabolism in Surgically Stressed Rats Treated with GH and IGF-I," part 1, *American Journal of Physiology* 270, no. 6 (June 1996): E968–74.

D. H. Kang, "Metabolic Acidosis as a Catabolic Factor in Peritoneal Dialysis Patients," *Peritoneal Dialysis International* 19, supplement 2 (1999): S304–8.

18. A. Sebastian et al., "Improved Mineral Balance and Skeletal Metabolism in Postmenopausal Women Treated with Potassium Bicarbonate," *New England Journal of Medicine* 330 (1994): 1776–81.

19. K. A. Steinmetz et al., "Vegetables, Fruit, and Colon Cancer in the Iowa Women's Health Study," *American Journal of Epidemiology* 139, no. 1 (January 1, 1994): 1–15.

20. J. Sabate, "Nut Consumption, Vegetarian Diets, Ischemic Heart Disease Risk, and All-Cause Mortality: Evidence from Epidemiologic Studies," *American Journal of Clinical Nutrition* 70, no. 3, supplement (September 1999): 500–503S.

21. G. A. Clawson, "Protease Inhibitors and Carcinogenesis: A Review," *Cancer Investigation* 14, no. 6 (1996): 597–608.

22. Y. Pan, M. Anthony, and T. B. Clarkson, "Effect of Estradiol and Soy Phytoestrogens on Choline Acetyltransferase and Nerve Growth Factor mRNAs in the Frontal Cortex and Hippocampus of Female Rats," *Proceedings of the Society for Experimental Biology and Medicine* 221, no. 2 (June 1999): 118–25.

E. D. Lephart et al., "Phytoestrogens Decrease Brain Calcium-Binding Proteins but Do Not Alter Hypothalamic Androgen Metabolizing Enzymes in Adult Male Rats," *Brain Research* 859, no. 1 (March 17, 2000): 123–31.

23. L. R. White et al., "Association of Mid-life Consumption of Tofu with Late Life Cognitive Impairment and Dementia: The Honolulu-Asia Aging Study" (paper presented at the Fifth International Conference on Alzheimer's Disease, no. 487, Osaka, Japan, July 27, 1996).

L. R. White et al., "Brain Aging and Midlife Tofu Consumption," *Journal of the American College of Nutrition* 19, no. 2 (April 2000): 242–55.

24. "Soy Infant Formula Could Be Harmful to Infants: Groups Want It Pulled," *Nutrition Week* 29, no. 46 (December 10, 1999): 1–2.

25. K. D. Setchell et al., "Exposure of Infants to Phyto-estrogens from Soy-Based Infant Formula," *Lancet* 350, no. 9070 (July 5, 1997): 23–27.

26. Y. Miyagi et al., "Trypsin Inhibitor Activity in Commercial Soybean Products in Japan," *Journal of Nutritional Science and Vitaminology* 43, no. 5 (October 1997): 575–80.

27. R. L. Divi, H. C. Chang, and D. R. Doerge, "Anti-thyroid Isoflavones from Soybean: Isolation, Characterization, and Mechanisms of Action," *Biochemical Pharmacology* 54, no. 10 (November 15, 1997): 1087–96.

28. T. H. Shepard, "Soybean Goiter," *New England Journal of Medicine* 262 (1960): 1099–1103.

CHAPTER 9: WATER: LIFESPRING OF THE METABOLIC PLAN

1. J. Shannon et al., "Relationship of Food Groups and Water Intake to Colon Cancer Risk," *Cancer Epidemiology Biomarkers and Prevention* 5, no. 7 (July 1996): 495–502.

2. D. Haussinger, F. Lang, and W. Gerok, "Regulation of Cell Function by the Cellular Hydration State," part 1, *American Journal of Physiology* 267, no. 3 (September 1994): E343–55.

3. G. N. Ling, "Solute Exclusion by Polymer and Protein-Dominated Water: Correlation with Results of Nuclear Magnetic Resonance (NMR) and Calorimetric Studies and Their Significance for the Understanding of the Physical State of Water in Living Cells," *Scanning Microscopy* 2, no. 2 (1988): 871–84.

4. J. S. Clegg, "On the Physical Properties and Potential Roles of Intracellular Water," in *Organization of Cell Metabolism,* ed. G. R. Welsh and J. S. Clegg (New York: Plenum Press, 1987).

5. D. K. Srivastava and S. A. Bernhard, "Metabolite Transfer via Enzyme-Enzyme Interactions," *Science* 234 (1986): 1081–84.

6. M. Rodbell, "The Role of GTP-Binding Proteins in Signal Transduction: From the Sublimely Simple to the Conceptually Complex," *Current Topics in Cellular Regulation* 32 (1992): 1–47.

J. G. Waterson, "A Model Linking Water and Protein Structures," *Biosystems* 22, no. 1 (1988): 51–54.

7. S. Katayama, "Aging Mechanism Associated with a Function of Biowater," *Physiological Chemistry and Physics and Medical NMR* 24 (1992): 43–50.

8. J. M. Brensilver and E. Goldberger, *A Primer of Water, Electrolyte and Acid-Base Syndromes* (New York: Oxford University Press, 1996).

9. N. J. Hoxie et al., "Cryptosporidiosis-Associated Mortality Following a Massive Waterborne Outbreak in Milwaukee, Wisconsin," *American Journal of Public Health* 87, no. 12 (December 1997): 2032–35.

10. K. Waller et al., "Trihalomethanes in Drinking Water and Spontaneous Abortion," *Epidemiology* 9, no. 2 (March 1998): 134–40.

CHAPTER 10: METABOLIC ISSUES FOR WOMEN AND MEN

1. G. Ravaglia et al., "The Relationship of Dehydroepiandrosterone Sulfate (DHEAS) to Endocrine-Metabolic Parameters and Functional Status in the Oldest-Old: Results from an Italian Study on Healthy Free-Living over-Ninety-Year-Olds," *Journal of Clinical Endocrinology and Metabolism* 81, no. 3 (March 1996): 1173–78.

2. R. Sands and J. Studd, "Exogenous Androgens in Postmenopausal Women," *American Journal of Medicine* 98, no. 1A (January 16, 1995): 76–79S.

3. S. H. Kennedy et al., "Antidepressant-Induced Sexual Dysfunction during Treat-

ment with Moclobemide, Paroxetine, Sertraline, and Venlafaxine," *Journal of Clinical Psychiatry* 61, no. 4 (April 2000): 276–81.

4. P. S. Masand and S. Gupta, "Selective Serotonin-Reuptake Inhibitors: An Update," *Harvard Review of Psychiatry* 7, no. 2 (July–August 1999): 69–84, review.

5. S. Rubino et al., "Neuroendocrine Effect of a Short-Term Treatment with DHEA in Postmenopausal Women," *Maturitas* 28, no. 3 (January 12, 1998): 251–57.

6. É.-É. Baulieu et al., "Dehydroepiandrosterone (DHEA), DHEA Sulfate, and Aging: Contribution of the DHEAge Study to a Sociobiomedical Issue," *Proceedings of the National Academy of Sciences of the United States of America* 97, no. 8 (April 11, 2000): 4279–84.

W. Arlt et al., "Dehydroepiandrosterone Replacement in Women with Adrenal Insufficiency," *New England Journal of Medicine* 341 (1999): 1013–20.

7. G. K. Gouras et al., "Testosterone Reduces Neuronal Secretion of Alzheimer's ß-Amyloid Peptides," *Proceedings of the National Academy of Sciences* 97, no. 3 (2000): 1202–5.

8. S. N. Ameratunga and P. M. Brown, "Commentary: Older People's Perspectives on Life after Hip Fracture," *British Medical Journal* 320 (2000): 346.

9. S. R. Cummings et al., "Epidemiology of Osteoporosis and Osteoporotic Fractures," *Epidemiologic Reviews* 7 (1985): 178.

10. A. D. Martin and C. S. Houston, "Osteoporosis, Calcium and Physical Activity," *Canadian Medical Association Journal* 136, no. 6 (March 15, 1987): 587–93.

11. R. P. Heaney, "Effect of Calcium on Skeletal Development, Bone Loss, and Risk of Fractures," *American Journal of Medicine* 91, no. 5B (November 25, 1991): 23–28S.

12. M. S. Deehr et al., "Effects of Different Calcium Sources on Iron Absorption in Postmenopausal Women," *American Journal of Clinical Nutrition* 51, no. 1 (1990): 95–99.

J. A. Harvey, M. M. Zobitz, and C. Y. Pak, "Dose Dependency of Calcium Absorption. A Comparison of Calcium Carbonate and Calcium Citrate," *Journal of Bone and Mineral Research* 3, no. 3 (June 1988): 253–58.

J. A. Harvey et al., "Superior Calcium Absorption from Calcium Citrate Than Calcium Carbonate Using External Forearm Counting," *Journal of the American College of Nutrition* 9, no. 6 (December 1990): 583–87.

A. Pines et al., "Clinical Trial of Microcrystalline Hydroxyapatite Compound in the Prevention of Osteoporosis Due to Corticosteroid Therapy," *Current Medical Research and Opinion* 8 (1984): 734–39.

A. Stellon et al., "Microcrystalline Hydroxyapatite in Prevention of Bone Loss in Corticosteroid Treated Patients with Chronic Active Hepatitis," *Postgraduate Medicine* 61 (1985): 791–97.

13. R. M. Angus et al., "Dietary Intake and Bone Mineral Density," *Bone and Mineral* 4, no. 3 (July 1988): 265–77.

14. S. M. Kleiner, "Bone Up on Your Diet," *Physician and Sportsmedicine* 21, no. 5 (1993): 27–28.

15. "Nationwide Food Consumption Survey: Continuing Survey of Food Intakes by Individuals," USDA Report 85–1, Human Nutrition Information Service, CSF II (Washington, D.C.: U.S. Department of Agriculture, 1994–96).

"Ten State Nutrition Survey, 1978–1990," HSM 72–8130 through 8134, U.S. Dept. of Health, Education and Welfare, Health Services and Mental Health Administration (Atlanta, Ga.: Centers for Disease Control).

16. K. J. Morgan and G. L. Stampley, "Dietary Intake Levels and Food Sources of

Magnesium and Calcium for Selected Segments of the US Population," *Magnesium* 7, nos. 5–6 (1988): 225–33.

17. L. L. Hardwick et al., "Comparison of Calcium and Magnesium Absorption: In Vivo and in Vitro Studies," part 1, *American Journal of Physiology* 259, no. 5 (November 1990): G720–26.

D. W. Watkins et al., "Magnesium and Calcium Absorption in Fischer-344 Rats Influenced by Changes in Dietary Fibre (Wheat Bran), Fat and Calcium," *Magnesium Research* 5, no. 1 (March 1992): 15–21.

18. A. Halabe, B. M. Lifschitz, and J. Azuri, "Liver Damage Due to Alendronate," *New England Journal of Medicine* 343, no. 5 (August 3, 2000): 365–66.

R. J. Lieverse, "Hepatitis after Alendronate," *Netherlands Journal of Medicine* 53 (1998): 271–72.

19. D. Y. Graham and H. M. Malaty, "Alendronate Gastric Ulcers," *Alimentary Pharmacology and Therapeutics* 13 (1999): 515–19.

20. P. Diamond et al., "Metabolic Effects of 12 Month Percutaneous Dehydroepiandrosterone Replacement Therapy in Postmenopausal Women," *Journal of Endocrinology* 150 (1996): S43–50.

21. Baulieu et al., "Dehydroepiandrosterone (DHEA), DHEA Sulfate, and Aging."

22. C. M. Gordon et al., "Changes in Bone Turnover Markers and Menstrual Function after Short-Term Oral DHEA in Young Women with Anorexia Nervosa," *Journal of Bone and Mineral Research* 14, no. 1 (January 1999): 136–45.

23. S. T. Haden et al., "Effects of Age on Serum Dehydroepiandrosterone Sulfate, IGF-I, and IL-6 Levels in Women," *Calcified Tissue International* 66, no. 6 (June 2000): 414–18.

24. A. S. Ryan et al., "Resistive Training Maintains Bone Mineral Density in Postmenopausal Women," *Calcified Tissue International* 62, no. 4 (April 1998): 295–99.

25. F. Li and R. C. Muhlbauer, "Food Fractionation Is a Powerful Tool to Increase Bone Mass in Growing Rats and to Decrease Bone Loss in Aged Rats: Modulation of the Effect by Dietary Phosphate," *Journal of Bone and Mineral Research* 14, no. 8 (August 1999): 1457–65.

26. L. J. Vatten et al., "Androgens in Serum and the Risk of Prostate Cancer: A Nested Case-Control Study from the Janus Serum Bank in Norway," *Cancer Epidemiology Biomarkers and Prevention* 6, no. 11 (November 1997): 967–69.

P. H. Gann et al., "A Prospective Study of Plasma Hormone Levels, Nonhormonal Factors, and Development of Benign Prostatic Hyperplasia," *Prostate* 26, no. 1 (January 1995): 40–49.

27. É.-É. Baulieu, "Dehydroepiandrosterone (DHEA): A Fountain of Youth?" *Journal of Clinical Endocrinology and Metabolism* 81, no. 9 (1996): 3147–51.

28. S. S. Yen, A. J. Morales, and O. Khorram, "Replacement of DHEA in Aging Men and Women: Potential Remedial Effects," *Annals of the New York Academy of Sciences* 774 (December 29, 1995): 128–42.

29. O. Khorram, L. Vu, and S. S. Yen, "Activation of Immune Function by Dehydroepiandrosterone (DHEA) in Age-Advanced Men," *Journal of Gerontology* 52A, no. 1 (1997): M1–7.

30. C. W. Cutting et al., "Serum Insulin-like Growth Factor-1 Is Not a Useful Marker of Prostate Cancer," *BJU International* 83, no. 9 (June 1999): 996–99.

31. D. L. McCormick and K. V. Rao, "Chemoprevention of Hormone-Dependent Prostate Cancer in the Wistar-Unilever Rat," *European Urology* 35, nos. 5–6 (May 1999): 464–67.

32. R. Nelson et al., "Dehydroepiandrosterone and 7-Keto DHEA Augment Interleukin 2 (IL2) Production by Human Lymphocytes," *Proceedings: 5th Conference on Retroviruses and Opportunistic Infections,* February 1–5, 1998.

33. M. Davidson et al., "Safety and Endocrine Effects of 7-Keto DHEA," *Proceedings of the Society for Experimental Biology,* San Francisco, April 19–22, 1998.

34. H. W. Baker et al., "Changes in the Pituitary-Testicular System with Age," *Clinical Endocrinology* (Oxford) 5, no. 4 (July 1976): 349–72.

L. E. Carlson and B. B. Sherwin, "Steroid Hormones, Memory and Mood in a Healthy Elderly Population," *Psychoneuroendocrinology* 23, no. 6 (August 1998): 583–603.

35. K. Suzuki et al., "Endocrine Environment of Benign Prostatic Hyperplasia: Prostate Size and Volume Are Correlated with Serum Estrogen Concentration," *Scandinavian Journal of Urology and Nephrology* 29, no. 1 (March 1995): 65–68.

K. M. Lau et al., "Expression of Estrogen Receptor (ER)-Alpha and ER-Beta in Normal and Malignant Prostatic Epithelial Cells: Regulation by Methylation and Involvement in Growth Regulation," *Cancer Research* 60, no. 12 (June 15, 2000): 3175–82.

36. S. Gupta et al., "Over-expression of Cyclooxygenase-2 in Human Prostate Adenocarcinoma," *Prostate* 42, no. 1 (January 2000): 73–78.

37. M. Cuendet and J. M. Pezzuto, "The Role of Cyclooxygenase and Lipoxygenase in Cancer Chemoprevention," *Drug Metabolism and Drug Interactions* 17, nos. 1–4 (2000): 109–57.

38. J. Zhao, Y. Sharma, and R. Agarwal, "Significant Inhibition by the Flavonoid Antioxidant Silymarin against 12-O-Tetradecanoylphorbol 13-Acetate-Caused Modulation of Antioxidant and Inflammatory Enzymes, and Cyclooxygenase 2 and Interleukin-1alpha Expression in SENCAR Mouse Epidermis: Implications in the Prevention of Stage I Tumor Promotion," *Molecular Carcinogenesis* 26, no. 4 (December 1999): 321–33.

CHAPTER 11: KEEPING SCORE, STAYING MOTIVATED, AND TAKING ACTION

1. E. Furuya, M. Maezawa, and O. Nishikaze, "17-KS Sulfate as a Biomarker in Psychosocial Stress," *Rinsho Byori* 46, no. 6 (June 1998): 529–37.

2. O. Nishikaze, "17-KS sulfate as a Biomarker in Health and Disease," *Rinsho Byori* 46, no. 6 (June 1998): 520–28.

O. Nishikaze and F. Furuya, "Stress and Anticortisols: 17-Ketosteroid Sulfate Conjugate as a Biomarker in Tissue Repair and Recovery," *Sangyo Ika Daigaku Zasshi* 20, no. 4 (December 1, 1998): 273–95.

3. Q. Jia et al., "Quantification of Urine 17-Ketosteroid Sulfates and Glucuronides by High-Performance Liquid Chromatography—Ion Trap Mass Spectroscopy," *Journal of Chromatography B* 750 (2001): 81–91.

4. D. Carmelli and T. Reed, "Stability and Change in Genetic and Environmental Influences on Hand-Grip Strength in Older Male Twins," *Journal of Applied Physiology* 89, no. 5 (November 2000): 1879–83.

5. C. M. Beard et al., "The Epidemiology of Ovarian Cancer: A Population-Based Study in Olmsted County, Minnesota, 1935–1991," *Annals of Epidemiology* 10, no. 1 (January 2000): 14–23.

J. Wohlfahrt et al., "Reproductive History and Stage of Breast Cancer," *American Journal of Epidemiology* 150, no. 12 (December 15, 1999): 1325–30.

6. W.L.D.M. Nelen et al., "Homocysteine and Folate Levels as Risk Factors for Recurrent Early Pregnancy Loss," *Obstetrics and Gynecology* 95 (2000): 519–24.

M. F. Picciano, "Is Homocysteine a Biomarker for Identifying Women at Risk of Complications and Adverse Pregnancy Outcomes?" *American Journal of Clinical Nutrition* 71 (2000): 857–58.

7. Lipid Research Clinics Program, "The Lipid Research Clinics Coronary Primary Prevention Trial Results: II. The Relationship of Reduction in Incidence of Coronary Heart Disease to Cholesterol Lowering," *JAMA—Journal of the American Medical Association* 251 (1984): 365–74.

CHAPTER 12: CONCLUSION: A QUESTION OF BALANCE, THE NATURE OF TIME

1. Neil Postman, *Amusing Ourselves to Death* (New York: Viking Press, 1986): 65.

2. Bill McKibben, *The Age of Missing Information* (New York: Plume, 1993): 200, 244.

3. Ibid.

Index

About the Author

STEPHEN CHERNISKE, M.S., is a nutritional biochemist with more than thirty years of academic, research, and clinical experience. Cherniske directed the nation's first FDA-licensed clinical laboratory specializing in nutrition testing, advised the U.S. Olympic team, and served on the faculty of the American College of Sports Medicine. He currently serves as president and chief scientific officer for Oasis Wellness Network in Broomfield, Colorado. He is the author of *The DHEA Breakthrough* and *Caffeine Blues*.